INFLAMMATORY BOWEL DISEASE

Edited by **Imre Szabo**

Inflammatory Bowel Disease
http://dx.doi.org/10.5772/46222
Edited by Imre Szabo

Contributors

Hyunjo Kim, Rahul Anil Sheth, Michael Gee, Valeriu Surlin, Adrian Saftoiu, Catalin Copaescu, Diehl, Yves-Jacques Schneider, Alina Martirosyan, Madeleine Polet, Alexandra Bazes, Thérèse Sergent, Ladislava Bartosova, Michal Kolorz, Milan Bartos, Katerina Wroblova, Michael Wannemuehler, Albert E. Jergens, Amanda E. Ramer-Tait, Anne-Marie C. Overstreet, Brankica Mijandrusic Sincic, Ana Brajdić

Published by InTech

Janeza Trdine 9, 51000 Rijeka, Croatia

Publishing Process Manager Danijela Duric
Technical Editor InTech DTP team
Cover InTech Design team

Additional hard copies can be obtained from orders@intechopen.com

Inflammatory Bowel Disease, Edited by Imre Szabo
p. cm.
ISBN 978-953-51-0879-5

For EU product safety concerns:
IN TECH d.o.o., Prolaz Marije Krucifikse Kozulić 3, 51000 Rijeka, Croatia,
info@intechopen.com or visit our website at intechopen.com.

Meet the editor

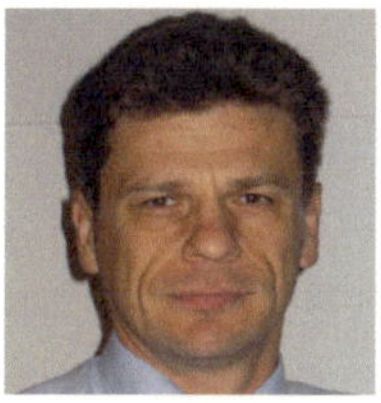

Dr. Imre Laszlo Szabo is a medical doctor holding a Ph. D. degree in Gastroenterology from the University of Pécs (Hungary, 2004), where he studied the mechanisms of cytoprotection and mucosal healing processes in different regions of human gastrointestinal system. He currently works as an Assistant Professor at the First Department of Medicine, University of Pécs and has 10 years of experience in teaching Internal Medicine and Gastroenterology at graduate and postgraduate level. His research in the United States included the study of ulcer healing, nonsteroidal gastroenteropathy in animal models and their molecular mechanisms in isolated cells. He has published his work in several peer reviewed journals and given oral and poster presentations at national and international conferences. In addition he has authored Hungarian grants and participated in grants from U.S. Veteran's Administration. His fields of special expertise include gastrointestinal mucosal injury, defensive and healing mechanisms.

Contents

Preface

Inflammatory bowel disease (IBD) is a term for a two very different and yet in many characteristics congruent chronic inflammatory disorder of the intestinal tract. Crohn's disease (CD) and ulcerative colitis are two principal components of IBD. Both CD and ulcerative colitis are considered as multifactoral diseases. For long period of time we keep these inflammatory intestinal disorders as the result of environmental factors and immunological disturbances manifested in persons with genetic predisposition. The pathogenesis of IBD has remained largely unknown, but surely involves environmental factors, immunological factors in a complex form. Increasing disease prevalence and gathered lot of new research data on IBD suggested the pretence for review.

Epidemiological studies have shown that prevalence of IDB has dramatically increases in western world probably due to western lifestyle. Environmental factors are suggested to have major role in development of diseases connected to westernalization of the lifestyle. These factors include smoking, use of antibiotics and non-steroidal anti-inflammatory drugs, stress, various infections and diet. The initiating mechanisms of their actions are still not understood. Research has revealed several genetic factors contributing to IDB pathogenesis; more than a hundred IDB genes, loci and their allele variation have been defined (e.g. NOD2/CARD15, IL23, ATG16L1, IRGM, ICAM-1, CCR5, TLR4, TNFα).

Intestinal stricture is a serious and late complication of CD. Recent studies have identified certain disease specific characteristics that may be used in identifying individuals having higher risk for stricture development. These are lower age at initial diagnosis of CD, need for steroid therapy at the diagnosis, perianal fistulizing disease or small intestinal localized disease. Anti-Saccharomyces cerevisiae antibody (ASCA) levels were also found to be correlated to fibrostenosing or penetrating disease behaviour. Recently, other serological markers (anti-I2 and anti-CBir1), fibronectin, bFGF and YKL-40 glycoprotein of the chitinase family have been shown to lead to the hyperplasia of the intestinal muscle layers and deposition of collagen.

Determination of gene polymorphism can also be important in regarding the prediction of therapy response. Since no curative therapy for IBD exists, pharmacological therapy mainly focuses on inflammation control. IBD pharmacotherapy utilizes a wide scale of drugs for inflammation reduction including aminosalicylates, glicocorticoids, immunomodulators and biological therapy. Their pharmocodinamics and pharmacokinetics can be altered by polymorphisms of certain gene coding proteins resulting faster drug elimination, tolerance or more side affect development. Namely, the form of N-acetyltransferase in slow acetylators can develop more side effects for sulfasalazine, mutation of glucocorticoid receptor-β lead to decreased affinity to exogenous glucocorticoids, mutations of thiopurine

S-methyltransferase defining allelic variations determine the likeliness of leucopenia and thrombocytopenia development during azathioprine or 6-mercaptopurine treatment. Patients who are homozygous for certain standard alleles of NOD2, TLR4 and TNFα are more often resistant to infliximab therapy.

The role of altered composition in intestinal microbiota has also been emphasized in the development of IBD over the years. The gut microbiota composition varies upon individual but remains highly stable containing large amount of *Bacteroidetes, Firmicutes, Acinetobacter, Proteobacteria and Fusobacteria* containing 150 times larger genetic information than the human genome. This changed composition in IBD surely affects normal barrier function, cell metabolism, antibiotic function and inflammatory responses. This book is trying to give further research data to answer the main question whether altered microbiota composition is a cause of or a consequence of the inflammatory state.

In the first part of this book you can read chapters for outstanding researchers on the ethiopathogenesis of IBD including a reviews on environmental factors, genetic predisposition (including gene polymorphisms influencing disease development, efficacy of therapy with standard aminosalicylates, glucocorticoids and immunomodulators as well as biological therapy), altered immune response effecting various components of the innate and acquired immune system leading to loss of tolerance to commersal enteral bacteria and to gut dysbiosis.

In the second part of the book clinicians show the management of IBD including the presentation of use of modern radiological diagnostic modalities in the diagnosis and identification of extent and activity of IBD. The place of surgical therapy in the management of IBD patients will be discussed by showing up-to-date minimally invasive techniques along with the long-term results of classical surgical options.

The last part of the book focuses on future directions of IBD therapy utilizing new pharmacological methods for more effective drug delivery. Potential role of liposomes and nanoparticules (NP) will be highlighted in the treatment of IBD and colon cancer. Data will show that certain nanopaticules, like Ag-NPs or chitosan, may enhance the epithelial permeability and could therefore serve as an effective carrier for drug delivery, but also might favour the systemic absorption of toxins or other NPs that would likely cause immune activation. You can find more interesting data on the beneficial role and night-side of colon targeting drug delivery systems in this last part of the book.

I am sure together with the Commissioning Editors and the Publisher that all readers, researcher, clinicians and novice readers, will receive lot of new scientific information by reading this book.

I wish to thank the outstanding work of all authors, the invitation to the publisher and the excellent support throughout the publishing process to the commissioning editors, Ms. Ivona Lovric, Ms. Danijela Duric and Mr. Vedran Greblo.

Imre Szabo MD, PhD
Division of Gastroenterology
First Department of Medicine
University of Pécs
Hungary

Section 1

Pathogenesis of Inflammatory Bowel Disease

Chapter 1

Insights to the Ethiopathogenesis of the Inflammatory Bowel Disease

Ana Brajdić and Brankica Mijandrušić-Sinčić

Additional information is available at the end of the chapter

http://dx.doi.org/10.5772/52970

1. Introduction

Inflammatory bowel disease (IBD) is a term that refers to two very different yet in many ways related phenotypes, Crohn's disease (CD) and ulcerative colitis (UC). It is well known that both of the two primary human inflammatory bowel diseases are characterized by chronic inflammation of the intestinal tract, yet their etiology still remains unclear.

CD and UC are considered to be multifactorial diseases and the underlying pathological process seems to be a combination of genetic predisposition and immunologic disturbances. Being the largest surface in the human body and since it is constantly colonized by a highly diverse community of microbes that are in normal circumstances either commensal or beneficial to human health, the role of the intestinal microbiota in development of IBD has been thoroughly investigated over the years. It is now generally accepted that the commensal flora plays a central role in triggering and perpetuating the disease process. [1] Even though there are several logical arguments contributing to the theory that the intestinal microbiota plays a major role in the IBD development, the types of microbes involved have not been adequately described. Studies of experimental animal models of IBD uncover that the presence of gut bacteria is essential in inflammation initiation and there is no disease onset in germ-free mice [2]. Furthermore, decreasing bacterial numbers in the intestine by using antibiotics, can lead to clinical improvement and decreased inflammation in both humans [3] and animal models of IBD [4, 5].

Pathogenesis of the IBD is characterized by various genetic abnormalities that lead to overly aggressive altered immune response, triggered by heterogeneous environmental factors under the influence of the commensal intestinal microbiota. There is no single abnormality of the gastro intestinal tract that would lead to development of CD or UC. Only in correlation of those four mentioned main factors a dysbalance of the gastrointestinal tract develops, leading to chronic inflammation with all its consequences and complications. Schematized and simplified pathogenesis involving correlation between environmental factors, genetic predisposition, host immune response and intestinal microbiota is shown in Figure 1.

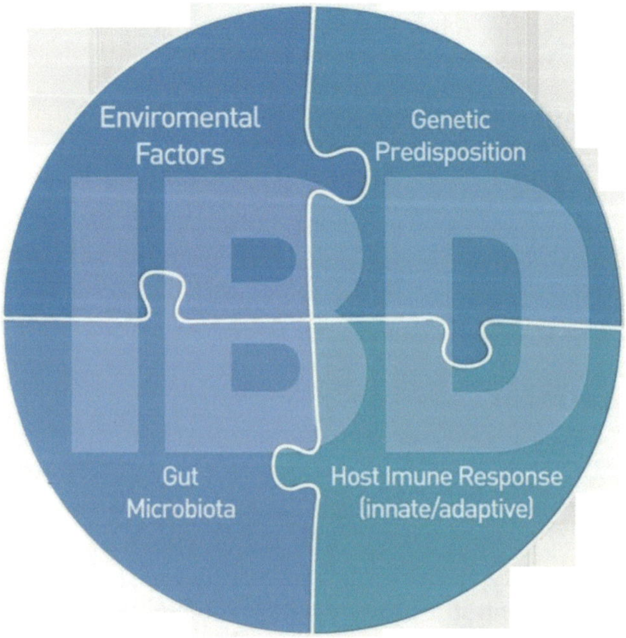

Figure 1. Schematized correlation of main factors involved in the IBD pathogenesis. Each of the mentioned factors fit together as separate pieces of puzzle, together creating a complex clinical and pathological image of the IBD.

In this review, we discuss recent insights in the ethiopathogenesis of the inflammatory bowel diseases.

2. Etiology and pathophysiology

2.1. Environmental factors

Epidemiological studies show that the prevalence of IBD dramatically increased in northern Europe, the United Kingdom and North America in the second half of the twentieth century and is also increasing in the rest of the world, proportionally to the adoption of western lifestyle [6]. This process, known as "westernization" of lifestyle [7], includes environmental triggers such as smoking (shown to be protective in UC but detrimental in CD), use of antibiotics and nonsteroidal anti-inflammatory drugs (NSAIDs), stress, infection and diet. Studies have also reported an association between early life exposure to antibiotics (in the first year of subject's life) and CD development due to early childhood dysbiosis [8].

The mechanisms by which these factors initiate the onset of IBD are still not well understood. There is some evidence that infection and NSAIDs can transiently initiate nonspecific inflammation, break the mucosal barrier and activate innate immune response [9]. This process may lead to enhanced uptake of commensal bacterial antigens and in combination with genetic susceptibility, in this way stimulate protracted T-cell mediated inflammation. Up until now, only smoking and appendectomy have been clearly linked with the risk of developing IBD. A recent cohort study concerning autophagy-related genes and granuloma formation in surgically treated CD patients has showed that there is a significant association between smoking and granuloma formation [10]. This observation could be a result of inflammation promoting effects of smoking, resulting in more severe inflammation with granulomas in smokers with CD [10]. Appendectomy and smoking reduce risk for UC but on the other hand, active smoking increases risk for CD [11]. Even though proven to be valid, these facts cannot be held answerable for all variations in IBD incidence and prevalence.

There is also a hypothesis known as the "hygiene hypothesis", that could be the fundamental reason for the switch from infectious to chronic inflammatory diseases. This hypothesis proposes that there has been a lifestyle change from one with high microbial exposure to one with low microbial exposure [12]. There are numerous environmental factors that could be assigned to the hygiene hypothesis, some of which being better housing, safer food, cleaner water, vaccines, dietary changes, fewer infections, improved hygiene and sanitation and widespread use of antibiotics [12].

Even though there are many firm epidemiological studies and evidence linking certain environmental factors to greater probability of developing IBD, it is still widely believed that there is no one simple environmental factor that could alone cause CD or UC. Based on the fact that differences in geographic distribution combined with changes in incidence over time within one observed area could provide insights into possible etiologic factors, a prospective population based study investigated the incidence of UC and CD in Primorsko-goranska County, Croatia (January 2000 to December 2004) was performed by the authors [13]. The study included a total of 170 patients residing a county with a stable, ethnic and racially homogeneous population and the results showed an increase in UC and CD incidence, in comparison to an earlier prospective study for the county of Zagreb, with a similar population and similar environmental circumstances [13]. It is considered that the rapid "westernization" of the country combined with the improved awareness of the disease play a role in the reported increase. Annual age-standardized incidence rate was $4{,}3/10^5$ for UC and $7{,}0/10^5$ for CD. Croatian results concerning UC were similar to those reported in Belgium, Northern France and Germany and those concerning CD reach the mean incidence value reported in European multicentric study of CD [13].

2.2. Genetic predisposition

There have recently been great advances in understanding the very complex genetics of the IBD, from studies based on single nucleotide polymorphism and candidate gene approaches to studies based on transgenic and deletion techniques [14]. It is thought that UC and CD may be heterogeneous polygenic disorders, sharing some but not all susceptibility loci and there are most likely several factors determining the disease phenotype [15]. Presence of a mutated gene in a host does not guarantee that IBD will develop and we cannot use it as a predicting factor for later development of IBD.

In order to prove that genetic factors contribute to the pathogenesis of IBD, studies have shown that the concordance rate between twins is much lower for UC than for CD, which may indicate that the genetic penetrance in CD is much greater than in UC. Reported concordance rate for UC in monozygotic twins is 15,4% vs. 3,9% in dizygotic twins and for CD 30,3% in monozygotic vs. 3,6% in dizygotic twins [16]. These findings may be considered valuable evidence that there is genetic susceptibility for IBD, particularly CD. Also, studies have shown that there is linkage between certain genetic disorders and incidence of IBD. In infants born to consanguineous parents there is a risk of developing extremely rare autosomal recessive mutations in genes encoding interleukin (IL)-10 receptor and the IL-10 cytokine [17, 18]. IL-10 is an anti-inflammatory cytokine and its primary purpose is to limit and ultimately terminate inflammatory responses [19]. Disturbance in either IL-10 or IL-10 receptor function via autosomal, recessive mutations are sufficient to cause severe forms of CD, which have been successfully treated by bone marrow transplantation [20].

There have been over a hundred IBD genes and loci defined and one of the most important genes associated with CD is *nucleotide binding oligomerization domain protein 2* (NOD 2), also known as the *caspase recruitment domain family member 15* (CARD15) gene [21, 22]. The NOD2 gene is expressed mainly in monocyte/macrophage cell lines where it plays an important role in host-signaling pathways. One of its main effects is the activation of the NF-κB protein, a transcription factor involved in cellular inflammatory pathways and an important regulator in cell fate decisions, such as programmed cell death and proliferation control, and also a critical factor in tumorigenesis.

The NOD2 mutations have been observed in individuals of European and African-American ancestry and studies have shown that in individuals of European ancestry heterozygous carriage of one of the major risk alleles bargain a 2,4-fold increase in risk for CD while homozygous or compound heterozygous carriage bargains 17,1-fold increase in risk for CD [22]. In those of African American origin, mutations are only heterozygous with similar risk for CD among carriers as mentioned above. When it comes to Asian populations, studies show that NOD2 mutation has not been associated with CD in studies of IBD patients form Hong Kong, China, Japan and Korea [23]. Mutations in the NOD2 gene, unexpectedly, reduce macrophage activation of NF- κB protein, which is why one would expect inflammation to weaken, instead of the increase of inflammation, which can be seen in IBD. In the absence of NOD-2 expression by epithelial cells, microbial products that normally induce these cells to secrete chemokines fail to do so, leading to potential loss of barrier function [7].

It is known that in about 70% of patients suffering from CD, the disease affects the small intestine. The human intestinal epithelial wall exceeds all other tissues of the human organism in its cell-renewal rate [24]. The intestinal adult stem cells self-renew and produce daughter cells. Daughter cells form an adjacent zone of rapidly cycling progenitors and undergo 4-6 rounds of division before differentiating into multiple lineages, fabricating up to

300 cells/crypt per day [25]. In this way, post-mitotic cells covering the biggest area of the intestinal epithelium are formed.

Besides absorptive cells, there are three classes of secretory cells: goblet cells (secrete mainly mucus), enteroendocrine cells (secreting different hormones) and Paneth cells [26]. Currently, the most acceptable role of Paneth cells in the small intestine is the production of a stream of antibacterial secretions, responsible for the sterile environment of the small intestinal lumen and in this way, protection of the vital stem cells in the neighborhood. Two most frequent defensins found in Paneth cells are the α defensins, human defensin 5 and 6 (DEFA5 and DEFA6) and in addition to DEFA5 and DEFA6, Paneth cells store several other antibiotic peptides (for example regenerating islet-derived 3-γ and phospholipase A2group IIA) [27]. Investigations on human α defensins have shown that DEFA5 has a very effective antibacterial activity against *S. aureus,* while DEFA6 expressed some antibacterial potential in vitro and there are ongoing investigations on their antiviral potential [28, 29]. There is numerous evidence for a link between the Paneth cell and ileal Crohn's disease. It is reported that NOD 2 is heavily expressed in Paneth cells and ileal CD is associated with a diminished synthesis of Paneth cell defensins [30, 31]. The role of NOD2 as an intracellular receptor for bacterial dipeptide in regulating Paneth cell defensin formation was confirmed in NOD-2 knockout mice and in patients after small intestinal transplantation [32, 33].

Being a genetically complex system, pathogenesis of IBD can be closely linked to numerous other genomic regions. Autophagy 16-like 1 (ATG16L1) is responsible for encoding a protein component of the autophagy complex and it has been strongly related to CD [34]. ATG16L1 is extensively expressed, including in Paneth cells, where it has a role in exocytosis of secretory granules containing antimicrobial products [35].

Other genes that regulate autophagy and that have been closely related to CD in genome-wide association studies are immunity-related guanosine triphosphotase M (IRGM) and leucine-rich repeat kinase 2 (LRRK2) [36, 37]. A recent study by Brinar et al. [10] investigated a relationship between variants in autophagy genes and granuloma formation in CD. The authors hypothesized that genetic variants in autophagy genes in CD patients may lead to impaired processing of intracellular bacterial components, thus contributing to granuloma formation. [10]. This cohort study detected an association in four autophagy genes, ATG4A, ATG4D, FNBP1L and ATG2A. The study has also shown that granuloma positive patients were significantly younger at diagnosis, that they had surgery at significantly younger age after a shorter duration of the disease. These findings suggest that there is a significant relationship between earlier mentioned variants in autophagy genes and granuloma formation, which could be a marker of a more aggressive disease course. [10]

After variants in NOD2, most significantly associated with CD is the amino acid change Arg381Gln variant in the IL-23 receptor (IL23). In comparison to Arg381 carriers, Glutamine 381 reduces risk for IBD by nearly 3-fold and studies on the proinflammatory role of IL-23 prioritize its signaling pathway as a therapeutic target in inflammatory bowel disease [38]. Many genes that encode factors in the IL-23 pathway have been associated with both psoriasis and IBD and numerous loci have been associated with both IBD and celiac disease [39,

40]. Studies show that neither IL23 nor ATG16L1 genes are associated with CD in Japanese and Korean patients [41].

There are numerous other loci associated with both CD and UC and the number of potential IBD genes continues to increase and searching for other genotype-phenotype correlations in the matter of IBD continues to be an important step in future studies. Despite all the facts specified, indications for genetic tests in everyday clinical practice still do not exist.

2.3. Host immune response

In order to develop IBD, both innate (macrophage, neutrophil) and acquired (T and B cells) immune responses combined with loss of tolerance to enteric commensal bacteria need to be activated in a host.

2.3.1. Innate immune responses

Studies have shown that there is an increase in the absolute number of macrophages and dendritic cells in both forms of IBD, with an enhanced production of proinflammatory cytokines and chemokines and an increase in the expression of adhesion molecules and co-stimulatory molecules [41].

Adhesion molecules (such as intracellular cell adhesion molecule 1, *ICAM1*) are crucial when it comes to binding circulating cells to the activated endothelium [42]. These molecules also have an important role in later mediation of migration of the extravagated immune cells through the stroma to the source of optimum chemokine production as well as through the epithelium to the lumen [43]. Mucosal dendritic cells are activated, express higher levels of the toll like receptors (TLR) 2 and 4, (which have an important role in recognition of bacterial products) and CD40, all of which is followed by increased production of IL-12 and IL-6 [44]. TLRs are profusely expressed on the surface of monocytes, macrophages, dendritic and epithelial cells and are responsible in identification of the commensal microflora as well as maintenance of the intestinal homeostasis [45]. Like NOD2, they selectively bind to specific microbial adjuvants and initiate signaling through nuclear factor kappa-light-chain-enhancer of activated B cell, *NF-κB.* Activation of NF-κB triggers expression of various molecules involved in the inflammatory response (such as IL-1β, TNF, IL-6, IL-8, ICAM1, CD 40, CD 80 and other chemokines, adhesion molecules and co-stimulatory molecules), all of which have an increased expression in IBD [41]. NF-κB is activated in tissues of IBD patients and its inhibition can attenuate experimental colitis [46].

In both forms of IBD, alterations of TLR 3 and 4 have been described, suggesting that abnormal bacterial sensing has a role in the disease pathogenesis [47]. As explained earlier, ileal Paneth cells also express the NOD-2 protein, and their production of mucosal α-defensins is decreased in CD patients with NOD-2 mutations.

2.3.2. Adaptive immune responses

Adaptive immune responses should be considered separately for CD and UC, due to their distinct profiles in those two entities.

2.3.2.1. Crohn's disease

Crohn's disease is predominantly T_H1 and T_H17 mediated process. Antigen presenting cells produce IL-12, which is responsible for stimulation of IFN-γ. IFN-γ then mediates traditional T_H1 responses. As the inflammatory response matures, in several models T_H1 responses can change into T_H2 responses [48]. On the other hand, IL-17 mediates T_H17 responses [49]. The production of IL-17 is impacted by innate immune cells and antigen presenting cells, which produce Il-6, IL-23 and TGFB [50].

When it comes to estimating the importance between T_H1 and T_H17 responses in CD development, studies have shown that even though Th17 responses play a role in the inflammation, the Th1 response is quantitatively greater [51]. This conclusion agrees with the intestinal pathologic effects of IFN-γ and the relation of Th1 responses to granulomatous disease [51]. In contribution, double blinded clinical trial of anti IL-17 in patients with CD has been carried out recently and the study showed that blockage of IL-17A is ineffective in tested subjects [51]. The role of IL-17 in patients suffering from CD is still under intense investigation.

2.3.2.2. Ulcerative colitis

Ulcerative colitis is considered to have an atypical T_H2 response, mediated by natural killer T cells that secrete IL-13 and IL-5 [52]. The T_H2 response is an atypical one due to the fact that concentrations of IL-4 and IL-5, which are normally elevated in T_H2 response, have been found to be variable in UC tissues [53]. Recent studies have shown an increase in IL-17 levels in UC (in compare to control groups), but that increase was found to be far less than the one found in CD patients. T-cell subsets are stimulated by antigen presenting cells, particularly dendritic cells, which have a unique capacity to activate naïve T cells. Dendritic cells are found in the lamina propria and Peyer's patches of normal intestine. Interaction between antigen presenting cells and T cells occurs by presenting an antigen on the surface of the major histocompatibility complex, which is then recognized by the appropriate T-cell receptor, followed by secretion of cytokines (such as IL-6, IL-10, IL-12, IL-23, TGF β).

The results of this pathway are increased levels of dendritic cells in patients with active IBD and in experimental colitis models [44, 54]. Peyer's patches, which can be considered as the immune senses of the intestine, seem to play a key organ in the relationship between innate and adaptive immunity in the human gut [55].

2.4. Intestinal microbiota

The understanding of the development of gastrointestinal (GI) tract microbiota has greatly developed, due to decreased costs of DNA sequencing and evolution of bioinformatics.

The human intestinal microbiota can be defined as a community of microbes that is either commensal or beneficial to human health. The adult human gut contains around 10^{14} bacterial cells and up to a 1000 different bacterial species [56]. The most abundant bacterial phyla in the healthy human large intestine are *Firmicutes, Bacteroidetes, Actinobacteria, Proteobacteria,*

Fusobacteria and *Verrucomicrobia* [56]. The gut microbiota composition varies between individuals and remains highly stable over time. A recent study performed by Arumugam et al. combined 22 newly sequenced faecal metagenomes of individuals from Denmark, France, Italy and Spain, resulting in three distinctive enterotypes. Furthermore, these results were combined with existing gut data-sets, 13 Japanese and four American, returning the same three clusters. These isolated bacterial communities were dominated by one of the three main distinct bacterial genera – *Bacteroides, Prevotella* and *Ruminococcus* [56]. In terms of function, it is indicated that drivers of each of the three enterotypes use different routes to generate energy from substrates available in the colon. *Bacteroides* seem to derive energy primarily from carbohydrates and proteins through fermentation, *Prevotella* is a known mucin degrader and *Ruminococcus* is linked to both mucin and sugar [56].

Numerous studies have shown that colonization of the GI tract in infants depends upon delivery mode and that the vagina has evolved to serve the fundamental inoculum for all mammals [57]. If a baby is exposed to vaginal microbes during birth, its initial gut bacteria will consist dominantly of *Lactobacillus* and *Prevotella* spp [58]. The bacteria, acquired from their mother's vaginal canal, can be found in the skin and mouth and the meconium of the baby. Many babies are not exposed to their mother's vaginal flora, due to the cesarean section-birth method (C-section). In contrast to vaginally delivered babies, those delivered by C-section accommodate bacterial communities that resemble bacteria of the skin: *Staphylococcus, Corynebacterium* and *Propionibacterium* spp [59]. In early childhood, the initial strains of GI bacteria are outcompeted by other bacterial strains, of a less certain origin, which rapidly increase in diversity and shift in response to dietary changes and/or illness [60, 61]. During early childhood, when peas and other plant-derived foods are introduced, the bacterial phyla of the GI tract changes and *Firmicutes* and *Bacteroidetes* are now dominant [62]. Microbial community can change, but the changes are now of a much slower rate than in early childhood and with unknown effects on health. The mentioned data and the development of the GI tract colonization in infants and early childhood can be seen in Table 1.

	INFANTS		EARLY CHILDHOOD
PREDOMINANT BACTERIAL COMMUNITES	Vaginal birth	C-section	Firmicutes Bacteroidetes
	Lactobacilus Prevotella spp.	Staphylococcus Corynebacterium Propionibacterium spp	

Table 1. Development of the GI tract colonization in infants and early childhood

Children from different parts of the world have different gut microbiota (for example Burkina Faso and Italy) [63], and when it comes to elderly, their GI tract microbiota is substantially different than in young adults [64]. According to Zoetendal et al., the gut microbiota composition of spouses showed the least degree of species similarity, while siblings showed increased degree of similarity in species make up [65].

The gut microbiota acts as a metabolic organ via production of short chain fatty acids and vitamins and it contributes to the barrier effect by preventing colonisation by pathogens. Recent studies have shown that a modulation of a gut microbiota using prebiotics increases epithelial barrier integrity by increasing expression of tight junction proteins [66]. The gut microbiota also helps to shape and maintain normal mucosal immunity.

The human gut microbiome consists of 150x more genes than the human genome [67]. In 2010, initiative called Meta-HIT (Metagenomics of the Human Intestinal Tract) published a catalogue of the microbial genomes strained from 124 faecal samples. The results found that the gene set was approximately 150 times larger than the human gene complement with 3,3 million different microbial genes [68]. Recent studies have shown that the intestine is home to specialized dendrytic cells, whose function is to induce a highly tolerogenic response from T and B cells, through induction of regulatory T cells and secretion of IgA [69]. Activated immune cells, such as mucosal dendrytic cells, constantly sample luminal microbial antigens and present them to adaptive immune cells [70]. There are three main ways by which flagellin from commensal microbes may play a role in IBD. Flagellin from commensal microbes may cross the altered epithelial barrier that occurs in IBD. Such flagellin can, via Toll-like receptor 5 (TLR5), induce the epithelium to secrete cytokines that recruit polymorphonuclear neutrophils (PMN) [71]. Such cytokines may promote adaptive immunity and/or, alternatively, flagellin may activate dendritic cells and directly promote adaptive immune immunity. Flagellin is also targeted by the CD-associated adaptive immune response [71].

In healthy hosts the pro-inflammatory pathways associated with TLR and NLR are suppressed by inhibitory molecules of both human and bacterial origin, such as COX-2 inhibitors, NF-κβ inhibitor, IL-10, TGF-β, IFN-α/β etc. [72, 73]. A disruption of this homeostasis threatens the state of immune tolerance and may result in gut inflammation. How the host tolerates resident bacteria whilst being able to mount an effective inflammatory response to invading pathogens is still not fully understood.

Gut microbiota and activity in IBD patients are proven to be abnormal. IBD patients are characterized by a reduced abundance of dominant members of the gut microbiota. According to *Frank et al.*, mucosal biopsies taken from CD and UC patients showed reduced abundance of *Firmicutes* and *Bacteroidetes* and a concomitant increase of *Proteobacteria* and *Actinobacteria*, compared to non-IBD control [74]. As a consequence of this dysbiosis, the relative abundance of *Enterobacteriaceae* was increased in IBD patients compared to healthy control [75, 76]. Significantly lower counts of *Bifidobacterium* populations were found in rectal biopsies of patients with UC [77]. Study performed by *Macfarlane et al.* showed that *Clostridium leptum (Firmicutes)* is less abundant in fecal samples of CD patients (Table 2) [77].

Clostridium and *Bacteroides* species are the cardinal producers of short chain fatty acids (SCFA) in the human colon [66]. There were decreased SCFA concentrations found in fecal samples of IBD patients, which could be explained by decreased clostridia of groups IV and XIVa (a broad phylogenetic classification comprised of several genera and species of gram positive bacteria). Among the SCFA produced upon carbohydrate fermentation, butyrate has an important role as a major source of energy for colonic epithelial cells, an inhibitor of pro-inflammatory cytokine expression in the intestinal mucosa and an inductor of production of mucin and antimicrobial peptides, thus strengthening epithelial barrier [66, 78]. A decrease of butyrate levels could be involved in the increased inflammatory state characteristic of IBD. Stimulation of butyric acid production could be achieved through repopulation of clostridial clusters IV and XIVa, or even through probiotic therapy with lactic acid bacteria [79]. Some evidence has indicated a promising therapeutic effect of pro, pre and synbiotics in IBD.

	BACTERIAL COMMUNITIES
MOST ABUNDANT BACTERIAL PHYLA IN HEALTHY HUMAN LARGE INTESTINE	Firmicutes Bacteroidetes Actinobacteria Proteobacteria Fusobacteria Verrucomicrobia
ALTERED INTESTINAL MICROBIOTA IN IBD	↓Firmicutes, Bacteroidetes ↑Proteobacteria, Actinobacteria ↓Clostridium leptem (Firmicutes) in CD ↓Bifidobacterium in UC

Table 2. Most abundant bacterial communities in healthy human large intestine and its alterations in IBD

Paneth cells of the small intestine also have an important role in the human gut microbiota, as they are a source of α defensins 5 and 6, which may regulate and maintain microbial balance in the intestinal lumen. The α defensins 5 and 6 are efficacious against *Enterobacteriaceae* and *Bacteroides* vulgatus and studies have shown their levels are increased in chronic inflammatory conditions [80, 81]. In association with ileal CD, they are significantly reduced, particularly in patients with NOD-2 mutations. Colonic CD (but not UC) is associated with β defensins 2 and 3, which are secreted by leukocytes and epithelial cells of many kinds [82].

As explained above, it is a widely accepted hypothesis that the bacteria play an important role in the pathogenesis of IBD. There are several ways in which the microbiota might be linked to IBD. The microbiota as a whole could act as a surrogate pathogen, or specific members of the microbiota could be overt pathogens.

It remains unclear whether the altered gut microbiota composition is a cause of the disease or a consequence of the inflammatory state, but it is most likely that microbial dysbiosis and lack of beneficial bacteria, together with genetically predisposed increased epithelial permeability, bacterial translocation into the lamina propria, defective innate immunity and loss of tolerance to the resident microbiota eventually lead to IBD.

3. Conclusion

Chronic intestinal inflammation in inflammatory bowel disease develops under the influence of environmental triggers in genetically susceptible individuals with an altered im-

http://dx.doi.org/10.5772/52970

mune response. The role of the intestinal microbiota in the pathogenesis of IBD still remains unclear, but even though some enteric bacteria are detrimental and some are protective, their involvement in the pathogenesis of IBD is unquestionable. Table 3 lists main factors associated with IBD development, including known differences between UC and CD ethiopathogenesis.

Since we currently lack complete understanding of the mechanisms leading to the disease, this topic remains to be exceedingly interesting and enigmatic and most certainly a challenging clinical entity that yet remains to be further investigated and unraveled.

	ULCERATIVE COLITIS	**CROHN'S DISEASE**
ENVIRONMENTAL FACTORS	'westernization of lifestyle'	
	Smoking (protective in UC , detrimental in CD) Use of antibiotics Use of NSAIDs Stress Infection Diet Appendectomy	
GENETIC PREDISPOSITION	Major histocompatibility complex region (6p21)	mutations in genes encoding interleukin (IL)-10 receptor and the IL-10 cytokine
	genes mediating epithelial defense function	NOD2 mutations
		ATG16L1 expression
HOST IMMUNE RESPONSE	Higher level of TLR2, 4 and CD 40, followed by increased production of IL-12 and IL-6	
Innate immune responses	↓ Activation of NF-κB ↓ Expression of IL-1β, TNF, IL-6, IL-8, ICAM1, CD 40, CD 80 and other chemokines, adhesion molecules and co-stimulatory molecules	
Adaptive immune responses	atypical T_H2 response, mediated by NK-T cells that secrete IL-13 and IL-5	predominantly TH1 and TH17 (mediated by IL 12 and IL17)
INTESTINAL MICROBIOTA **see table 1 and 2 for further information*	microbiota as a whole acts as a surrogate pathogen, or specific members of the microbiota could be overt pathogens*	

Table 3. Interaction of environmental factors, genetic predisposition, host immune response and intestinal microbiota, main factors associated with CD and UC ethiopathogenesis

Author details

Ana Brajdić and Brankica Mijandrušić-Sinčić*

*Address all correspondence to: bsincic@gmail.com

Department of Internal Medicine, School of Medicine, University of Rijeka, Croatia

References

[1] Wehkamp J, Stange F E. Paneth's Disease. Journal of Crohn's & colitis 2010;4(5): 523-531.

[2] Nell S, Suerbaum S, Josenhans C. The Impact of the Microbiota on the Pathogenesis of IBD: Lessons from Mouse Infection Models. Nature Reviews Microbiology 2010;8(8):564-577.

[3] Sartor RB. Therapeutic Manipulation of the Enteric Microflora in Inflammatory Bowel Diseases: Antibiotics, Probiotics, and Prebiotics. Gastroenterology 2004;126(6): 1620-1633.

[4] Rath HC, Schultz M, Freitag R, Dieleman LA, Li F, Linde HJ, Scholmerich J, Sartor RB. Different Subsets of Enteric Bacteria Induce and Perpetuate Experimental Colitis in Rats and Mice. Infect Immun 2001;69(4):2277-2285.

[5] Hoentjen F, Harmsen HJM, Braat H, Torrice CD, Mann BA, Sartor RB, Dieleman LA. Antibiotic with a Selective Aerobic or Anaerobic Spectrum have Different Therapeutic Activities in Various Regions of the Colon in Interleukin 10 Gene Deficient Mice. Gut 2003;52(12):1721-1727.

[6] Loftus EV Jr. Clinical Epidemiology of Inflammatory Bowel Disease: Incidence, Prevalence, and Environmental Influences. Gastroenterology 2004;126(6):1504-1517.

[7] Hanauer BS, Inflammatory Bowel Disease: Epidemiology, Pathogenesis, and Therapeutic Opportunities, Inflamm Bowel Dis.2006;12(1):3-9.

[8] Shaw SY, Blanchard JF, Bernstein CN., Association Between the Use of Antibiotics in the First Year of Life and Pediatric Inflammatory Bowel Disease. Am J Gastroenterol. 2010;105(12):2687-2692.

[9] Berg DJ Zhang J, Weinstock JV, Ismail HF, Earle KA, Alila H, Pamukcu R, Moore S, Lynch RG. Rapid Development of Colitis in NSAID Treated IL-10 Deficient Mice. Gastroenterology;2002 123(5):1527-1542.

[10] Brinar M, Vermeire S, Cleynen I, Lemmens B, Sagaert X, Henckaerts L, Van Assche G, Geboes K, Rutgeerts P, De Hertogh G. Genetic Variants in Autophagy-related

Genes and Granuloma Formation in a Cohort of Surgically Treated Crohn's Disease Patients. J Crohn's Colitis 2012;6(1):43-50

[11] Cosnes J, Gower-Rousseau C, Seksik P, Cortot A. , Epidemiology and Natural History of Inflammatory Bowel Diseases. Gastroenterology 2011;140(6):1785-1794.

[12] Bach JF. The Effect of Infections on Susceptibility to Sutoimmune and Allergic Diseases. N Engl J Med 2002;347(12):911-920.

[13] Sinčić Mijandrušić B, Vucelić B, Peršić M, Brnčić N, Eržen Jurišić D, Radaković B, Mićović V, Štimac D., Incidence of Inflammatory Bowel Disease in Primorsko-goranska County, Croatia, 2000-2004: A prospective Population-based Study. Scand J Gastroenterol. 2006;41(4):437-44.

[14] Newman B, Siminovitch KA. Recent Advances in the Genetics of Inflammatory Bowel Disease. Curr Opin Gastroenterol. 2005;21(4):401-7.

[15] Judy H. Cho, Steven R. Brant. Recent Insights Into the Genetics of Inflammatory Bowel Disease. Gastroenterology 2011;140(6):1704-1712.

[16] Brant SR. Update on the Heritability of Inflammatory Bowel Disease: The Importance of Twin Studies. Inflammatory Bowel Diseases 2011;17(1):1-5 .

[17] Glocker EO, Kotlarz D, Boztug K, Gertz EM, Schäffer AA, Noyan F, Perro M, Diestelhorst J, Allroth A, Murugan D, Hätscher N, Pfeifer D, Sykora KW, Sauer M, Kreipe H, Lacher M, Nustede R, Woellner C, Baumann U, Salzer U, Koletzko S, Shah N, Segal AW, Sauerbrey A, Buderus S, Snapper SB, Grimbacher B, Klein C. Inflammatory Bowel Disease and Mutations Affecting the Interleukin-10 Receptor. N Engl J Med 2009;361(21):2033-2045.

[18] Glocker EO, Frede N, Perro M, Sebire N, Elawad M, Shah N, Grimbacher B. Infant Colitis - It's in the Genes. The Lancet 2010; 376(9748) 1272

[19] Moore KW, de Waal Malefyt R, Coffman RL, O'Garra A. Interleukin-10 and the Interleukin-10 Receptor. Annu Rev Immunol. 2001;19:683-765.

[20] Hugot JP, Chamaillard M, Zouali H, Lesage S, CeÂzard JP, Belaiche J, Almerk S, Tysk C, O'Morain CA, Gassull M, Binder V, Finkel Y, Cortot A, Modigliani R, Laurent-Puig P, Gower-Rousseau C, Macrykk J, Colombel JF, Sahbatou M, Thomas G. Association of NOD2 leucine-rich repeat variants with susceptibility to Crohn's disease. Nature. 2001;411(6837):599-603.

[21] Ogura Y, Bonen DK, Inohara N, Nicolae DL, Chen FF, Ramos R, Britton H, Moran T, Karaliuskas R, Duerr RH, Achkar JP, Brant SR, Bayless TM, Kirschner BS, Hanauer SB, Nuñez G, Cho JH. A Frameshift Mutation in NOD2 Associated with Susceptibility to Crohn's Disease. Nature 2001;411(6837):603-606.

[22] Economou M, Trikalinos TA, Loizou KT, Tsianos EV, Ioannidis JP. Differential Effects of NOD2 Variants on Crohn's Disease Risk and Phenotype in Diverse Populations: A Metaanalysis. Am J Gastroenterol. 2004;99(12):2393-404.

[23] Ahuja V, K Tandon R. Inflammatory Bowel Disease in the Asia–Pacific Area: A Comparison with Developed Countries and Regional Differences. Journal of Digestive Diseases 2010;11(3):134–147.

[24] Gregorieff A, Clevers H. Wnt Signaling in the Intestinal Epithelium: from Endoderm to Cancer. Genes Dev 2005; 19(8):877-890.

[25] Barker N. The Canonical Wnt/beta-Catenin Signaling Pathway. Methods Mol Biol 2008;468:5-15.

[26] Crosnier C, Stamataki D, Lewis J. Organizing Cell Renewal in the Intestine: Stem Cells, Signals and Combinatorial Control. Nat Rev Genet 2006;7(5):349-59.

[27] Wehkamp J, Schmid M, Stange EF. Defensins and Other Antimicrobial Peptides in Inflammatory Bowel Disease. Curr Opin Gastroenterol 2007;23(4):370-378.

[28] Ericksen B, Wu Z, Lu W, Lehrer RI. Antibacterial Activity and Specificity of the Six Human α-Defensins. Antimicrob Agents Chemother. 2005;49(1):269–275.

[29] Klotman ME, Chang TL. Defensins in Innate Antiviral Immunity. Nat Rev Immunol 2006;6(6) 447-456.

[30] Lala S, Ogura Y, Osborne C, Hor SY, Bromfield A, Davies S, Ogunbiyi O, Nuñez G, Keshav S. Crohn's Disease and the NOD2 Gene: A Role for Paneth Cells. Gastroenterology. 2003;125(1):47-57.

[31] Rosenstiel P, Fantini M, Bräutigam K, Kühnbacher T, Waetzig GH, Seegert D, Schreiber S. Gastroenterology. 2003;124(4):1001-1009.

[32] Kobayashi KS, Chamaillard M, Ogura Y, Henegariu O, Inohara N, Nuñez G, Flavell RA. Nod2-Dependent Regulation of Innate and Adaptive Immunity in the Intestinal Tract. Science. 2005;307(5710):731-734.

[33] Fishbein T, Novitskiy G, Mishra L, Matsumoto C, Kaufman S, Goyal S, Shetty K, Johnson L, Lu A, Wang A, Hu F, Kallakury B, Lough D, Zasloff M. NOD2-Expressing Bone Marrow-Derived Cells Appear to Regulate Epithelial Innate Immunity of the Transplanted Human Small Intestine. Gut. 2008;57(3):323-330.

[34] Levine B, Deretic V. Unveiling the Roles of Auotphagy in Innate and Adaptive Immunity. Nat Rev Immunol 2007;7(10):767-777.

[35] Cadwell K, Liu JY, Brown SL, Miyoshi H, Loh J, Lennerz JK, Kishi C, Kc W, Carrero JA, Hunt S, Stone CD, Brunt EM, Xavier RJ, Sleckman BP, Li E, Mizushima N, Stappenbeck TS, Virgin HW 4th. A Key Role for Autophagy and the Autophagy Gene Atg16l1 in Mouse and Human Intestinal Paneth Cells. Nature. 2008;456(7219): 259-263.

[36] Barrett JC, Hansoul S, Nicolae DL, Cho JH, Duerr RH, Rioux JD, Brant SR, Silverberg MS, Taylor KD, Barmada MM, Bitton A, Dassopoulos T, Datta LW, Green T, Griffiths AM, Kistner EO, Murtha MT, Regueiro MD, Rotter JI, Schumm LP, Steinhart AH,

Targan SR, Xavier RJ; NIDDK IBD Genetics Consortium, Libioulle C, Sandor C, Lathrop M, Belaiche J, Dewit O, Gut I, Heath S, Laukens D, Mni M, Rutgeerts P, Van Gossum A, Zelenika D, Franchimont D, Hugot JP, de Vos M, Vermeire S, Louis E; Belgian-French IBD Consortium; Wellcome Trust Case Control Consortium, Cardon LR, Anderson CA, Drummond H, Nimmo E, Ahmad T, Prescott NJ, Onnie CM, Fisher SA, Marchini J, Ghori J, Bumpstead S, Gwilliam R, Tremelling M, Deloukas P, Mansfield J, Jewell D, Satsangi J, Mathew CG, Parkes M, Georges M, Daly MJ. Genome-Wide Association Defines More than 30 Distinct Susceptibility Loci for Crohn's Disease. Nat Genet. 2008;40(8):955-962.

[37] Parkes M, Barrett JC, Prescott NJ, Tremelling M, Anderson CA, Fisher SA, Roberts RG, Nimmo ER, Cummings FR, Soars D, Drummond H, Lees CW, Khawaja SA, Bagnall R, Burke DA, Todhunter CE, Ahmad T, Onnie CM, McArdle W, Strachan D, Bethel G, Bryan C, Lewis CM, Deloukas P, Forbes A, Sanderson J, Jewell DP, Satsangi J, Mansfield JC; Wellcome Trust Case Control Consortium, Cardon L, Mathew CG. Sequence Variants in the Autophagy Gene IRGM and Multiple Other Replicating Loci Contribute to Crohn's Disease Susceptibility. Nat Genet. 2007;39(7):830-832.

[38] Duerr RH, Taylor KD, Brant SR, Rioux JD, Silverberg MS, Daly MJ, Steinhart AH, Abraham C, Regueiro M, Griffiths A, Dassopoulos T, Bitton A, Yang H, Targan S, Wu Data L, Kistner EO, Schumm LP, Lee AT, Gregersen PK, Barmada MM, Rotter JI, Nicolae DL, Cho JH. A Genome-Wide Association Study Identifies IL23R as an Inflammatory Bowel Disease Gene. Science 2006;314(5804):1461- 1463.

[39] Cargill M, Schrodi SJ, Chang M, Garcia VE, Brandon R, Callis KP, Matsunami N, Ardlie KG, Civello D, Catanese JJ, Leong DU, Panko JM, McAllister LB, Hansen CB, Papenfuss J, Prescott SM, White TJ, Leppert MF, Krueger GG, Begovich AB. A Large-Scale Genetic Association Study Confirms IL12B and Leads to the Identification of IL23R as Psoriasis-risk Genes. Am J Hum Genet. 2007;80(2):273-290.

[40] Franke A, McGovern DP, Barrett JC, Wang K, Radford-Smith GL, Ahmad T, Lees CW, Balschun T, Lee J, Roberts R, Anderson CA, Bis JC, Bumpstead S, Ellinghaus D, Festen EM, Georges M, Green T, Haritunians T, Jostins L, Latiano A, Mathew CG, Montgomery GW, Prescott NJ, Raychaudhuri S, Rotter JI, Schumm P, Sharma Y, Simms LA, Taylor KD, Whiteman D, Wijmenga C, Baldassano RN, Barclay M, Bayless TM, Brand S, Büning C, Cohen A, Colombel JF, Cottone M, Stronati L, Denson T, De Vos M, D'Inca R, Dubinsky M, Edwards C, Florin T, Franchimont D, Gearry R, Glas J, Van Gossum A, Guthery SL, Halfvarson J, Verspaget HW, Hugot JP, Karban A, Laukens D, Lawrance I, Lemann M, Levine A, Libioulle C, Louis E, Mowat C, Newman W, Panés J, Phillips A, Proctor DD, Regueiro M, Russell R, Rutgeerts P, Sanderson J, Sans M, Seibold F, Steinhart AH, Stokkers PC, Torkvist L, Kullak-Ublick G, Wilson D, Walters T, Targan SR, Brant SR, Rioux JD, D'Amato M, Weersma RK, Kugathasan S, Griffiths AM, Mansfield JC, Vermeire S, Duerr RH, Silverberg MS, Satsangi J, Schreiber S, Cho JH, Annese V, Hakonarson H, Daly MJ, Parkes M. Genome-Wide Meta-Analysis Increases to 71 the Number of Confirmed Crohn's Disease Susceptibility Loci. Nat Genet. 2010;42(12):1118-1125.

[41] Sartor RB, Hoentjen F. Proinflammatory Cytokines and Signaling Pathways in Intestinal Innate Immune Cells. Mucosal Immunology London: Elsevier Academic Press; 2005. pp. 681–701.

[42] Siew C Changing Epidemiology and Future Challenges of Inflammatory Bowel Disease in Asia. Intestinal Research 2010;8(1)1-8.

[43] Reaves TA, Chin AC, Parkos CA. Neutrophil Transepithelial Migration: Role of Toll-like Receptors in Mucosal Inflammation. Mem Inst Oswaldo Cruz. 2005;100(1): 191-198.

[44] Hart AL, Al-Hassi HO, Rigby RJ, Bell SJ, Emmanuel AV, Knight SC, Kamm MA, Stagg AJ. Characteristics of Intestinal Dendritic Cells in Inflammatory Bowel Diseases. Gastroenterology. 2005;129(1):50-65.

[45] Rakoff-Nahoum S, Paglino J, Eslami-Varzaneh F, Edberg S, Medzhitov R. Recognition of Commensal Microflora by Toll-Like Receptors is Required for Intestinal Homeostasis. Cell. 2004;118(2):229-241.

[46] Neurath MF, Pettersson S, Meyer zum Büschenfelde KH, Strober W. Local Administration of Antisense Phosphorothioate Oligonucleotides to the p65 Subunit of NF-kappa B Abrogates Established Experimental Colitis in Mice. Nat Med. 1996;2(9): 998-1004.

[47] Cario E, Podolsky DK. Differential Alteration in Intestinal Epithelial Cell Expression of Toll-Like Receptor 3 (TLR3) and TLR4 in Inflammatory Bowel Disease. Infect Immun. 2000;68(12):7010-7017.

[48] Barnias G, Martin CIII, Mishina M, Ross WG, Rivera Nieves J, Marini M, Cominelli F. Proinflammatory Effects of T_H2 Cytokines in a Murine Model of Chronic Small Intestinal Inflammation. Gastroenterology 2005;128(3):654-666.

[49] Kolls JK, Linden A. Interleukin -17 Family Members and Inflammation. Immunity 2004;21(4):467-476.

[50] Fujino S, Andoh A, Bamba S, Ogawa A, Hata K, Araki Y, Bamba T, Fujiyama Y. Increased Expression of IL-17 in Inflammatory Bowel Disease. Gut 2003;52(1):65-70.

[51] Strober W, Fuss IJ. Proinflammatory Cytokines in the Pathogenesis of Inflammatory Bowel Diseases. Gastroenterology 2011;140(6):1756-1767.

[52] Fuss IJ Heller F, Boirivant M, Leon F, Yoshida M, Fichtner-Feigl S, Yang Z, Exley M, Kitani A, Blumberg RS, Mannon P, Strober W. Nonclassical CD1d-Restricted NK T Cells that Produce IL-13 Characterize an Atypical Th2 Response in Ulcerative Colitis. J Clin Invest. 2004;113(10):1490–1497.

[53] Liu Z, Geboes K, Heremans H, Overbergh L, Mathieu C, Rutgeerts P, Ceuppens JL. Role of Interleukin-12 in the Induction of Mucosal Inflammation and Abrogation of Regulatory T cell Function in Chronic Experimental Colitis. European Journal of Immunology 2001; 31(5):1550-1560.

[54] Smythies LE, Shen R, Bimczok D, Novak L, Clements RH, Eckhoff DE, Bouchard P, George MD, Hu WK, Dandekar S, Smith PD. Inflammation anergy in human intestinal macrophages is due to Smad-induced IkappaBalpha expression and NF-kappaB inactivation..J Biol Chem 2010;285(25):19593–19604.

[55] Jung C,Hugot JP, Barreau F. Peyer's Patches: The Immune Sensors of the Intestine. International Journal of Inflammation 2010 Article ID 823710, 12 pages, doi: 10.4061/2010/823710.

[56] Arumugam M, Raes J,nPelletier E, Le Paslier D, Yamada T, Mende1 DR, Fernandes GR, Tap J, Bruls T, Batto JM, Bertalan M, Borruel N, Casellas F, Fernandez L, Gautier L, Hansen T, Hattori M, Hayashi T, Kleerebezem M, Kurokawa K, Leclerc M, Levenez F, Manichanh C, Nielsen BH, Nielsen T, Pons N, Poulain J, Qin J, Sicheritz-Ponten T, Tims S, Torrents D, Ugarte E, Zoetendal EG, Wang J, Guarner F, Pedersen O, de Vos WM, Brunak S, Dore J, MetaHIT Consortium, Weissenbach J, Ehrlich SD, Bork P Enterotypes of the human gut microbiome. Nature 2011;473:174–180. http://www.nature.com/nature/journal/v473/n7346/full/nature09944.html

[57] Dominguez-Bello MG, Blaser M, Ley RE, Knight R. Development of the Human Gastrointestinal Microbiota and Insights From High -Throughput Sequencing. Gastroenterology 2011;140(6):1713-1719.

[58] Domínguez-Bello MG, Costtello EK, Contreras M, Magris M, Hidalgo G, Fierer N, Knight R. Delivery Mode Shapes the Acquisition and Structure of the Initial Microbiota Across Multiple Body Habitats in Newborns. Proc Natl Acad Sci U S A. 2010;107(26):11971–11975.

[59] Mackie RI, Sghir A, Gaskins HR. Developmental Microbial Ecology of the Neonatal Gastrointestinal Tract. Am J Clin Nutr. 1999;69(5):1035–1045.

[60] Vaishampayan PA, Kuehl JV, Froula JL, Morgan JL, Ochman H, Pilar Francino M. Comparative Metagenomics and Population Dynamics of the Gut Microbiota in Mother and Infant. Genome Biol Evol. 2010;6(2):53–66.

[61] Matsumiya Y, Kato N, Watanabe K, Kato H.. Molecular Epidemiological Study of Vertical Transmission of Vaginal *Lactobacillus* Species from Mothers to Newborn Infants in Japanese, by Arbitrarily Primed Polymerase Chain Reaction. J Infect Chemother. 2002;8(1):43–49.

[62] Koenig JE, Spor A, Scalfone N, Fricker AD, Stombaugh J, Knight R, Angenent LT, Ley RE. Microbes and Health Sackler Colloquium: Succession of Microbial Consortia in the Developing Infant Gut Microbiome. Proc Natl Acad Sci U S A. 2011;108(1): 4578–4585

[63] Filippo C, Cavalieri D, Di Paola M, Ramazzotti M,Poullet JB, Massart S, Collini S, Pieraccini G, Lionetti P. Impact of Diet in Shaping Gut Microbiota Revealed by a Comparative Study in Children from Europe and Rural Africa. Proc Natl Acad Sci U S A. 2010;107(33):14691–14696

[64] Rajilic-Stojanovic M, Heilig HG, Molenaar D, Kajander K, Surakka A, Smidt H, de Vos WM. Development and Application of the Human Intestinal Tract Chip, a Phylogenetic Microarray: Analysis of Universally Conserved Phylotypes in the Abundant Microbiota of Young and Elderly Adults. Environ Microbiol. 2009;11(7):1736–1751.

[65] Zoetendal EG, Akkermans ADL, Akkermans-van Vliet WM, de Visser JAGM, de Vos WM. The Host Genotype Affects the Bacterial Community in the Human Gastronintestinal Tract. Microb Ecol Health Dis. 2001;13(3):129-134.

[66] Fava F., Danese S. Intestinal Microbiota in Inflammatory Bowel Disease: Friend of Foe? World J Gastroenterol. 2011;17(5):557-566.

[67] Baoli Zhu, Xin Wang, Lanjuan Li. Human Gut Microbiome: The Second Genome of Human Body. Protein Cell 2010;1(8):718-725.

[68] Qin J, Li R, Raes J, Arumugam M, Burgdorf KS, Manichanh C, Nielsen T, Pons N, Levenez F, Yamada T, Mende DR, Li J, Xu J, Li S, Li D, Cao J, Wang B, Liang H, Zheng H, Xie Y, Tap J, Lepage P, Bertalan M, Batto JM, Hansen T, Le Paslier D, Linneberg A, Nielsen HB, Pelletier E, Renault P, Sicheritz-Ponten T, Turner K, Zhu H, Yu C, Li S, Jian M, Zhou Y, Li Y, Zhang X, Li S, Qin N, Yang H, Wang J, Brunak S, Doré J, Guarner F, Kristiansen K, Pedersen O, Parkhill J, Weissenbach J; MetaHIT Consortium, Bork P, Ehrlich SD, Wang J. A Human Gut Microbial Gene Catalogue Established By Metagenomic Sequencing. Nature 2010;464(7285):59-65.

[69] Coombes JL, Siddiqui KR, Arancibia-Cárcamo CV, Hall J, Sun CM, Belkaid Y, Powrie F. A Functionally Specialized Population of Mucosal CD103+ DCs Induces Foxp3+ Regulatory T Cells via a TGF-Beta and Retinoic Acid-Dependent Mechanism. J Exp Med. 2007;204(8):1757-1764.

[70] Tezuka H, Abe Y, Iwata M, Takeuchi H, Ishikawa H, Matsushita M, Shiohara T, Akira S, Ohteki T. Regulation of IgA Production by Naturally Occurring TNF/iNOS-Producing Dendritic Cells. Nature. 2007;448(7156):929-933

[71] Gewirtz AT. TLRs in the Gut. III. Immune Responses to Flagellin in Crohn's Disease: Good, Bad, or Irrelevant? Am J Physiol Gastrointest Liver Physiol 2007;292(3): 706-710.

[72] Neish AS, Gewirtz AT, Zeng H, Young AN, Hobert ME, Karmali V, Rao AS, Madara JL. Prokaryotic Regulation of Epithelial Responses by Inhibition of IkappaB-alpha Ibiquitination. Science. 2000;289(5484):1560-1563.

[73] Fukata M, Chen A, Klepper A, Krishnareddy S, Vamadevan AS, Thomas LS, Xu R, Inoue H, Arditi M, Dannenberg AJ. Cox-2 is Regulated by Toll-Like Receptor-4 (TLR4) Signaling: Role in Proliferation and Apoptosis in the Intestine. Gastroenterology. 2006;131(3):862-877.

[74] Frank DN, St. Amand AL, Feldman RA, Boedeker EC, Harpaz N, Pace NR. Molecular-Phylogenetic Characterization of Microbial Community Imbalances in Human In-

flammatory Bowel Diseases. Proceedings of the National Academy of Sciences of the United States of America. 2007;104(34):13780–13785.

[75] Gophna U, Sommerfeld K, Gophna S, Doolittle WF, Veldhuyzen van Zanten SJ. Differences Between Tissue-Associated Intestinal Microfloras of Patients with Crohn's Disease and Ulcerative Colitis. J Clin Microbiol. 2006;44(11):4136-4141.

[76] Manichanh C, Rigottier-Gois L, Bonnaud E, Gloux K, Pelletier E, Frangeul L, Nalin R, Jarrin C, Chardon P, Marteau P. Reduced Diversity of Faecal Microbiota in Crohn's Disease Revealed by a Metagenomic Approach. Gut. 2006;55(2):205-211.

[77] Macfarlane S, Furrie E, Cummings JH, Macfarlane GT. Chemotaxonomic Analysis of Bacterial Populations Colonizing the Rectal Mucosa in Patients With Ulcerative Colitis. Clin Infect Dis. 2004;38(12):1690-1699

[78] Vanhoutvin SA, Troost FJ, Hamer HM, Lindsey PJ, Koek GH, Jonkers DM, Kodde A, Venema K, Brummer RJ. Butyrate-Induced Transcriptional Changes in Human Colonic Mucosa. PLoS One. 2009;4:e6759. doi:10.1371/journal.pone.0006759 http://www.plosone.org/article/info%3Adoi%2F10.1371%2Fjournal.pone.0006759

[79] Duncan SH, Louis P, Flint HJ. Lactate-Utilizing Bacteria, Isolated from Human Feces, that Produce Butyrate as a Major Fermentation Product. Appl Environ Microbiol. 2004;70(10):5810-5817.

[80] Nuding S, Fellermann K, Wehkamp J, Stange EF. Reduced Mucosal Antimicrobial Activity in Crohn's Disease of the Colon. Gut. 2007;56(9):1240-1247.

[81] Wehkamp J, Harder J, Weichenthal M, Schwab M, Schäffeler E, Schlee M, Herrlinger KR, Stallmach A, Noack F, Fritz P. NOD2 (CARD15) Mutations in Crohn's Disease are Associated with Diminished Mucosal Alpha-Defensin Expression. Gut. 2004;53(11):1658-1664.

[82] Wehkamp J, Harder J, Weichenthal M, Mueller O, Herrlinger KR, Fellermann K, Schroeder JM, Stange EF. Inducible and Constitutive Beta-Defensins are Differentially Expressed in Crohn's Disease and Ulcerative Colitis. Inflamm Bowel Dis. 2003;9(4): 215-223.

Chapter 2

Gene Polymorphisms and Inflammatory Bowel Diseases

Bartosova Ladislava, Kolorz Michal,
Wroblova Katerina and Bartos Milan

Additional information is available at the end of the chapter

http://dx.doi.org/10.5772/53465

1. Introduction

1.1. What is it a gene polymorphism?

Every protein is coded by a gene and every human gene exists in several allelic variants, which occur due to mutations and are inherited together with other genetic characteristics from parents to children. If a certain allelic variant occurs within the population with at least a 1% frequency, it is known as a common gene polymorphism. However, if the frequency in the given population is below 1%, it is referred to as a rare allelic variant.

An allele having a majority within a population is called a wild type or standard. Allele(s), which are a minority within a population, are known as a variant, non-standard or sometimes a mutant allele.

Percentage frequencies of individual alleles for the same gene polymorphisms in various populations are often significantly different, which makes many clinical studies complicated. For example, variant allele asterisk *10 of gene coding for cytochrome CYP2D6 codes an unstable enzyme with decreasing activity. It can result in the slower metabolism of some drugs, e.g. antidepressants. The frequency of this variant allele is from 1 - 2% in the Caucasian population but 51% in the Asian population. The gene CYP2D6 can also be duplicated or multiplicated. The amount of enzyme is from 2 to 13 times higher compared to the standard gene allele, which leads to ultra rapid metabolism. The occurrence of this polymorphism differs. For example, in Central Europe, the occurrence is 4% and in Saudi Arabia it is 29%.

1.2. Molecular biological basis of gene polymorphism

The molecular biological basis of gene polymorphism is a mutation of the given gene, in which individual variant alleles occur. Mutations can have a form of replacement or substitution when one or more nucleotides in a gene are replaced by another one; or they can have a form of frameshift mutations, including deletions or insertions, when one or more nucleotides in a gene are missing (=deletion) or are redundant (=insertion). Frameshift mutations lead to frameshift changes, and from the position of the mutation other amino acids can be incorporated in the protein chain or a stop codon is generated, which prematurely terminates transcription of the protein chain.

The most common mutation in gene polymorphisms is the replacement of a single nucleotide, or the so-called single nucleotide polymorphism or SNP.

SNP represents 90% of all gene polymorphisms in humans. There is a freely accessible database (http://www.ncbi.nlm.nih.gov/SNP/index.html), which lists over 38 million identified and validated SNPs, and their number grows every day. SNPs are also associated into blocks - haplotypes, which are usually inherited together. Therefore, the identification of a single SNP can theoretically identify the whole haplotype.

1.3. Methods of gene polymorphisms detection

Presently, the basic method of molecular diagnostics is a polymerase chain reaction, PCR. A basic PCR reaction contains two primers and serves for the detection of one specific locus in the form of amplicon of a pre-calculated size.

For the purposes of finding simple nucleotide polymorphisms, the products of amplification can be further digested by restriction endonuclease, and this arrangement is marked PCR-REA (PCR-restriction enzyme analysis), PRA (primer restriction analysis) or PCR-RFLP (PCR-restriction fragment length polymorphism) [1]. This method allows for the analysis of any gene up to a length of approximately 5 kbp. Amplicons of the same length are the result of PCR amplification. These amplicons are further digested by a suitable restriction endonuclease and the resulting products analyzed by gel electrophoresis. It is a very simple, fast and highly sensitive detection method for single gene polymorphisms. However, it can only be used for determining gene polymorphism when two alleles in the given locus differ in such a way that one contains a restriction locus for the given endonuclease and the other does not.

DNA sequencing is the determination of the primary structure of nucleotide chain, i.e. the sequence of nucleotides in DNA molecules. It is a final and definite determination of the basic information which DNA carries. Knowledge of the DNA sequence allows to find the reading frames of potential genes, to analyse exons and introns in structural genes, and to determine the sequences of amino acid-coded proteins, and is usable for the detection of regulatory genes and regulatory areas, repetitive sequences and all simple nucleotide polymorphisms. There are two fundamentally different methods which are commonly used for sequencing. The first method is based on terminating DNA chains using chemical substances and is called Maxam-Gilbert Sequencing [2]. The second method uses the inhibition of the enzymatic synthesis of DNA by dideoxyterminators, and is known as Sanger's Sequencing Method [3]. Both methods use the same original material, i.e. DNA fragments obtained, for example, by restriction or cloned in vector. They can also be products of polymerase chain reaction. The most recent development in sequencing methods has been the introduction of devices for automatic sequencing. This method uses enzymatic Sanger's method and allows for the determination and processing of DNA sequences at a much faster rate as well as being more economical than standard techniques [4].

1.4. Clinical consequences of gene polymorphism

The clinical consequences of mutations on the function and the amount of coding protein (phenotype) depend on their localization and can influence the development of certain diseases or a patient's response to a particular drug regarding their effectiveness, as well as the safety of a chosen pharmacotherapy.

A mutation can be located in the coding areas of a gene (exons), in the regulatory areas (promoter or generally in the 5′ region of gene) or at the exon–intron interface, i.e. in the exon-intron primary transcript splicing site.

Mutation in the exon area (the coding part of a gene), is manifested by the substitution of amino acids or from a change of the amino acid sequence in the protein chain.

If a gene codes for an enzyme, the result of the mutation is a change in the pharmacokinetic parameters at the drug metabolization level, i.e. leading to the altered activity of this enzyme, or to its complete inactivation and consequent acceleration or deceleration of the metabolic processes leading to the degradation of the active substance in the drug or, on the other hand, to the formation of the active substance in case of the "prodrug". If a gene codes for a receptor protein, the mutation can lead to a change of the receptor's ability to bind a ligand and to activate the signaling cascade. This can cause changes in the pharmacodynamic parameters of the drug. Membrane carriers, protein and P-glycoprotein transporters coded by a variant allele of a gene can have an altered affinity to its substrates; variant channel proteins can create channels with different electrical and chemical characteristics, and this can result in a change of ionic homeostasis.

Mutation in the regulatory areas of a gene leads to changes in gene expression, i.e. to either upregulation or downregulation. It is manifested by the lack or excess of protein coded by this gene. If the mutation is located in the interface area between intron and exon in the primary transcript splicing site, this can result in the faulty splicing of the primary transcript, and can cause a shortening or lengthening of a protein chain, which leads to the loss or restriction of functions of the coding protein.The splicing site is distinguishable by specific ribonucleoproteins. If the nucleotide sequences in this area differ from the standard gene as a result of mutation, incorrect splicing of primary transcript hnRNA to mRNA occurs.

The presence of variant alleles can have an impact not only on metabolic processes (absorption, distribution and drug elimination), it can also influence the effectiveness and safety of the chosen pharmacotherapy. Furthermore, it represents an increased risk of the development of certain diseases due to the changing structures or functions of several regulatory proteins, which influence the physiological processes of the body. Disease development is caused by both genetic and environmental factors. Additionally, a patient's sensitivity to external factors is varied and this variability is again, genetically conditioned.

2. The role of candidate genes in etiopathogenesis of inflammatory bowel diseases

Inflammatory bowel diseases (IBD) are chronic inflammatory diseases of the gastrointestinal tract. The term covers two specific conditions – Crohn's disease (CD) and ulcerative colitis (UC), which differ in their anatomic location, intensity and the scope of their affect on the intestinal mucosa. The etiopathogenesis of these two conditions is not fully understood to date. However, several studies have confirmed that there are external factors, together with genetic predisposition, which contribute to the diseases' onset [5]. The significant role of genetic predisposition is supported by a relatively high familial occurrence of Crohn's disease, a high concordance in monozygotic twins up to 67% a connection with patients' ethnic or racial character, and parallel incidences of other rare genetic syndromes. The risk of Crohn's disease is 3–5 times higher in the first degree relatives, and a familial occurrence was found in 15–20% of cases. However, genetic predisposition is more important in CD than in UC [6–8]. Genes whose products somehow influence the development of the inflammatory reaction are called "candidate genes," and they are located at different places on the genome marked from IBD1 to IBD9 [9]. These candidate genomic loci include *NOD2/CARD15, ICAM-1, CCR5, MDR1, TLR4* and other genes [10–12]. At present, the correlation between the genetic makeup of an individual and the predisposition to contract a disease has been studied as well as its connection with the clinical characteristic of a disease.

2.1. NOD2/CARD15 gene

NOD2 (nucleotide-binding oligomerization domain) is a protein expressed by several immune system cells (monocytes, macrophages and dendritic cells). It is a key molecule that reacts to the intracellular presence of peptidoglycans of bacterial origin [13]. The binding of peptidoglycans initiates the signalling cascade, ending with NF-κB activation and the expression of pro-inflammatory genes including *TNFα* [14,15]. In the gene for the protein NOD2, several polymorphisms were described. Substitutions at positions 702Arg>Trp, 908Gly>Arg and the frameshift mutation (cytosine nucleotide insertion) at position 1007 (3020fsinsC) are most often linked with the disruption of receptor functions. These three mutations represent 81% mutations of *NOD2* in CD patients [16]. The presence of the latter mutation leads to the disruption of the reading frame during the transcription and to the termination of proteosynthesis due to a newly formed stop codon [17]. For the polymorphisms at positions 702 and 908 was described a comparable or just a slightly increased NF-κB induction [18]. Furthermore, the presence of the frameshift mutation at position 1007 limits the structure and function of the NOD2 protein to such an extent that the NF-κB activation in the presence of peptidoglycan is (MDP used as a standard inductor) undetectable [15] and

TNFα expression is decreased [19–21]. The described polymorphisms have a relatively high frequency in the Caucasian population. Carriers of one mutant allele have a 2 to 4 times higher risk of CD outbreak and recessive homozygotes at 20–40 times higher [20]. An association between the occurrence of the 1007fs frameshift mutation in the *NOD2* gene and the IBD incidence has also been confirmed. A similar association, somewhat less significant, was also discovered in the 908Gly>Arg polymorphism [21]. Patients with mutations in the gene *CARD15/NOD2* also showed a decreased expression of defensines [22]. Mutations can therefore be predisposed to CD not only directly, but indirectly as well, i.e. by obstructing the natural antimicrobial immunity mediated by defensines.

2.2. ICAM-1 gene

Lately, the association between IBD and the *ICAM-1* gene has also been intensively studied. This gene codes for the intracellular adhesive molecule ICAM-1 which performs many physiological functions. It controls the migration of inflammatory elements, participates in the presentation of antigen, and because it is expressed by various cell types, it is involved in many signalling cascades [23]. Its significantly increased expression in the intestinal mucosa was observed in inflammatory bowel diseases. In the ICAM-1 gene, at least 20 SNPs were identified. A SNP marked 469Lys>Glu has also been linked with IBD [24]. A substitution of nucleotides leads to the substitution of amino acid in the 5th immunoglobulin domain of ICAM-1, which is important for the adhesion of B cells and dendritic cells [25]. An altered function of the protein ICAM-1 potentially contributes to the genetic predisposition for inflammatory diseases and immunity disorders. The prevalence of the 469Lys>Glu polymorphism has also been linked with multiple sclerosis [26], Behcet's disease [27], psoriatic and rheumatic arthritis [28] and other chronic inflammatory diseases [29].

2.3. CCR5 gene

Another gene, which intervenes in the reactions of the immune system, is the gene that codes for the receptor CCR5, whose ligands are CC chemokines. The endogenous functions of this receptor include the mobilization of the relevant immune system cells and the targeting of their chemotaxis into the inflamed area. The CCR5 receptor is responsible for the transport of chemokine CC and participates in the entering of virus particles of the human immunodeficiency virus (HIV-1) into macrophages [30].

Its regulatory role lies in the preference of the Th1 immune response and suppression of the Th2 immune pathway. It participates, for example, in the immune defence against *Mycobacterium tuberculosis*, [31]. In the 1990s, it was discovered that the gene for this receptor occurs in various allelic forms in the population. In particular, a 32 base pairs deletion in the gene *CCR5* was studied because it leads to the expression of a shorter, and therefore non-functional receptor in the cell membrane and consequently to the disrupted communication between cells of the immune system. This deletion mutation is associated with the onset of pathological inflammatory conditions, such as sarcoidosis [32], rheumatoid arthritis [33] and periodontitis [34]. A cellular immunity disorder caused by the non-functional receptor CCR5 could play some role in IBD development.

2.4. TLR4 gene

The Toll receptor was originally described in Drosophila, where its function lies in the immune defence against fungal and yeast infections in adults. It was found that the intracellular part of this receptor molecule often resembles parts similar to a completely different receptor – for cytokine interleukin-1 (IL-1). In humans, a total of 10 receptors have been described in which their amino acid sequence is similar to the original Toll receptor of Drosophila [35]. Thus, they were named Toll-like receptors. Individual TLR receptors differ in their presence in various cell populations and in their affinity for various ligands. TLR4 in particular is a model ligand of lipopolysaccharide (LPS), which activates the NF-κB expression after binding to the extracellular domain of a receptor, and, in the next step, the expression of pro-inflammatory cytokines (TNFα, IL). The gene for TLR4 is located on chromosome 9, in the area 9q32-33, and is expressed by monocytes, macrophages, mastocytes and immature dendritic cells, as well as by intestinal cells in a small amount in the apical part of epithelium, and also by renal, corneal and pulmonary epithelial cells [36]. A substitution of adenine for guanine at position 896 (896A>G) was detected by direct sequencing. This substitution is manifested on the amino acid sequence level by the substitution of a conservative aspargic acid with glycine at position 299 (299Asp>Gly). This single nucleotide polymorphism (SNP) is located in exon 4 of the gene for TLR4 and results in production of an altered extracellular domain of this receptor.

Another SNP was found at position 399 of the amino acid sequence, where non-conservative threonine was replaced by isoleucine (399Thr>Ile). This mutation cosegregates with mutation 299Asp>Gly [37]. Polymorphisms in the gene for TLR4 are linked with various diseases such as chronic periodontitis [38], COPD [39], Behcet's disease [40], septic shock [41] or IBD [42] and are associated with the disruption of intracellular processes leading to NF-κB induction and TNFα expression.

2.5. TNFα gene

Several SNPs have been described in the *TNFα* gene sequence; in the promoter, intron, as well as exon areas. In the promoter area, the following polymorphisms have been described: substitutions at nucleotide positions –1031T>C, –863 C>A, –857 C>A, –851C>T, –419 G>C, –376 G>A, –308 G>A, –238 G>A, –163 G>A, and –49 G>A. In the intron 1 sequence, there is the substitution of 488G>A [43]. The mutation in the gene *TNFα* results in a changed level of the gene expression and therefore a different amount of active cytokine. As was mentioned before, the physiological or pathological manifestations of its effect are based on TNFα quantity. In this context, the polymorphisms in the promoter area of the gene, which interacts with the transcription factors, are highlighted. Nucleotide polymorphisms at positions –376, –308 and –238 are most often mentioned in connection with the change of the gene expression level.

2.5.1. Polymorphism –376G>A

Transcription factor OCT-1 binds at position –376. It was proved that the transcription factor binds with a higher preference to the variant allele –376A [44].

2.5.2. Polymorphism –308G>A

This polymorphism is most often mentioned in connection with increased TNFα production. At the same time, it is the most closely studied predisposition factor for chronic inflammatory diseases including IBD. Braun et al. [45] as well as Sashio et al. [46] confirmed *in vitro* a higher transcription activity of the variant allele –308A. In his study of the Czech population, Sykora et al. [47] stated that a statistically significant association existed between the –308G>A polymorphism and the occurrence of UC in child patients. He also discovered that patients who were carriers of at least one variant allele, i.e. carriers of the genotype G/A or A/A, had significantly higher levels of C-reactive protein (CRP) compared with carriers of the standard G/G genotype [47]. A study of the Mexican population confirmed that there was a significantly higher frequency of the variant allele –308A in the gene for TNFα in patients with UC, compared with a healthy population [48,49] found a significantly higher risk of pancolitis in carriers of the variant allele –308A. The risk is 1.91 times higher in comparison with carriers of the standard genotype [49]. A meta-analysis of 27 studies confirmed a significantly higher risk of the onset of ulcerative colitis and Crohn's disease in carriers of the non-standard A/A genotype polymorphism –308G>A in the European population [50].

2.5.3. Polymorphism –238G>A

Some authors stated that the variant allele –238A is associated with a high expression of TNFα, but other groups of scientists have not confirmed this statement [51,52]. It is also assumed that the levels of the TNFα transcription are influenced by DNA sections situated outside the promoter area.

3. Gene polymorphisms associated with inflammatory bowel diseases: Differences between CD and UC patients

At present, it is generally considered that IBDs have a genetic background and that there are environmental factors which can trigger the disease [53].

The locus IBD1 is the most often linked with a genetic predisposition to IBD. It is situated, along with others, in the gene *NOD2/CARD15*. In our study, we studied three polymorphisms in this gene (702Arg>Trp, 908Gly>Arg and 1007fs insC) in 101 patients with CD, 35 patients with UC and 78 healthy volunteers. At least one variant allele was found in 56.3% of the patients with CD, whereas in patients with UC it was found in only 14.6%, and in healthy volunteers, 20%. Recessive homozygotes (carriers of two non-standard alleles in the gene *NOD2/CARD15*) were found only in the group of patients with CD. The most serious clinical impact and therefore the strongest association with CD, was confirmed in the frameshift mutation (Leu1007fs insC) in this gene – see Table 1. Similar results were reported by other authors [5, 54 - 56] and also by our research team in their previous works [21,8]

The second monitored mutation in this gene (702Arg>Trp) was significantly less frequent in patients with UC compared with patients with CD. In the third mutation of the gene, substitution 908Gly>Arg, we did not find any statistical association with CD or UC. The frequency of this allele in Czech and Slovak populations is very low; the allele frequency in the group of healthy volunteers was 2%. Brant et al. [54], unlike our results, found a significant connection between Crohn's disease and the mutation Gly908Arg in a larger set of patients.

Gene	Variant allele	Patients with CD	Patients with UC	Health volunteers
NOD2/CARD15	702Trp	9.90•	2.86•	8.97
	908Arg	3.96	1.43	1.92
	Leu1007fs	16.83*	8.57	5.77*
ICAM-1	469Glu	48.02**	37.14Δ	26.28**, Δ
CCR5	Δ32	8.91•	17.14•	14.74

Table 1. Frequency (in %) of variant allele of all tested genes and statistically significant differences among groups. Statistical analysis by Fisher test $^{*}P<0.01$; $^{**}P<0.05$ - statistical significant differences between group of CD patients and group of healt volunteers $^{\Delta}P<0.01$; $^{\Delta\Delta}P<0.05$ - statistical significant differences between group of UC patients and group of healt volunteers $^{\bullet}P<0.01$; $^{\bullet\bullet}P<0.05$ - statistical significant differences between group of CD patients and UC patients.

All present studies imply that the genetic predisposition to IBD is polygenic, i.e. the process of pathogenesis includes more genes, and the presence of individual mutations is cumulative, which means that the occurrence of a larger number of mutations in the same gene increases the probability of a phenotype change, or, i.e., the loss of function of a protein coded by this particular gene. We found a highly significant difference between the group of patients with Crohn's disease and the control group ($P = 0.0019$) in the total number of monitored mutations. Our results also confirmed that the average number of mutations in the gene *NOD2/CARD15* calculated in one person is significantly ($P < 0.05$) higher in the group of patients with CD, when compared with UC or the control group. Furthermore, patients with UC revealed a lower frequency of these mutations than the control group, but the result was not significant. It seems that the occurrence of variant alleles in the gene *NOD2/CARD15* is really typical for patients with Crohn's disease [5].

The *ICAM-1* gene plays a key role in the migration of neutrophils to the inflammation area and is connected with several inflammatory diseases. Matsuzawa [29] reported a significantly increased frequency of the variant allele for the polymorphism 469Lys>Glu in this gene among Japanese patients with CD. We also confirmed a strong association between the occurrence of a non-standard allele for this polymorphism and CD ($P = 0.0002$) in our set (patients of Caucasian population). Carriers of two non-standard alleles in this gene were up to 83% in patients with Crohn's disease, but only 0.6% in patients with UC and less than one percent in healthy individuals. The odds ratio implies that the risk of CD in these recessive homozygotes is 10.6 times (95% CI = 2.9–38.7) higher than in people with standard alleles in the gene *ICAM-1*, and the risk of UC is 3.1times (95% CI = 0.55–17.35) higher.

Herfarth et al. [57] suggested that the mutation in chemokine receptors CCR5 could play a key role in the regulation of the intestinal immune response in CD. They did not succeed in finding a higher frequency of the deletion allele Δ32 in patients with CD, but they found out that the polymorphism in the gene for the CCR5 receptor can contribute to the disease progression and its location. The results of our study suggest that patients with CD have a deletion allele Δ32 in the gene *CCR5* significantly less often compared with patients having UC. The deletion allele is found in patients with UC insignificantly more often compared with healthy volunteers.

Polymorphism –308G>A in the gene for TNFα is most often mentioned in connection with the increased production of this cytokine, therefore it is studied as a predisposition factor for chronic inflammatory diseases, including IBD. The highest frequency of the non-standard allele of this polymorphism (25%) was found in the group of patients with indeterminated colitis. In the groups of patients diagnosed with CD and UC, the allele frequency was almost identical – 13.96% and 14.29%. To compare the occurrence of the variant allele in the evaluated group of patients, a control group of healthy individuals was used. The overall frequency of the variant allele for the polymorphism –308G>A in the control group of healthy individuals reached 8.46%. When comparing the allele frequencies in both groups, i.e. healthy volunteers to the group of patients with IBD, it is obvious that the variant allele of the monitored polymorphism occurs 1.86 times more frequently in the group of patients compared with the group of healthy individuals, and this probability is highly significant ($P = 0.0002$). In the group of patients with indeterminate colitis, the variant allele occurs 3.95 times more often compared with the group of healthy volunteers.

The allelic frequency of the monitored polymorphism in the entire Caucasian population is generally about 11% [58]. The results indicate a possible role of the variant allele of the polymorphism –308G>A in the gene *TNFα* as a predisposing factor for the onset of IBD. An increased level of TNFα can lead to a predisposition to a more intense inflammatory reaction and represents one of the risk factors contributing to the development of this disease [49,50].

From the available data it is obvious that genetic factors can determine the IBD character, especially in case of CD. In monozygous twins with CD, 7 out of 9 cases showed a correspondence to the disease location, and in 6 out of 9 cases the disease was diagnosed within 2 years. However, the disease behaviour did not reveal any correspondence [60]. Available data imply that the mutation in the gene *CARD15/NOD2* can be connected with the affected ileum, or preferential occurrence of inflammation in the ileocaecal area [6] and with the stenotic form of the disease [59,60]. There has also been a discussion regarding the impact of mutation in this gene on the onset age of Crohn's disease [61]. Herfarth [57] reported that carriers of the deletion mutation Δ32 in the gene *CCR5* are less often affected in the upper part of gastro intestinal tract (GIT), but they are more susceptible to the development of strictures. Due to the absence of CCR5 receptors and decreased ability of a cell to initiate an inflammatory response [57], carriers of the deletion mutation Δ32 experience less often the aggressive progress of the disease (perforating or fistula type of CD) [57].

However, our results revealed that the perforating type of CD occurs significantly more often in patients with the deletion allele Δ32, compared with patients with the non-stenotic form of the disease, in whom the occurrence of this deletion allele was significantly lower. Therefore we did not confirm the results of Herfarth et al. [57].

Statistical analyses of our results confirmed an association between the polymorphism in the gene *ICAM-1* and CD outbreak. The occurrence of the variant allele 469Glu in the gene *ICAM-1,* both in heterozygous and homozygous state, is statistically significantly higher in patiens, in whom CD broke out before 16 years of age, compared with patients, in whom the disease broke out between 16 and 40 years of age [8] – see Figure 1. However, we did not confirm the results of Hradský et al. [56] that the frameshift mutation 1007fs in the gene *NOD2/CARD15* occurs more often in child patients with CD than in adult patients. This was probably caused by the fact that the group of patients with a very early clinical manifestation of the disease consisted of only 10 individuals. Nevertheless, even our results imply that the greater the genetic predisposition is, the earlier the age of manifestation and disease diagnosis. For example, three or more mutations in all of the monitored candidate genes were detected in 46.2% of young patients, in whom the clinical manifestations of the disease appeared before 16 years of age, but only in 26.3% of patients did the disease manifested from 16 to 40 years of age and in 0% of patients with CD after 40 years of age [8].

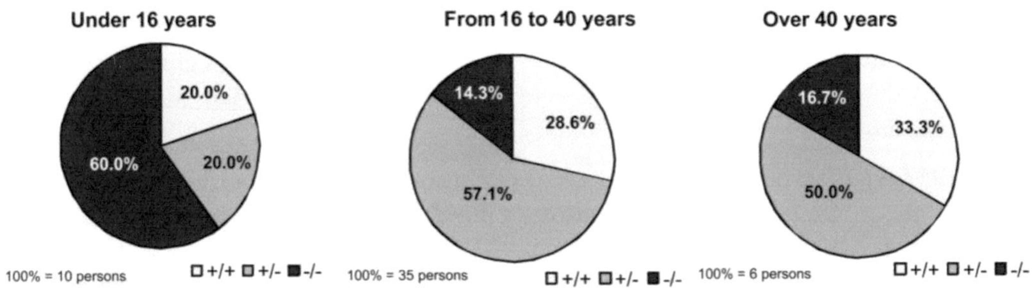

Figure 1. Influence of ICAM-1 gene mutation on the age of CD manifestation. Note: +/+: standard homozygote (carrier of two wild type alleles); +/- : heterozygote (carrier of one variant allele); -/- : variant homozygote (carrier of two variant alleles).

4. Pharmacotherapy of inflammatory bowel diseases and genes affecting drug metabolism, the occurrence of adverse effects and response to therapy

At the present time, there is no curative therapy and hence the pharmacological treatment focuses on inflammation control, eliminating disease symptoms and improving of the quality of life. IBD pharmacology utilises a wide scale of drugs including salicylates, glucocorticoids, and immunosuppressives (e.g. thioguanine derivatives, methotrexate and cyclosporine).

In clinical practice, IBD therapy, using a step-by step system, is influenced by the intensity of the disease and the effectiveness of previous therapy.

At present, aminosalicylates constitute the substantial part of the conservative treatment of IBD. When this therapy is insufficient, corticoid or immunosuppressive therapy is applied, either separately or combined. The highest level is biological therapy. Many authors indicate that TNFα as a pro-inflammatory cytokine plays a crucial role in the pathogenesis of many diseases, including IBD. The use of monoclonal antibodies, which neutralize TNFα, seems to be a very effective method of treatment. IBD requires long-term treatment. It is also necessary to mention surgical resection of the affected part of the intestine, which is used as an alternative method or pharmacotherapy supplement.

Patients are potentially exposed to the side effects of many drugs. Some toxic effects could be caused by overdose induced by a low metabolism and the elimination of effective substances. However, mechanisms of metabolism and elimination are complex; there are some crucial enzymatic proteins whose activity affects metabolism on an important therapeutical level. Single nucleotide polymorphisms (SNPs) of these genes affect enzyme structure and activity and are therefore, therapeutically significant.

4.1. Aminosalicylates

Aminosalicylates has been used in IBD therapy since the 1940s. Historically, the first preparation in this drug group was Sulfasalazine. It is a prodrug, which is dissociated in the intestine by bacteria into the active substance 5-ASA and pharmacologically inactive sulfapyridine.

During this therapy, adverse effects develop in 5 to 50% of individuals (most common are nausea, vomiting, general asthenia, headache, abdominal discomfort and rarely haemolytic anaemia and rash), in which some patients require termination of the therapy. The cause of these undesired effects is considered to be the sulfonamide component of the substance. Sulfapyridine released in the intestine is absorbed into the systemic circulation and acetylated in the liver by N-acetyltransferase (NAT) into N-acetylsulfapyridine. N-acetyltransferase is a cytosol enzyme with broad distribution into various tissues. The highest activity was observed in liver cells, intestinal epithelium and the urinary bladder. In contrast, an insignificant activity of this enzyme was found in plasma, brain and muscle [62]. N-acetyltransferase exists in two different and independently regulated isoforms: NAT1 and NAT2, which differ in their affinity to various substrates. The NAT2 isoenzyme in the liver is a lot more important for sulfapyridine acetylation than NAT1 present in the liver and gut.

4.1.1. Polymorphisms influencing aminosalicylates therapy

The genes for NAT1 and NAT2 are located on chromosome 8p22. The *NAT2* gene is polymorphous and to date, several allelic variants have been identified with various impacts on the acetylation activity of these enzymes. Any population can be divided into fast, intermediate and slow acetylators, where over 50% of the Caucasian population represent the slow acetylator phenotype. Slow acetylators, unlike the fast ones, have higher concentrations of plasma sulfapyridine and its elimination half-time is longer. Sulfapyridine is responsible for various adverse effects; therefore, the NAT2 acetylation phenotype/genotype could be important for the prediction of toxicity. Several studies confirmed higher incidences of adverse effects in slow acetylators [63–65]. Nevertheless, acetylation status is not the only factor regulating plasma concentration. Sulfapyridine is not only acetylated, it is also metabolised by the hydroxylation of an unknown polymorphous enzyme [66,67] and the high hydroxylation capacity can, in some individuals, compensate for the low level of acetylation. Due to the frequent occurrence of adverse effects, Sulfasalazine has been replaced by the active component alone, i.e. 5-aminosalicylic acid (5-ASA). 5-ASA is acetylated by polymorphous *NAT1* into the pharmacologically inactive metabolite, therefore, there is a hypothesis that the increased acetylation capacity of NAT1 could be causing the decreased effectiveness of 5-ASA. Studies in patients with ulcerous colitis did not confirm the correlation between the *NAT1* and *NAT2* genotypes and the therapeutic response to aminosalicylates [68,69].

4.2. Glucocorticoids

Glucocorticoids (GCs) play an important role in the IBD therapy but like other drug groups, they are now used not in the causal therapy but in the symptomatic therapy. Glucocorticoids (GCs) are broadly used to inhibit common inflammatory and autoimmune reactions of the body. They play a crucial role in the CD therapy, especially during the high activity of the disease. GCs are effective for the treatment of active inflammation but not for the maintaining of remission and prevention of relapses. Despite the massive boom of other drugs, they keep their position of golden standard in the IBD therapy.

Corticosteroids have anti-inflammatory and immunomodulating properties – mainly immunosuppressive. Their anti-inflammatory effect is partly immediate; peaking within 6 hours of the GCs injection application and subsiding within 24 hours. This is connected with quantitative changes in circulating leucocytes. GCs are at high doses affecting B-lymphocytes. Furthermore, they can lead to the decreased production of IgA and IgG 2-3 weeks after the onset of the therapy. Anti-inflammatory effect, which starts later, is a long-term with an impact on T-lymphocytes, especially Th-lymphocytes, and substantially less on Ts-lymphocytes [70]. However, quite limiting factors in the therapeutic use of GCs are various adverse effects during a long-term use, which are mainly connected with their numerous physiological functions in the body. The toxicity of corticosteroids is insignificant and physiological doses are administered during the substitution therapy, adverse effects do not develop. They only occur after administering of high doses during anti-inflammatory and immunosuppressive therapy.

GCs are highly lipophilic substances, which easily penetrate membranes of target cells and bind to specific glucocorticoid receptors. GCs complexes + receptor form homodimers, which are transported into the cell nucleus. Here they bind to specific responsive DNA structures of various genes. The result of this interaction is a changed gene transcription. The inhibition of promoters for the *AP-1* gene (activator protein 1) or NF-κB (nuclear factor kappa B), which are transcription factors for pro-inflammatory cytokines, and then induction of IκBα (inhibitor kappa B alfa), which is able to bind and therefore inhibit NF-κB, are important for the immunosuppressive and anti-inflammatory effect of GCs.

Terminating of the corticoidsteroid therapy leads in a part of patients to the disease relapse. To maintain the remission state, their long-term administering is therefore necessary; we talk about the so-called corticodependence. The opposite problem is corticoresistance, i.e. condition, when administering of GCs does not lead to the calming down of the disease or remission. Corticoresistance occurs in 16-20% of patients; corticodependence in 28-36% of treated patients [71,72]. Corticoresistance is not only the problem of Crohn's disease and has been intensively studied [73].

4.2.1. Polymorphisms influencing glucocorticoid therapy

Corticoresistance is mainly associated with polymorphisms in the *MDR1* gene (multidrug resistance gene). P-glycoprotein (P-gp) coded by this gene is a membrane protein serving as an ATP-dependent transporter of xenobiotics from cells. Polymorphism in this gene was described for the first time in tumour cells in connection with the occurrence of the multidrug resistance of anticancer drugs [74]. However, the *MDR1* gene is also present in normal tissue with excretion functions, i.e. the intestines, liver, kidneys, placenta and testes. It is also formed in brain capillary endothelial cells, where it participates in the function of the blood-brain barrier [75]. P-glycoprotein in these tissues is probably formed as a defence mechanism against xenobiotics. It is an important regulator of the biological activity and tissue distribution of various drugs, and it participates in their transport from cells into the extracellular environment. The increased activity of the P-glycoprotein pump is one of the reasons for the multidrug resistance of cancer cells to cytostatic drugs, and it is assumed that it could cause the non-responsiveness to glucocorticoids.

MDR1 gene is located on the 7q chromosome and consists of 28 exons. Farrell et al. proved the increased expression of this gene in T-lymphocytes and in the cells of the intestinal epithelium in patients with UC and CD, who had to undergo an intestine resection after the failure of drug therapy [76]. Therefore, the level of the *MDR1* gene expression significantly influences the therapeutic response to the administered glucocorticoides (GCs). An indirect dependence between the cells' sensitivity to GCs and MDR1 expression was also described [77].

The presence of polymorphisms in the *MDR1* gene can influence the gene expression, its amount and also the function of the P-glycoprotein pump, based on the mutation place and character. Substitutions of amino acids in the primary protein structure can result in changes of the substrate spectrum and the effectiveness of transport or pump sensitivity to specific inhibitors. These two mechanisms can also be combined.

Polymorphism in the *MDR1* gene was described for the first time in 1989 [78]. *MDR1* variants and their functional impact are still being studied intensively. To date, 50 SNP and 3 deletion and insertion mutations has been described [79,80]. From the perspective of the biological availability of glucocorticoids, mutations in exon 12 (e.g. 1236C>T), exon 21 (2677G>T/A) and exon 26 (3435C>T) have been studied more predominantly [81].The most frequent polymorphisms have a character of substitution at position 2677, where guanine usually occurs, or possibly thymine and less frequently, alanine (2677G>T/A).

Some authors assume that the reason for the increased transport activity of MDR1 is because of this polymorphism [83]. In contrast, mutation 3435C>T in exon 26 is connected with a low expression of P-glycoprotein in the small intestine. The frequency of this mutation in the Caucasian population reaches 28.6% [83]. Carriers of the homozygous variant genotype TT showed a lower production of intestinal P-glycoprotein, when compared with standard homozygotes of the CC genotype. Several studies imply that the frequency of the CC genotype is significantly higher in African populations, when compared with Caucasian and Asian populations [84,85]. It could be speculated that it might provide the African population with a certain selective advantage against GIT infections, which are endemic in tropical regions, because P-glycoprotein plays a crucial role in the defence against bacterial and viral infections. The physiological role of P-glycoprotein lies in the protection against entering bacterial toxins into the intestinal mucosa. This hypothesis is supported by Panwala [86], who demonstrated that knockout mice are sensitive to the development of severe spontaneous intestinal inflammations.The ambiguous results of the studies focusing on the impact of individual SNPs on the expression or function of the P-glycoprotein pump were brought into consonance by the results of haplotype analysis, which found a correlation between mutations 3435C>T, 2677G>T and 1236C>T. Potocnik [87] demonstrated a significantly higher risk of resistance to glucocorticoids in carriers of the haplotype marked as T/T/T.

The *MDR1* gene is also included in the group of so-called candidate genes for IBD. At present, the relationship is being studied between the polymorphism 3435C>T, which results in the decreased expression of P-glycoprotein and the increased susceptibility to the development of IBD... Another cause of corticoresistance is examined on the level of the glucocorticoid receptor (GR). It could be because of the disturbed receptor function or the change of its expression.

Glucocorticoid receptor (GR) exists in two isoforms (GR-α, and GR-β), which are formed by an alternate splicing of hnRNA to mRNA. Only the GR-α isoform, whose expression many times exceeds the expression of GR-β, is able to bind glucocorticoids and mediate their effect. Corticoresistant patients showed a higher expression of the GR-β isoform, but when compared with GR-α, this amount was still very little [88,89]. *In-vitro* obtained data imply that the formation of GR-β isoform is inducible and can be influenced by cytokines IL-2 and IL-4 [90,91] as well as by glucocorticoids [92]. The question is, how GR-β participates in modulating the sensitivity of an organism to glucocorticoids.

Polymorphisms ER22/23EK, located in exon 2, consist of two point mutations - substitutions in codons 22 and 23. The first mutation is silent, changing codon 22 from GAG to GAA (both code glutamic acid). The consequent mutation in codon 23, AGG→AAG, leads to the substitution of arginine for lysine [93]. ER22/23EK is associated with the decreased sensitivity (relative resistance) to glucocorticoids [94]. Its mechanism probably lies in the changed ratio between the forming translation isoforms GR-α and GR-β, in favour of the weaker transactivator GR-A α [93]. Two other polymorphisms in the gene *GR*, 363Asn>Ser in exon 2 and *Bcl* I, are associated with hypersensitivity to GCs [95–97]. A study in 119 IBD patients observed a more frequent occurrence of the *Bcl* I polymorphism in individuals responsive to GCs therapy [97].

Mutation 641Arg>Val and 729Ile>Val, that lead to the expression of receptors with a decreased affinity for exogenously supplemented corticosteroids, including Dexametasone, were described in the binding domain for the glucocorticoid receptor. The negative feedback induced by glucocorticoid resistance leads to the increased production of cortisol in the adrenal gland. This increased adrenal activity also leads to an increased production of androgens and mineralocorticoids [95,98,99]. In contrast, a polymorphism (363Asn>Ser) in exon 2 leading to an increased sensitivity to dexamethasone was also observed [100]. Yet another potential predictor of glucocorticoids' effectiveness from the group of polymorphisms of the gene for the corticoid receptor seems to be polymorphism *BcI* I, in which an association between hypersensitivity and glucocorticoids [97].

Since corticoresistance is most often observed in severely afflicted patients, it is still unclear whether corticoresistance is a singular phenomenon or whether it is caused by an exhaustion of the anti-inflammatory capacity of glucocorticoids due to an excessive production of pro-inflammatory cytokines, which, in turn, is caused by the excessive activity of several intracellular transcription factors that can also reduce the affinity of the glucocorticoid receptor for its intracellular ligands [101]. The results of several studies imply that the relative corticoresistance of T-lymphocytes could possibly be conditioned by their contact with pro-inflammatory cytokines and the consequential decrease of GR affinity for ligands [91]. However, this explanation of corticoresistance is not satisfactory because state of remission can be achieved in a substantial number of patients with a severe form of the disease by corticotherapy, even though their T-lymphocytes are exposed to the same conditions as the non-responders.

So far, no clinical or genetic marker exists which could be used to predict whether glucocorticoid therapy would lead to the desired therapeutic response, or that the inflammation would be corticoresistant.

4.3. Thiopurines

Thiopurine analogues (azathioprine, 6-mercaptopurine) were therapeutically used as immunosuppressives in the early 1950s for the first time. They are chemical thiol analogues of endogenous purine compounds. Azathioprine is one of the most commonly used drug in this group. The effect of azathioprine, just like its potential toxicity, depends on the amount of its active metabolites or the administered dose. Azathioprine metabolism is so complex that it is obvious that the levels of active and inactive metabolites correlate with the activity of metabolic enzymes. Scientific teams focused on the research of variant alleles of the genes for TPMT, ITPA and XDH, which are key enzymes for the metabolism of thiopurines, in which it is possible to expect an impact on the phenotype or on the decreased enzymatic activity of the native protein. Variant alleles can indirectly influence azathioprine's effect and incidence of its toxicity manifestations by this mechanism.

Azathioprine has a wide therapeutic spectrum and therefore it is considered to be a relatively safe drug. Despite this, adverse effects are common during therapy. Pharmacovigilance studies have noted them in up to 15-25% of patients [102]. Thiopurines are associated with two types of adverse effects, i.e. reactions, which are independent of the dosage and occur in up to 25% patients (nausea, fever, rash, flu-like syndrome, arthralgia), or adverse effects which are connected with the drug dosage and induced by a different mechanism. The latter is represented mainly by thiopurine-induced myelosupression, which is usually manifested by leukopenia and thrombocytopenia [102]. Basically it is a manifestation of the therapy toxicity caused by a high level of active metabolites when exceeding the therapeutic dose or due to ineffective metabolization and elimination processes. Myelosupression induced by these drugs is reversible; however, for a patient, in whom the therapeutic objective was only immunosuppression, this means a risk of life-threatening infection. Another problem is the fact that the thiopurine-induced myelosupression is manifested after a certain latency period and in most cases it also means termination of the azathioprine medication. However, some works state that a moderate myelosupression is associated with better clinical results from the therapy [103].

4.3.1. Polymorphisms influencing the thiopurines therapy

4.3.1.1. The gene for thiopurine S-methyltransferase (TPMT)

In the 1960s, this enzyme, which catalyzes the methylation of the thiol functional group, was described in several cell populations. Activity of S-adenosyl-L-methionine: thiopurin S-methyltransferase (TPMT; EC 2.1.1.67) was demonstrated in cytoplasm of prokaryotic as well as eukaryotic cells. In humans, the activity of this enzyme was mainly described in erythrocytes, leukocytes, renal parenchyma, hepatocytes and intestinal cells. Its occurrence was also confirmed in mammalian placenta [104].

The human gene for TPMT is located in the short arm of chromosome 6 (6p22.3). It consists of 9 exon and 8 intron regions [105]. Its length (including introns) is about 25 kbp [106]. In the sequence of this gene, there were 21 SNPs identified, which facilitated the formation of 22 variant allelic form of the gene. In compliance with the agreed rules, nomenclature of the non-standard *TPMT* alleles is marked by a number, or a number and a letter. Variant alleles are listed in Table 2.

Even though the differences in the catalytic activity of the TPMT enzyme has been known for several decades, the first proof of the association of this phenotype with gene polymorphism was provided by Krynetski [107]. It was evidence that a variant allele TPMT*2 is present in individuals with low enzymatic activity [107].

Since then, many gene alleles for TPMT have been discovered. They differ not only in the nucleotide sequence but also in the activity of enzymes transcribed from such sequence. The fact that many variant alleles lead to a decreased enzymatic activity resulted in the belief that gene polymorphisms of this gene substantially influence pharmacokinetic parameters of the drug with a thiopurine structure.

Allele	SNP	Substitution of AA	Reference
TPMT*1	Standard allele - wild type (wt)		
TPMT*1S	474T>C	Silent	[108]
TPMT*1A	-178C>T		[108]
TPMT*2	238G>C	Ala80Pro	[107]
TPMT*3A	460G>A	Ala154Thr	[109]
	719A>G	Tyr240Cys	
TPMT*3B	460G>A	Ala154Thr	[110]
TPMT*3C	719A>G	Tyr240Cys	[111]
TPMT*3D	460G>A	Ala154Thr	[110]
	719A>G	Tyr240Cys	
	292G>T	Glu92Stop	
TPMT*4	_1G>A (intron 9)	Splicing defect	[111]
TPMT*5	146T>C	Leu49Ser	[110]
TPMT*6	539A>T	Tyr180Phe	[110]
TPMT*7	681T>G	His227Gln	[110]
TPMT*8	644G>A	Arg215His	[112]
TPMT*9	356A>C	Lys119Thr	[110]
TPMT*10	430G>C	Gly144Arg	[110]
TPMT*11	395G>A	Cys132Tyr	[113]
TPMT*12	374C>T	Ser125Leu	[110]
TPMT*13	83A>T	Glu28Val	[110]
TPMT*14	1A>G	Met1Val	[110]
TPMT*15	_1G>A (intron 7)	Splicing defect	[114]
TPMT*16	488G>A	Arg163His	[115]
TPMT*17	124C>G	Gln42Glu	[110]
TPMT*18	211G>A	Gly71Arg	[110]
TPMT*19	365A>C	Lys122Thr	[115]

Table 2. Listing of variant alleles of the gene for TPMT including the location of the nucleotide polymorphism and changes in the protein primary structure.

Variant TPMT alleles occurring in Caucasian population and their phenotype

About 90% of the Caucasian population shows standard enzymatic activity. Medium enzymatic activity correlates with the heterozygous genotype, i.e. the presence of some variant alleles, and is found in less than 10% of the population. Enzymatic activity is virtually undetectable in one of 300 individuals. This condition is related with the occurrence of a homozygous genotype for variant alleles [116]. It is sufficient to administer to these patients just 6-10% of the standard azathioprine dose. In heterozygotes, the activity of an enzyme transcribed according to the matrix of a standard allele is metabolically sufficient. In these patients, however, it is necessary to consider the increased hematotoxicity of the therapy.

Allele TPMT*1 (wt)

Marking TPMT*1 belongs to the standard allele (wild type, wt), which is the most frequent in population. Enzymatic protein, which is expressed on the basis of this nucleotide sequence, has a high, which means standard activity.

Allele TPMT*2 (238G>C; 80Pro>Ala)

Allele TPMT*2 carries a substitution 238G>C (exon 5). This nucleotide transversion leads to a change of the primary structure of the protein, in which the rigid amino acid proline (at position 80) is substituted for alanine, an amino acid which is chemically more flexible. This results in altered intermolecular interactions, a disturbed tertiary structure and also the catalytic activity and stability of the protein [107], and a decreased enzymatic activity of up to a 100 times is expected [116].

Allele TPMT*3A (460G>A, 719A>G; 154Ala>Thr, 240Tyr>Cys)

Allele TPMT*3A includes two nucleotide substitutions in the gene sequence. Substitutions at positions 460G>A (exon 7) and 719A>G (exon 10) lead to the substitution of alanine for threonine at position 154, and tyrosine for cysteine at position 240 of the peptide chain. Based on this mutation, a very unstable protein is formed during the protein synthesis [110]. Enzymatic activity is decreased up to 200 times [116].

Allele TPMT*3B (460G>A; 154Ala>Thr)

Allele TPMT*3B carries only one nucleotide substitution, at position 460G>A, resulting in the change of the primary protein structure due to the substitution of alanine for theonine at position 154. The expressed protein has an extremely unstable structure and is rapidly degraded by cell proteases.

Allele TPMT*3C (719A>G; 240Tyr>Cys)

The nucleotide substitution at position 719 (exon 10) and the consequential amino acid substitution at position 240 have a similar effect on protein stability [111].

The above variant alleles are present in 85-90% of individuals with a low enzymatic activity of the TPMT enzyme. Other gene polymorphisms occur in the Caucasian population with such a low frequency that their low incidence in the population makes them quite difficult to detect, and the possibility to use them in clinical practice is minimal.

Among non-standard alleles of the gene for TPMT, variant alleles TPMT*3A, TPMT*3C and TPMT*2 have the highest frequency. Population testing revealed substantial racial and ethnic differences in the occurrence of variant alleles. For example, the inhabitants of South Asia (India, Pakistan) reveal a smaller incidence of variant alleles – from detected non-standard alleles, only the TPMT*3A was confirmed [117]. On the other hand, the African population has an overall frequency of variant alleles comparable with Caucasian population, but the highest representation among non-standard alleles has TPMT*3C [118]. This allele (TPMT*3C) represents 50% of variant alleles in Afro-Americans, compared with only 5% in Americans of European origin [104]. The most common variant allele in the Caucasian population is TPMT*3A (some papers state that up to 10% of the population carries the heterozygous genotype; [119]. The occurrence of individual variant alleles in various populations is shown in Table 3.

Ethnic group	TPMT*2	TPMT*3A	TPMT*3B	TPMT*3C	Reference
Caucasian - France	0.7	3	0	0.4	[119]
Caucasian - Germany	0.5	8.6	0	0.8	[113]
Caucasian - Norway	0	3.4	0	0.3	[120]
Caucasian - America	0.2	3.2	-	0.2	[112]
Afro - American	0.4	0	-	2.4	[112]
Afro - Kenya	0	0	-	5.4	[118]
African - Ghana	0	0	-	7.6	[121]
Asian - Southeast Asia	0	0	-	1	[122]
Asian - Japan	0	0	0	1.6	[123]
Asian - China	0	0	0	1	[124]

Table 3. Occurrence of variant alleles TPMT*2, TPMT*3A, TPMT*3B and TPMT*3C in various populations (in %). Legend: 0 – occurrence of alleles was not confirmed; - allele was not detected.

An important outcome of these population studies is that clinically significant variant alleles or their polymorphisms are present in all populations; therefore, the same diagnostic methods based on the determination of genotype can be used. [106]. From the phenotype perspective, the overall protein stability of TPMT is the most important. *In vitro* and *in vivo* studies confirm that the quantity of expression of variant alleles is comparable with the expression of the variant allele TPMT*1. It is the shorter biological halftime of the protein expressed on the basis of the variant allele which is responsible for the decreased metabolic activity of the enzyme [109]. Experiments assessing protein quality using the Western blot procedure imply that enzymatic protein produced by the transcription of the variant allele has a significantly shorter halftime compared with proteins translated according to the wt allele. Western blot analysis in cells with two copies of a variant allele did not confirm the presence of enzymatic protein. This fact directly correlates with the phenotype feature – undetectable TPMT activity. Tai et al. [109] determined protein quantity *in vitro* and found that the amount of enzymatic protein at a particular time after the expression decreased the most in the variant allele TPMT*3A, (200 times lower compared to TPMT*1). In the variant allele TPMT*2, the decrease of protein density was smaller by one order (20 times). In the allele

TPMT*3B, in which only one nucleotide substitution is present, the protein density was decreased 4 times; in the variant allele TPMT*3C, the density determined by Western blotting was comparable with the wt allele [109]. Furthermore, the amount of protein determined by Western blotting after 24-hour cultivation also corresponds with the results of degradation halftimes for native proteins. It was confirmed that the halftime of a protein expressed from a wt allele is about 18 hours. A comparable halftime can be observed in case of the protein, if it was expressed from the allele TPMT*3C Degradation halftimes in the alleles TPMT*3B (6h) and TPMT*2 (0.2h) are significantly shorter. The shortest degradation halftime detected in a protein expressed according to the sequence corresponds with the allele TPMT*3A (0.25h; [109]). These results imply that the lowest enzymatic activity, resulting from the fast degradation of a protein, is connected with the alleles TPMT*3A and TPMT*2. This hypothesis is supported by the phenotype-undetectable metabolic activity of enzymes in patients with the variant alleles TPMT*3A and TPMT*2 in their genotype.

4.3.1.2. The gene for Inosine Triphosphate Pyrophosphatase (ITPA)

Inosine triphosphate pyrophosphatase (ITPA; EC 3.6.1.19) is one of the ubiquitous cytosol enzymes. It catalyzes the reaction of inosine triphosphates hydrolysis to inosine monophosphate. Even though the activity in various types of cells is different and the role of the enzyme in the cell is not clearly understood; it is supposed that it prevents the accumulation of false nucleotides, which could be incorporated in the DNA and RNA molecules instead of standard nucleotides, and therefore damage these macromolecules. Another possible role of these nucleotides can be their competition with GTP during cell signalling processes [125]. The role of ITPA in azathioprine biotransformation lies in the hydrolytic breakdown of potentially hepatotoxic 6-thio-ITP.

The gene coding for ITPA is situated on the short arm of chromosome 20 (20p13) and contains 8 exon sequences [126]. Several nucleotide polymorphisms were identified in its sequence; in 5 of these polymorphisms, a correlation with a low activity of the native protein was proven [127]. The lowest enzymatic activity was discovered in individuals who carry the nucleotide substitution of cytosine for adenine at position 94 in the sequence of the exon 2 (94C>A). At the protein primary structure level, this substitution is manifested by the substitution of proline for threonine at position 32, which decreases its affinity for the production of active dimer in ITPA proteins, decreases the protein stability and leads to a non-specific mRNA splicing [128,125,129]. The heterozygous genotype for the variant allele 94A is from the phenotype perspective manifested by the decrease of ITPA activity up to 22.5% of the activity of a standard form. ITPA activity was not detectable in individuals who are homozygous for this variant allele [128]. The frequency of the variant allele 94A in the *ITPA* gene is 5–7% in the Caucasian population [130–133]. Another nucleotide substitution in which an impact on the enzymatic activity was confirmed, is the substitution of adenine for cytosine at the sequence of intron 2 (IVS2+21A>C). The presence of this substitution leads to a faulty mRNA splicing during post-transcriptional modifications and the formation of a protein, which reaches 61% activity in heterozygous individuals, when compared to the native form of the enzyme [134,125]. Homozygous carriers of this variant allele have their enzymatic activity at 30% of the activity of a standard form [132]. The frequency of this variant allele in the Caucasian population reaches 10-13% [128,134]. Individuals who have the variant allele 94A in their genome as well as the variant allele IVS2+21C, showed 10% activity of ITPA [128]. A connection between the decreased ITPA activity and the occurrence of pancreatitis, a rash, a flu-like syndrome and leukopenia was identified in patients treated by azathioprine [135,136].

4.3.1.3. The gene for Xanthine Dehydrogenase (XDH)

Xanthine dehydrogenase (XDH, XO; EC 1.17.1.4) also belongs among cytosol enzymes, which participate in the metabolism of endogenous purine and pyrimidine nucleotides, as well as exogenous substances with this chemical structure [137]. The enzyme activity has been observed mainly in hepatocytes, enterocytes and renal parenchyma cells. XDH catalyses the oxidation of hypoxanthine to xanthine and consequently to uric acid. This enzyme is a crucial element of the biological availability of drugs containing the thiopurine molecule [138]. XDH activity significantly fluctuates depending on the ethnicity, sex and tissue type [139–141]. The administering of the competitive XDH inhibitor allopurinol leads to a higher biological availability of 6-MP (6-mercaptopurine) and in some cases to a better therapeutic response to thiopurine therapy [138,142].

The gene coding for the enzyme XDH is situated on the short arm of chromosome 2 (2p23). In humans, several polymorphisms have been identified, which facilitate the formation of 21 allelic variants [143]. Several of these allelic variants are associated with the occurrence of adverse effects during azathioprine therapy and with higher levels of toxic metabolites 6-MP [133,144]. Several of the noted single nucleotide polymorphisms influence XDH enzymatic activity. However, many of these variant alleles have only been discovered within the Japanese or Asian populations. A potential clinical importance can be expected in example of polymorphisms 837C>T, which has a 6% frequency in the Caucasian population. At the primary protein structure level, there is no amino acid substitution. Nevertheless, this polymorphism somehow influences enzymatic activity and its occurrence correlates with higher levels of thiopurine metabolites. A possible explanation may be the coincidence with an unknown polymorphism [144] or RNA interferency. During the reaction of the catalyzed XDH, free oxygen radicals are generated, which are expected to participate in the hepatotoxic effect of thiopurines [145].

4.4. Biological therapy

Biological therapy represents a completely new therapeutic approach to chronic inflammatory diseases. This therapeutic approach has proved useful not only in IBD therapy, but also in the therapy of other chronic inflammatory diseases, such as rheumatoid arthritis, ankylosing spondylarthritis and psoriasis. In IBD, the most common drugs intervene in the TNFα cytokine-mediated signalling at the molecular level (infliximab, adalimumab and etanercept).The main mechanism of these "anti-TNFα" antibodies is the binding of a drug to the TNFα soluble form (sTNFα) and blocking biological functions, which are mediated by it. Some studies demonstrated that individual antibodies have a different neutralisation potential and that this ability is also dependent on the TNFα concentration. At high sTNFα concentrations, the neutralising potential of infliximab, adalimumab and etanercept is comparable [146]. However, if the sTNFα concentration in the tissue is small, etanercept is about 20 times more effective than other antibodies. Two mechanisms are employed during the binding of the antibody to the membrane-bound TNFα form (tmTNFα). The first is antagonism, preventing the interaction between tmTNFα and its receptor (TNFR). The second is agonism; the binding of the drug to tmTNFα activates the reverse signalling cascade which leads to the suppression of TNFα production, other pro-inflammatory cytokines and apoptosis [147].

The cytotoxicity of anti-TNFα antibodies is caused by two mechanisms. The first lies in the binding of antibodies to tmTNFα and the apoptosis activation. The second mechanism is based on the initiation of complement-dependent cytotoxicity through the antibody Fc fragment. The antibody Fc fragment has the function of effector mediated by the Fc receptor in immunocompetent cells of monocytes and macrophages, NK cells and some types of T lymphocytes. Activation initiates a cascade of intracellular processes leading to phagocytosis, degranulation, activation of the complement and cytokines release [148]. Monoclonal substances with an Fc fragment in its structure (infliximab, adalimumab, and etanercept) have the ability to interact with these receptors. The antibody or the complex anti-TNFα Ig-TNFα can bind to the receptor [147]. One of the major risks of biological therapy is the production of antibodies against the drug. No of anti-TNFα drugs, in which the sequences are fully human, have this undesired property suppressed. Infliximab is the most immunogenic chimeric antibody [149]. The production of antibodies targeted against the drug decreases its therapeutic effect and increases the drug clearance. Due to this, the anti-TNFα therapy is supplemented by immunosuppressives (MTX, AZA) with the goal to prevent the induction of immune reactions [150].

4.4.1. Polymorphisms, which influence the anti-TNFα antibodies therapy

Mutations in the gene *TNFα*, especially mutations in the promoter area of this gene, lead to an altered expression of the gene and subsequently to a change in the amount of active TNFα. Its increased level result not only in pathological manifestations of chronic inflammation, but also in the effectiveness of the biological therapy,which at the molecular level influence the TNFα cytokine-mediated signalling (infliximab, adalimumab and etanercept). Therefore, the gene coding for the cytokine TNFα is classified among candidate genes as well as therapeutic genes, whose protein products influence the effectiveness and safety of drug therapy. More information on polymorphisms in this gene can be found in Chapter 2.5.

TNFα production is strictly controlled. Most of the regulatory mechanisms are embedded into the post-transcription processes [148]. The amount of the TNFα active form (both s and tm forms) is therefore dependent not only on the presence of the above mentioned SNPs, but also on the stimulation of cytokine-producing cells, TACE activity (TNF-α-converting enzyme) and intracellular regulatory processes and mRNA stability [151]. The initiating factor is the presence of gram-negative and gram-positive microorganisms (lipopolysaccharide,LPS, is one of the strongest stimulators), viral antigens or tumour-transformed cells.

Receptor molecules such as NOD2/CARD15 (receptor for muramyl dipeptide, MDP) and transmembrane receptor structures of the TLR family (receptor for lipopolysaccharides, LPS) play a key role in this step. The system of gradual activation of intracellular elements of signal pathways leads to the activation of NF-κB, which is common for both of these pathways and leads to the activation of the expression of TNFα and other pro-inflammatory cytokines. Another area, which influences the level of TNFα expression, is the promoter area of the gene coding for this cytokine.

There are also other cytokines which influence TNFα production (e.g. IL-1, IL-17, GM-CSF and interferon-γ), the antigen-antibody complexes and complements. TNFα release is also stimulated by pathological damage to tissue due to trauma or ischemia/hypoxia [148].

Factors which quantitatively influence the TNFα expression as well as molecules, which are inductors of this expression, seem to be potential predictors of the therapeutic response to biological therapy. One of the key molecules which regulate the gene expression of many cytokines is the nuclear factor κB (NF-κB) [14,15]. Its activation is closely linked with complex intracellular processes, by which the immune system recognizes bacterial antigens and reacts to their presence. In mammalian cells, there are NOD proteins and Toll-like receptors (also the so-called pattern recognition receptors, PRRs), which recognize these bacterial structures. More information about polymorphisms in the *NOD2/CARD15* and *TLR4* genes is given in Chapters 2.1 and 2.4.

During the infliximab therapy, the growth of apoptosis was confirmed in immune cells. As described above, it is one of the effect mechanisms which lead to the suppression of the immune reaction. A Belgium group of scientists led by Mr. Hlavaty [152] based their research on this finding and demonstrated the possible impact of polymorphisms in genes for individual proteins of the pro-apoptotic pathway (Fas-ligand and caspase 9) on the infliximab therapy effectiveness in patients with Crohn's disease. Apoptosis can be induced in cells by the "extrinsic pathway", where TNFα molecules, Fas ligand and TRAIL (TNF-related apoptosis-inducing ligand) work as inductors of the apoptosis. There is also an intrinsic pathway, which includes the release of cytochrome c from mitochondria in a reaction to DNA damage. Both of these pathways are connected in the area of activation of cysteinyl-aspartate-specific protease (Caspase 3). Fas ligand is expressed in many immune system cells and, via the apoptosis induction, maintains the balance between the production and death of T lymphocytes and B lymphocytes. In this manner it contributes to immune tolerance [153]. The gene for Fas ligand is situated on the long arm of chromosome 1 (1q23). It consists of 4 exons and its length is approximately 8kb [153]. Polymorphism located in the promoter area (–844C>T) is at a position where a transcription enhancer has bonded. Variant allele T is responsible for the decreased binding affinity of this transcription factor. Individual homozygous for variant T allele have a decreased expression activity and a decreased quantity of the native protein in the membrane [154]. Patients with such polymorphism have a decreased activation of the pro-apoptotic pathway.

The intrinsic pathway for apoptosis activation is formed by individual cytosol proteases, which are activated in cascades. Caspase 9 (Casp9) is one of them. The primary stimulus for the activation of intrinsic pro-apoptotic pathway is damage to mitochondria and cytochrome c release. This, after binding to APAF-1, forms a complex with caspase 9 [155]. The consequential chain of reactions results in the activation of other proteases - caspase 3, 6 and 7, which cause the disruption of the nuclear membrane, the fragmentation of nucleic DNA and the production of apoptotic vesicles [156]. Even though there has been some research focusing on the possible association between the 93C>T polymorphism and infliximab therapy effectiveness or the predisposition to Crohn's disease and the disease activity [157], its role at the molecular level has not been exactly understood to date. However, it was demonstrated that this polymorphism does not result in the amino acid substitution at the level of the protein primary structure.

5. Gene polymorphisms and adverse effects of azathioprine treatment

During azathioprine therapy, about 10-28% of patients experience adverse effects [158–160]. The most serious of these is myelosupression, which is most often manifested as leukopenia. In their study, Katsanos [161] found the myelosupression incidence totalling 7%. Other common adverse effects, which may result in the termination of the therapy, are hepatotoxicity (9.7%), pancreatitis (10.5%) and digestive intolerance (17.5%), and to a lesser degree, extended infections (6.1%) or flu-like symptoms (5.7%) [162]. Most of these adverse effects are dose-dependent reactions.

The occurrence of myelosupression correlates with high levels of active azathioprine metabolites (6-thioguanine nucleotide, 6-TGN) [163], which result from a deficient azathioprine metabolism in individuals with a variant *TPMT* genotype. There are many experiments which confirm this dependence [136,164–167].

We tested a group of 188 patients treated with azathioprine for inflammatory bowel disease (IBD). During the therapy, 34 individuals experienced leukopenia (WBCs count $<4 \times 10^9$ /L), hepatotoxicity (alanine aminotransferase or aspartate aminotransferase > 3times upper limit of normal) was confirmed in 4 patients, digestive intolerance was revealed in 4 individuals (nausea, vomiting, abdominal pain associated with treatment; ceased after AZA withdrawal) and pancreatitis developed in 2 patients. The variant *TPMT* allele was confirmed in 8 (23.5%) patients with leukopenia. Within the group of patients who did not experience leukopenia, the variant *TPMT* allele was confirmed in 8 people (5.2%). Fisher test confirmed an association between the variant *TPMT* genotype and leukopenia (P=0.003) – see Figures 2, and 3.

Patients with a variant *TPMT* genotype (heterozygotes) were five times at risk of developing leukopenia than patients with a standard genotype (P = 0.003, CI 95%, 1.8058–13.8444) [168]. These findings comply with previously published findings [136,164–167].

The FDA recommends a large-scale *TPMT* genotype testing prior to the azathioprine therapy [169]. Nevertheless, the presence of the variant *TPMT* genotype does not imply an absolute azathioprine contraindication in these patients. There were even earlier works, which reported the desired therapeutic effects without the manifestation of myelotoxicity in patients with variant *TPMT* genotypes achieved by a proportionate decrease of the dose [170]. Carriers of variant *TPMT* alleles were recommended to decrease the AZA dosing to 30-70% or to 10% of standard doses in heterozygotes and in variant homozygotes, respectively [165,171]. In these patients, the dosage should be carefully subjected to titration and regular checking of WBCs counts [170,172 –174].

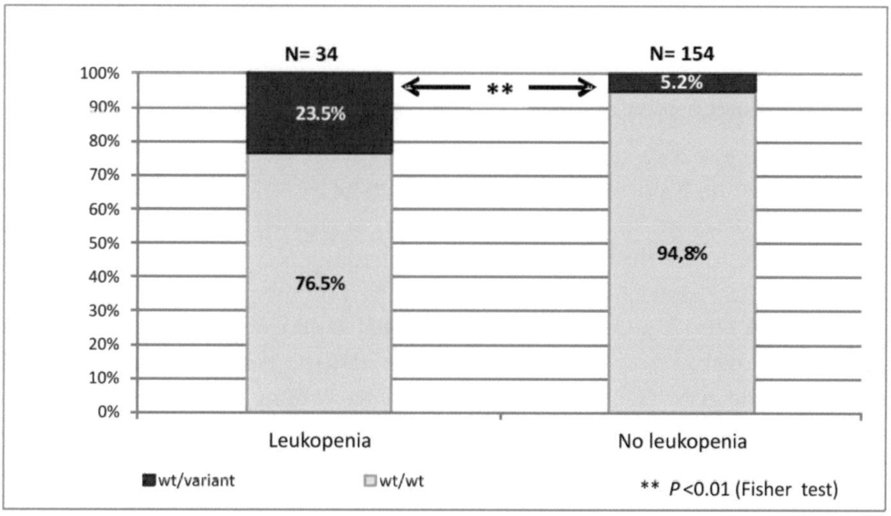

Figure 2. Occurence of leukopenia in patients with different genotypes. Note: +/+: carrier of two wild type alleles TPMT*1; +/- : carrier of one variant allele: TPMT*2 or *3A,*3B or *3C.

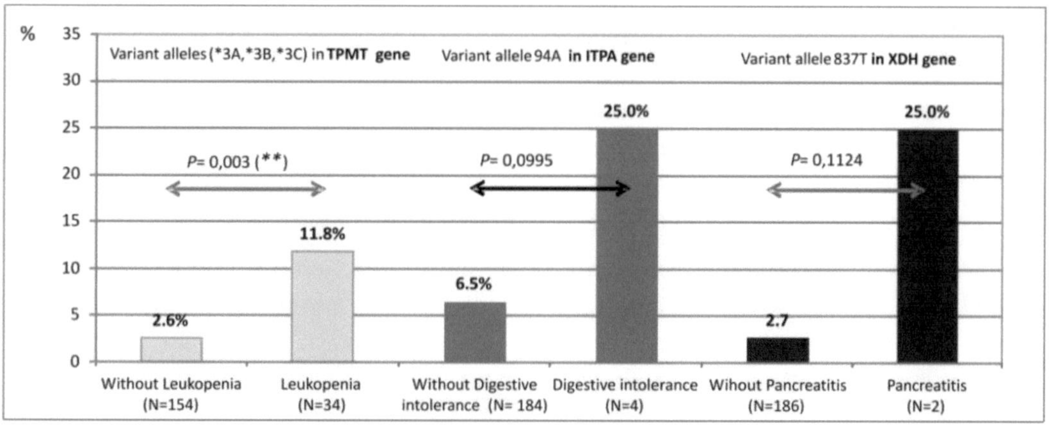

Figure 3. Frequency of variant alleles in patient with / without adverse effects

A similar association between deficient azathioprine metabolism and the occurrence of leukopenia can be expected in the case of the polymorphism in the gene for XDH. Even though our set revealed a tendency for a higher frequency of the variant allele 837T in patients with leukopenia (4.4%) compared with patients without this adverse effect (2.6%), this difference was not statistically significant [168,175]. Unlike the TPMT enzyme, whose activity is well described and quantified in individuals with standard and variant genotypes, the relationship between the genotype and phenotype activity of XDH is not so clear. It is supposed that despite the decrease of metabolic activity, this decrease is not as striking as in case of TPMT. Furthermore, the decreased XDH activity can be better compensated for by the activity of other enzymes, which participate in azathioprine metabolising. However, the situation is different if XDH is inhibited by allopurinol. In this case, there is probably an extensive competition that would result in the 6-TGN levels having a toxic effect (343 pmol/8x10^8) [163].

To date, no pathological condition connected with decreased ITPA activity has been described. Similarly, available data regarding the association between polymorphisms in the gene for this enzyme and the occurrence of adverse effects of azathioprine therapy are contradictory. Some studies describe the association between decreased ITPA activity and the occurrence of pancreatitis, rash, flu-like syndrome and leukopenia [135,136]. There are no other studies confirming the association between the ITPA polymorphism and the occurrence of adverse effects [166,176,177]. Our test group included 4 patients who experienced digestive intolerance during azathioprine therapy; 2 of these patients were heterozygous for the variant allele 94A in the gene *ITPA*. The frequency of the variant allele in patients with digestive intolerance reached 25% (compared with 6.5% in patients without digestive intolerance) but due to a low number of individuals its statistical interpretation is difficult – see Figure 3. However, we confirmed that patients, who are carriers of the variant allele, have a 3.33 times greater probability of digestive intolerance (CI 95%, 1.09-13.5) than patients with a standard allele [168,175]. The association between the variant allele 94A and the occurrence of digestive intolerance must be confirmed in a larger set of patients. The occurrence of pancreatitis was similarly rare (n=4) in our set. In these patients, the variant allele *XDH* 837T had a frequency of 25% (compared with 2.7% in patients without pancreatitis). It is expected that the presence of this variant allele leads to the decreased activity of the XDH enzyme [168,175] – see Figure 3. Because of this, 6-MP is subsequently metabolised and the levels of its cytotoxic metabolites increase, which can cause pancreatitis [133]. In the group of individuals, in whom the variant genotype was confirmed, there were 12.1 individuals with pancreatitis per one individual without this adverse effect (CI 95%; 1.15-126.4). However, even in this case it is necessary to confirm or disprove these results in a larger set of patients.

The most important polymorphisms with a significant impact on the azathioprine therapy are SNPs in the gene for TPMT. The impact of other genetic variants must be verified in a larger set of patients.

6. Gene polymorphisms as predictors of the effectiveness of infliximab therapy

Infliximab, a chimeric monoclonal antibody, was the first biological agent registered for the treatment of CD by FDA in 1998. Presently, infliximab, adalimumab and cetrolizumab pegol are used in the therapy of CD. Subsequently, the effectiveness of biological therapy was also confirmed in moderate to severe active UC [178–180].

The effect of biological therapy is based on the suppression of the anti-inflammatory effect of cytokines, which are inflammation mediators. In patients with IBD, it is assumed that TNFα has the main role in the induction and prolonging of the inflammatory reaction. The use of monoclonal antibodies inhibiting this cytokine has been a great therapeutic benefit to the therapy. Biotechnologically produced monoclonal antibodies have already demonstrated its significant position in the therapy of IBD as well as other chronic inflammatory diseases. Infliximab was firstly used for Crohn's disease therapy and later Rutgeerts et al. confirmed its effect in patients with UC [179]. Infliximab as a monoclonal antibody has an affinity for both soluble and membrane-bound forms of TNFα. Binding to soluble cytokine inhibits its pro-inflammatory effect, and the affinity for the membrane form of TNFα induces apoptosis. Today, biological therapy in IBD has a significant position in the treatment of patients who do not respond to the conventional pharmacological approach, or in corticoid-dependent patients and in patients with severely active Crohn's disease with fistulas and in serious active ulcerative colitis. The high therapeutic effectiveness of infliximab was confirmed by large-scale clinical studies [179,181,182].

During infliximab therapy, several adverse effects were described. However, except for the allergic reaction, which occurs immediately after the infliximab is administered, they occur with low frequency (183). Biological therapy can therefore be considered highly effective. Still, there are about 20-30% of patients in whom no therapeutic effect occurs. At first, it was thought that the reason for the absence of any clinical effect was the presence of autoantibodies against infliximab [184]. However, this hypothesis has not been fully confirmed. Other possible causes are the subject of the study [185,186]. Factors which quantitatively influence TNFα expression seem to be among the potential predictors for the therapeutic response. They are molecules, which participate in the activation of NF-κB, the inductor of the TNFα expression. Nuclear factor κB (NF-κB) is a key component in the regulation of expression in the area of genome-carrying genes for cytokines [14,15]. Its activation is closely connected with complex intracellular processes, by which the immune system responds to the presence of bacterial antigens. For example, the presence of muramyl dipeptide (MDP) is detected by the interaction with NOD2. This cytosol protein is a component of cascade, which leads to local activation of the immune system in response to the presence of pathogen, and consequently to the expression and release of cytokines including TNFα. The gene for NOD2 lies in the area of the genome, which was earlier associated with incidences of IBD and which is linked to the occurrence of IBD [21,8]. In the Caucasian population, there are two single nucleotide polymorphisms marked 702Arg>Trp and 908Gly>Arg and a frameshift mutation 1007fs (3020fsinsC), which occur with a relatively high frequency. *In vitro* studies confirmed that a cell, which carries in its genome an allelic form corresponding to variant alleles 702Trp and 908Arg, is able to release TNFα after the induction by muramyl dipeptide in a quantitatively comparable amount like a cell with wild alleles in these polymorphisms [187–189]. These nucleotide substitutions lead to the change of the primary structure, but not so significant a change at the level of the secondary and tertiary protein structures. Therefore, the impact on the biological functions of the coded protein is minimal [188]. The insertion of cytosine nucleotide in the case of the frameshift mutation leads to the shift of the reading frame during the translation and the formation of a premature stop codon [190]. The transcription of the variant allele results in the production of a protein, which is shorter by the area coded behind the stop codon. Due to this, the biological activity of the shortened protein NOD2 is strongly disturbed, which was confirmed by *in vitro* and *in vivo* studies, which discovered that the production of TNFα was not detected after the stimulation of MDP [187–189]. The presence of the frameshift mutation therefore results in the absence of the TNFα expression *via* NF-κB [15].

If we accept the hypothesis that a higher effectiveness of infliximab therapy correlates with lower levels of TNFα, then carriers of the alleles, which are connected with the lower expression of this cytokine, should also respond favorably to the therapy. Our results confirm this hypothesis, even though we did not study the phenotype (plasma or tissue levels of TNFα) but only the genotype. The frequency of variant alleles, in which the significant influence on the quantity of the TNFα expression (702W and 908R) was not confirmed *in vitro*, was comparable in patients with a therapeutic response and in patients resistant to the therapy. On the other hand, the frequency of the frameshift mutation, which leads to a significant decrease of the TNFα expression after the MDP induction, was statistically and significantly higher (15.2%) in patients who reacted positively to the therapy, compared to patients that were resistant to the therapy (3.6%). Patients, who are carriers of the frameshift mutation, have a 4.25 times higher probability that the infliximab therapy will be effective (CI 95%; 1.06-17.07). The frequency of the frameshift mutation (variant allele 1007fs) was virtually identical in patients who responded to the infliximab therapy by mucosal healing, and in patients who revealed only clinical improvement of parameters (15.15% and 15.22%, respectively).

The TNFα expression via NF-κB occurs also after the binding of a specific ligand, e.g. lipopolysaccharide (LPS), to the membrane TLR4 receptor. The activation of the intracellular signalling cascade and the expression of pro-inflammatory cytokines occur in cooperation with the molecule CD14 [191]. In the *TLR4* gene, there are nucleotide polymorphisms, which influence its biological functions [192,193]. One of these is a substitution of adenine by guanine at the position 896 of the nucleotide chain. The variant allele 896G has a lower ability to induce TNFα production in reaction to LPS stimulation in the *in vitro* experiments [192,193]. Analogically to the variant genotype *NOD2*, there is a possible hypothesis that the variant allele 896G is associated with a better therapeutic response. The occurrence of variant allele in our set was the highest in patients who responded best to infliximab therapy, i.e. those who showed both a clinical and morphological response to the therapy (9.9%). In patients with only a clinical response, the frequency of the variant allele was lower (3.6%), and among patients resistant to the therapy, there were only 1.8% of carriers of the variant allele. We can describe a certain tendency that a carrier of the variant allele has a greater probability that infliximab therapy will be effective. However, differences in the frequencies of the variant allele 896G in the *TLR4* gene between individual groups of patients were not statistically significant. According to the odds ratio, there are 2.59 patients with both a clinical and morphological reaction per one patient, with a clinical reaction in the group of patients with a variant allele 896G in the gene *TLR4* (CI 95%; 1.01-8.39) [175].

Several polymorphisms influencing the expression degree were described in the promoter area of the gene coding for TNFα. A single nucleotide substitution –308G>A is often mentioned. Production of TNFα can be increased by this mechanism even under the standard stimulation conditions. The variant allele –308A occurred with a 14.03% frequency in the set of patients. Even though according to the *in vitro* testing, this variant allele means a higher production of TNFα due to a higher transcription activity of the gene [194], it could be expected that it will be more frequent in patients resistant to the therapy. Our results did not confirm statistically significant differences between individual groups of patients.

Based on the above information, it can be concluded that a patient who is a carrier of a genotype containing variant allele 1007fs in the gene *NOD2,* variant allele 896A in the gene *TLR4* and the standard allele –308A in the gene *TNFα,* they will have the greatest probability that the infliximab therapy will be effective for them. Individuals who are homozygous for the standard (wild type) alleles of the listed polymorphisms in the gene *NOD2, TLR4* and *TNFα,* are more often resistant to the infliximab therapy. This standard genotype was in our study of 163 infliximab-administered patients confirmed in up to 75% of resistant patients, compared with 46.7% in the group with a therapeutic response. In patients with the best response to infliximab, (i.e. both clinical and morphological) the frequency of this allele combination was even lower (43.9%) – see Figure 4.

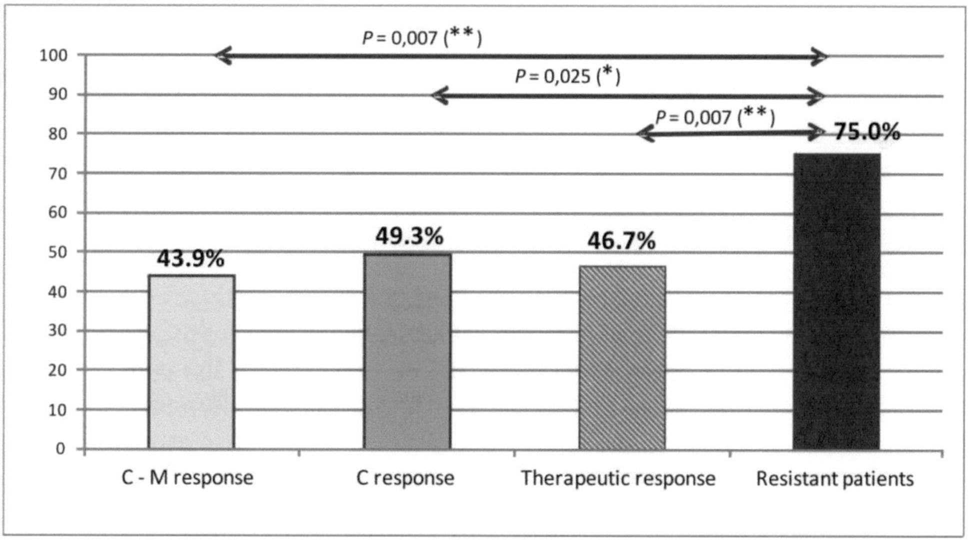

Figure 4. Occurrence (in %) of genotype consisted from wild type alleles in polymorphisms NOD2:1007fs, TLR4: 896A>G and TNFα: –308G>A in groups of patients with different response to infliximab therapy. Legend: C - M response - patients with clinical and morphological response to infliximab therapy; C response - patients with clinical response, but without morphological response; Therapeutic response - total number of patients in both groups (CM + C); Resistant patients = patients without clinical and without morphological response to infliximab therapy

Patients who are carriers of the standard genotype, are 2.13 times more probable to be resistant to the infliximab therapy (CI 95%; 1.10-4.13) compared with patients with other allele combinations [175].

In the group of patients with the genotype containing standard alleles of the monitored polymorphisms, there were 3.43% of individuals resistant to the therapy per one individual with a therapeutic response (CI 95%; 1.37-8.60). Patients, in whom the infliximab administering resulted in a therapeutic response, were also most often carriers of the combination 1007fs mut in *NOD2* gene, wt allele in *TLR4* gene and wt allele in *TNFα* gene (17%). The genotype containing standard alleles (wt) of *NOD2* and *TLR4* genes, i.e. the genotype corresponding to the standard expression activity of *TNFα*, was significantly more often presented in individuals resistant to the therapy (89.3%). The genotype composed of at least one variant allele responsible for the lower expression activity of TNFα was significantly more common in patients with a therapeutic response (32.6%; P=0.02).

In the group of patients with the greatest therapeutic benefits (clinical and morphological response), they most often represented carriers of at least one of the monitored variant alleles (39.4%) [175].

7. Conclusion of chapter – The potential of genotyping of IBD patients in clinical practice: The importance of gene polymorphisms for individualisation of IBD pharmacotherapy

Pharmacogenetics is a relatively young branch of pharmacology, which deals with the research of genetic backgrounds of individual differences in the patient's response to therapeutic drugs, both from the perspective of drug effectiveness and its safety. Its origin and development is closely connected with new knowledge in the area of the human genome and the development of molecular biology methods, which are used in this branch. The first, partly euphoric visions regarding the use of pharmacogenomic findings for pharmacotherapy individualisation and personalised medicine were later revised thanks to the empirical experience from applying theoretical hypotheses into medical practice. The difference between theoretical hypothesis and empirical findings results from the complicated biological system both at the level of genome and its regulatory mechanisms, and at the level of proteosynthesis, signalling pathways and interactions of intracellular molecules. The more we know about the human genome, the more we realise that we can only guess how many of its regions are activated in a decisive moment, and how complex the regulatory mechanisms are which influence the final effect, and resulted in phenotype.

The clinical application of pharmacogenetic findings can be limited by the existence of non-genetic factors. Even though genome cannot be influenced by external factors, the drug to drug interaction which occurs in the organism can influence not only the onset and development of a disease, but also the patient's response to the drug. Furthermore, it is necessary to remember that the patient's sensitivity to external factors is also a variable and that it is also

http://dx.doi.org/10.5772/53465

genetically conditioned. Because of this, pharmacogenetic information alone cannot predict exactly the effectiveness or safety of a drug. Despite this, pharmacogenetic studies have provided much significant information regarding the different rate of drug metabolisation in individuals as well as in populations, the effectiveness of various therapies and the development of serious adverse effects. Pharmacogenetics is a promising tool in the individualisation of the doctor-patient approach.

The characteristic presence of some polymorphisms in the "candidate genes" is connected with a predisposition to IBD. It seems that Crohn's disease is more genetically conditioned than ulcerative colitis. Some polymorphisms are typical for CD, others for UC. In patients with CD, the frameshift mutation is statistically more often present in the gene *NOD2/CARD15* (Leu1007fs insC) and the substitution mutation 469Lys>Glu in the gene *ICAM-1* than in a healthy population. Unlike patients with UC, they less often carry the substitution mutation 702Arg>Trp in the gene *NOD2/CARD15*. All three studied mutations in the gene *NOD2/CARD15* (Leu1007fs insC, 702Arg>Trp and 908Gly>Arg) are statistically more frequent in patients diagnosed with CD than in patients with UC. Genetic analysis could therefore help find individuals with a genetic predisposition that would require more frequent check-ups, or to inform physicians when to use additional endoscopic and laboratory tests or to help specify ambiguous diagnosis.

IBD therapy is lengthy; therefore it requires an individual choice of a drug with an aim to reduce or completely eliminate adverse effects, while at the same time maintain the therapy effectiveness. The aim is to achieve a maximum pharmacotherapeutic effect as well as the effective use of finance. The presence of variant alleles of polymorphisms in "therapeutic genes" can be of significant help in predicting the adverse effects of a given therapy. The relationship between myelosupression and the presence of variant alleles in the gene for TPMT is of the greatest interest. The frequency of variant alleles is significantly higher in patients who experience leukopenia during azathioprine therapy, than in patients in whom leukopenia does not develop. *TPMT* genotyping can therefore serve as a marker which will notify clinicians of a significantly increased potential risk in patients with a certain genotype, and on the necessity of increased surveillance over the patient or the need to adjust the dosage. In clinical practice, it is now common to determine variant alleles in the *TPMT* gene prior to the azathioprine therapy. This allows individualisation of the therapy and prevents serious complications.

Another desired goal is to find genetic markers which can potentially influence the effectiveness of pharmacotherapy, especially a therapy which is costly, such biological therapy for example. Our experimental data imply that patients who are carriers of a genotype composed from the variant allele 1007fs in the gene *NOD2*, variant allele 896A in the gene *TLR4* and standard allele –308A in the gene for TNFα will have the highest probability that infliximab therapy will be effective. On the other hand, individuals who are homozygous for standard (wild type) alleles of the given polymorphisms in the gene *NOD2, TLR4* and *TNFα*, are more often resistant to infliximab therapy. This standard genotype was confirmed in up to 75% of patients resistant to the therapy. Patients who are carriers of the standard genotype are 2.13 times more probable to be resistant to infliximab therapy (CI 95%; 1.10-4.13) than patients with different allelic combinations. A more complex genotyping of a larger set of patients could help define the "risk genotype", whose carriers have statistically and significantly decreased the probability of a full morphological response to anti-TNF therapy, or in contrast, to define a "positive genotype", where the probability of a successful therapy would be very high.

Abbreviations

AA - Amino acid

AP-1 - Activator protein 1

APAF-1 - Apoptotic protease activating factor 1

5-ASA - 5-aminosalicylic acid

AZA - Azathioprine

CARD15 - Caspase recruitment domain-containing protein 15

CCR5 - C Chemokine receptor type 5

CD - Crohn's Disease

CD-14 - Cluster of differentiation 14

COPD - Chronic obstructive pulmonary disease

CRP - C-reactive protein

DNA - Deoxyribonucleic acid

FDA - Food and Drug Administration

GCs - Glucocorticoids

GM-CSF - Granulocyte macrophage colony-stimulating factor

GR - Glucocorticoid receptor

GTP - Guanosine-5'-triphosphate

hnRNA - Heterogeneous nuclear RNA

IBD - Inflammatory Bowel Disease

ICAM-1 - Intercellular Adhesion Molecule 1

IκBα - Inhibitor kappa B alfa

IL-1 - Interleukin 1

ITPA - Inosine triphosphatase (nucleoside triphosphate pyrophosphatase)

LPS - Lipopolysaccharide

MDP - Muramyl dipeptide

MDR1 - Multidrug resistance protein 1

6-MP - 6-mercaptopurine

mRNA - Messenger RNA

MTX - Methotrexate

NAT - N-acetyl transferase

NF-κB - Nuclear factor kappa-light-chain-enhancer of activated B cells

NOD2 - Nucleotide-binding oligomerization domain

OCT-1 - Organic cation transporter 1

P-gp - P-glycoprotein

PCR - Polymerase chain reaction

PCR-REA - PCR-restriction enzyme analysis

PCR-RFLP - PCR-restriction fragment length polymorphism

PRA - Primer restriction analysis

SNP - Single-nucleotide polymorphism

sTNFα - Soluble TNFα

TACE - TNF-alpha converting enzyme

6-TGN - 6-thioguanine nucleotide

TLR4 - Toll-like receptor 4

tmTNFα - Transmembrane TNFα

TNFα - Tumor necrosis factor alpha

TNFR - Tumor necrosis factor alpha receptor

TPMT - Thiopurine S-methyl Transferase

TRAIL - TNF-related apoptosis-inducing ligand

UC - Ulcerative Colitis

WBCs - White blood cells

wt allele - Wild type allele

XDH - Xanthine dehydrogenace

XO - Xanthine oxidase

Acknowledgements

This work was supported by grant project no. NR9342-3/2007 of the Ministry of Health of the Czech Republic, grant project no. 2/2010 of the University of Veterinary and Pharmaceutical Sciences Brno, and grant project no. FR-TI2/075 of the Ministry of Industry and Trade of the Czech Republic (support for research and development).

Author details

Bartosova Ladislava[1], Kolorz Michal[2], Wroblova Katerina[3] and Bartos Milan[4]

*Address all correspondence to: kolorzm@vfu.cz

1 Department of Human Pharmacology and Toxicology, Faculty of Pharmacy, University of Veterinary and Pharmaceutical Sciences, Brno, Czech Republic

2 Department of Human Pharmacology and Toxicology, Faculty of Pharmacy, University of Veterinary and Pharmaceutical Sciences, Brno, Czech Republic

3 Department of Human Pharmacology and Toxicology, Faculty of Pharmacy, University of Veterinary and Pharmaceutical Sciences, Brno, Czech Republic

4 Department of Natural Drugs, Faculty of Pharmacy, University of Veterinary and Pharmaceutical Sciences, Brno, Czech Republic

References

[1] Sambrook J, Russell, DW. Molecular cloning. A laboratory manual. New York: Cold Spring Harbor Laboratory Press; 2001.

[2] Maxam AM, Gilbert W. A new method for sequencing DNA. Proceedings of the National Academy of Sciences of the U.S.A. 1977;74(2) 560-4.

[3] Sanger F, Nicklen S, Coulson AR. DNA sequencing with chain-terminating inhibitors. Proceedings of the National Academy of Sciences of the U.S.A. 1977;74(12) 5463-7.

[4] Hunkapiller T, Kaiser RJ, Koop BF et al. Large-scale and automated DNA sequence determination. Science 1991;254(5028) 59-67.

[5] Ogura Y, Bonen DK, Inohara N, et al. A frameshift mutation in NOD2 associated with susceptibility to Crohn's disease. Nature 2001;411(6837) 603–606.

[6] Podolsky, DK. Inflammatory bowel disease. The New England Journal of Medicine 2002;347(6) 417-429.

[7] Halme, L., Paavola-Sakki, P., Turunen, U. et al. Family and twin studies in inflammatory bowel disease. World Journal of Gastroenterology 2006;12(23) 3668-3672.

[8] Bartosova L., Kolorz M., Hosek J. et al. Genové polymorfismy jako predispoziční faktor IBD – jejich vztah ke klinické manifestaci a farmakoterapii onemocnění. Gene polymorphisms – IBD predisposing factor and their association with disease clinical manifestation and pharmacotherapy; Česká a Slovenská Gastroenterologie a Hepatologie 2009;63(6)265-274.

[9] Rodriguez-Bores L, Fonseca Gc, Villeda Ma, Yamamoto-Furusho Jk. Novel genetic markers in inflammatory bowel disease. World Journal of Gastroenterology 2007;13(42) 5560-5570.

[10] Hugot JP, Laurent-Pulg P, Gower-Rousseau C et al. Mapping of susceptibility locus for Crohn's disease on chromosome 16. Nature 1996;379(6568) 821–823.

[11] Hugot JP, Chamaillard M, Zouali H et al. Association of NOD2 leucine–rich repeat variants with susceptibility to Crohn's disease. Nature 2001;411(6837) 599–603.

[12] Aldhous MC, Nimmo ER, Satsangi J. NOD2/CARD15 and the Paneth cell: another piece in the genetic jigsaw of inflammatory bowel disease. Gut 2003;52(11) 1533–1535.

[13] Inohara N, Ogura Y, Fontalba A, Gutierrez O, Pons F, Crespo J, Fukase K, Inamura S, Kusumoto S, Hashimoto M, Foster SJ, Moran AP, Fernandez-Luna JL, Nuñez G. Host recognition of bacterial muramyl dipeptide mediated through NOD2. Implications for Crohn's disease. The Journal of Biological Chemistry 2003;278(8) 5509-5512.

[14] Barreiro-de Acosta M, Ouburg S, Morre SA et al. NOD2, CD14 and TLR4 mutations do not influence response to adalimumab in patients with Crohn's disease: a preliminary report. Revista Española de Enfermedades Digestivas 2010;102(10) 591-595.

[15] Linderson Y, Bresso F, Buentke E et al. Functional interaction of CARD15/NOD2 and Crohn's disease-associated TNF alpha polymorphisms. International Journal of Colorectal Disease 2005;20(4) 305-311.

[16] Lesage, S., Zouali, H., Cézard, J.-P. et al. CARD15/NOD2 mutational analysis and genotype-phenotype correlation in 612 patients with inflammatory bowel disease. The American Journal of Human Genetics 2002;70(4) 845-857.

[17] Beynon V, Cotofana S, Brand S et al. NOD2/CARD15 genotype influences MDP-induced cytokine release and basal IL-12p40 levels in primary isolated peripheral blood monocytes. Inflammatory Bowel Diseases 2008;14(8) 1033-1040.

[18] Li J, Moran T, Swanson E et al. Regulation of IL-8 and IL-1 beta expression in Crohn's disease associated NOD2/CARD15 mutations. Human Molecular Genetics 2004;13(16) 1715-1725.

[19] Kullberg BJ, Ferwerda G, de Jong DJ et al. Crohn's disease patients homozygous for the 3020insC NOD2 mutation have a defective NOD2/TLR4 cross-tolerance to intestinal stimuli. Immunology 2008;123(4) 600-605.

[20] Bonen, D. K., Cho, J. H. The genetics of inflammatory bowel disease. Gastroenterology 2003;124(2) 521-536.

[21] Hosek J, Bartosova L, Gregor P et al. Frequency of representative single nucleotide polymorphisms associated with inflammatory bowel disease in the Czech Republic and Slovak Republic. Folia Biologica 2008;54(3) 88-96.

[22] Wehkamp J, Harder J, Weichenthal M, et al. NOD2 (CARD15) mutations in Crohn's disease are associated with diminished mucosal {alpha}-defensin expression. Gut 2004;53(11) 1658–1664.

[23] Hubbard AK, Rothlein R. Intercellular Adhesion Molecule-1 (ICAM-1) expression and cell signalling cascades. Free radical biology and medicine 2000;28(9) 1379–86.

[24] Papa A, Pola R, Flex A et al. Prevalence of the K469E polymorphism of intercellular adhesion molecule 1 gene in Italian patients with inflammatory bowel disease. Digestive and Liver Disease 2004;36(8) 528–532.

[25] Nejentsev S, Laine AP, Simell O et al. Intercellular adhesion molecule–1 (ICAM–1) K469E polymorphism: no association with type 1 diabetes among Finns. Tissue Antigens. 2000;55(6) 568–570.

[26] Mycko MP, Kwinkowski M, Tronczynska E, et al. Multiple sclerosis, the increased frequency of the ICAM–1 exon 6 gene point mutation genetic type K469. Annals of Neurology 1998;44(1) 70–75.

[27] Verity DH, Vaughan RW, Kondeatis E, et al. Intercellular adhesion molecule 1 gene polymorphisms in Behcet´s disease. European Journal of Immunogenetics 2000;27(2) 73–76.

[28] Ho P, Bruce IN, Silman A et al. Evidence for common genetic control in pathways of inflammation for Crohn's disease and psoriatic arthritis. Arthritis & Rheumatism 2005;52(11) 3596–3602.

[29] Matsuzawa J, Sugimura K, Matsuda Y et al.Association between K469E allele of intercellular adhesion molecule 1 gene and inflammatory bowel disease in a Japanese population. Gut 2003; 52(1) 75–78.

[30] Hoffman TL, MacGregor RR, Burger H et al. CCR5 genotypes in sexually active couples discordant for human immunodeficiency virus type 1 infection status. The Journal of Infectious Diseases 1997;176(4) 1093-1096.

[31] Algood H, Flynn J. CCR5-deficient mice control Mycobacterium tuberculosis infection despite increased pulmonary lymphocytic infiltration. The Journal of Immunology 2004;173(5) 3287–3296.

[32] Katchar K, Eklund A, Grunewald J. Expression of Th1 markers by lung accumulated T cells in pulmonary sarcoidosis. Journal of Internal Medicine 2003;254(6) 564–571.

[33] Prahalad S, Bohnsack JF, Jorde LB, et al. Association of two functional polymorphisms in the CCR5 gene with juvenile rheumatoid arthritis. Genes and immunity 2006;7(6) 468–475.

[34] Garlet G, Martins W, Ferreira B, et al. Patterns of chemokines and chemokine receptors expression in different forms of human periodontal disease. Journal of Periodontal Research 2003;38(2) 210–217.

[35] Lee JY, Hwang DH. The modulation of inflammatory gene expression by lipids: Mediation through toll-like receptors. Molecules and Cells 2006;21(2) 174-185.

[36] Kumar MV, Nagineni CN, Chin MS et al. Innate immunity in the retina: Toll-like receptor (TLR) signaling in human retinal pigment epithelial cells. Journal of Neuroimmunology 2004;153(1-2) 7-15.

[37] Arbour NC, Lorenz E, Schutte BC et al. TLR4 mutations are associated with endotoxin hyporesponsiveness in humans. Nature Genetics 2000;25(2) 187-191.

[38] Schröder NWJ, Meister D, Wolff V et al. Chronic periodontal disease is associated with single-nucleotide polymorphisms of the human TLR-4 gene. Genes and Immunity 2005;6(5) 448-451.

[39] Speletas M, Merentiti V, Kostikas K et al. Association of TLR4-T399I Polymorphism with Chronic Obstructive Pulmonary Disease in Smokers. Clinical & Developmental Immunology 2009; doi:10.1155/2009/260286. http://www.ncbi.nlm.nih.gov/pmc/articles/PMC2822240/pdf/CDI2009-260286.pdf (accessed 18 August 2012).

[40] Horie Y, Meguro A, Ota M et al. Association of TLR4 polymorphisms with Behets disease in a Korean population. Rheumatology 2009;48(6) 638-642.

[41] Lorenz E, Mira JP, Frees KL et al. Relevance of mutations in the TLR4 receptor in patients with gram-negative septic shock. Archives of Internal Medicine 2002;162(9) 1028-1032.

[42] Gazouli M, Mantzaris G, Kotsinas A et al. Association between polymorphisms in the Toll-like receptor 4, CD14, and CARD15/NOD2 and inflammatory bowel disease in the Greek population. World Journal of Gastroenterology 2005;11(5) 681-685.

[43] D′Alfonso S, Richiardi PM. An intragenic polymorphism in the human tumor necrosis factor alpha (TNFA) chain-encoding gene. Immunogenetics 1996;44(4) 321-322.

[44] Hajeer AH, Hutchinson IV. TNF-alpha gene polymorphism: Clinical and biological implications. Microscopy Research and Technique 2000;50(3) 216-228.

[45] Braun N, Michel U, Ernst BP et al. Gene polymorphism at position -308 of the tumor-necrosis-factor-alpha (TNF-alpha) in Multiple Sclerosis and it's influence on the regulation of TNF-alpha production. Neuroscience Letters 1996;215(2) 75-78.

[46] Sashio H, Tamura K, Ito R et al. Polymorphisms of the TNF gene and the TNF receptor superfamily member 1B gene are associated with susceptibility to ulcerative colitis and Crohn's disease, respectively. Immunogenetics 2002;53(12) 1020-1027.

[47] Sýkora J, Šubrt I, Dědek P et al. Cytokine Tumor Necrosis Factor-alpha A Promoter Gene Polymorphism at Position -308 GA and Paediatric Inflammatory Bowel Disease: Implications in Ulcerative Colitis and Crohn´s Disease. Journal of Paediatric Gastroenterology and Nutrition 2006;42(5) 479–487.

[48] Yamamoto-Furusho JK, Uscanga LF, Vargas-Alarcón G et al. Polymorphism in the promoter region of tumor necrosis factor alpha (TNF-α) and the HLA-DRB1 locus in Mexican Mestizo patients with ulcerative colitis. Immunology Letters 2004;95(1) 31–35 .

[49] Ferguson LR, Huebner C, Petermann I et al. Single nucleotide polymorphism in the tumor necrosis factor-alpha gene affects inflammatory bowel diseases risk. World Journal of Gastroenterology 2008;14(29) 4652–4661.

[50] Fan W, Maoging W, Wangyang C et al. Relationship between the polymorphism of tumor necrosis factor-α-308 G>A and susceptibility to inflammatory bowel diseases and colorectal cancer: a meta analysis. European Journal of Human Genetics 2011;19(4) 432–437.

[51] Huizinga TWJ, Westendorp RGJ, Bollen ELEM et al. TNF-alpha promoter polymorphisms, production and susceptibility to multiple sclerosis in different groups of patients. Journal of Neuroimmunology 1997;72(2) 149-153.

[52] Pociot F, Briant L,Jongeneel CV et al. Association of Tumor-Necrosis-Factor (Tnf) and Class-Ii Major Histocompatibility Complex Alleles with the Secretion of TNF-Alpha and TNF-Beta by Human Mononuclear-Cells - A Possible Link to Insulin-Dependent Diabetes-Mellitus. European Journal of Immunology 1993;23(1) 224-231.

[53] Annese V, Latiano A, Palmieri O et al. NOD2/CARD15 in healthy relatives of IBD patients. European Review for Medical and Pharmacological Sciences 2006;10(1) 33–36.

[54] Brant SR, Picco MF, Achkar JP, et al. Defining complex contributions of NOD2/CARD15 gene mutations, age at onset and tobacco use on Crohn's disease phenotypes. Inflammatory Bowel Diseases 2003;9(5) 281–289.

[55] Kim YG, Shaw MH, Warner N et al. Cutting Edge: Crohn's Disease-Associated Nod2 Mutation Limits Production of Proinflammatory Cytokines To Protect the Host from Enterococcus faecalis-Induced Lethality. Journal of Immunology 2011;187(6) 2849-2852.

[56] Hradsky O, Lenicek M, Dusatkova P et al. Variants of CARD15, TNFA and PTPN22 and susceptibility to Crohn's disease in the Czech population: high frequency of the CARD15 1007fs. Tissue Antigens 2008; 71(6) 538–547.

[57] Herfarth H, Pollok-Kopp B, Goke M, et al. Polymorphism of CC chemokine receptors CCR2 and CCR5 in Crohn's disease. Immunology Letters 2001;77(2) 113–117.

[58] Reference SNP (refSNP) Cluster Report: http://www.ncbi.nlm.nih.gov/projects/SNP/snp_ref.cgi?rs=1800629 (accessed 30 July 2012)

[59] Peeters H, Vander Cruyssen B, et al. Radiological sarcoiliitis, a hallmark of spondylitis, is linked with CARD15 gene polymorphisms in patients with Crohn's disease. Annals of Rheumatic Diseases 2004;63(9) 1131–1134.

[60] Karban A, Dagan E, Eliakim R, et al. Prevalence and significance of mutations in the familial Mediterranean fever gene in patients with Crohn's disease. Genes and Immunity 2005;6(2) 134–139.

[61] Leshinsky-Silver E, Karban A, Buzhakor E et al. Is age of onset of Crohn's disease governed by mutations in NOD2/caspase recruitment domains 15 and Toll-like receptor 4? Evaluation of a pediatric cohort. Pediatr Research 2005;58(3) 499–504.

[62] Dostálek M, Janoštíková E, Juřica J et al. Farmakokinetika. Praha: Grada Publishing; 2006.

[63] Schröder H, Evans DA. Acetylator phenotype and adverse effects of sulphasalazine in healthy subjects. GUT 1972a;13(4) 278-284.

[64] Das KM, Eastwood MA, McManus JP et al. Adverse reactions during salicylazosulfapyridine therapy and the relation with drug metabolism and acetylator phenotype. The New England Journal of Medicine 1973;289(10) 491-495.

[65] Chen M, Xia B, Chen B et al. N-acetyltransferase 2 slow acetylator genotype associated with adverse effects of sulphasalazine in the treatment of inflammatory bowel disease. Canadian Journal of Gastroenterology 2007;21(3) 155-158.

[66] Schröder H, Evans DA. The polymorphic acetylation of sulphapyridine in man. Journal of Medical Genetics 1972b;9(2) 168-171.

[67] Goldstein PD Alpers DH, Keating JP. Sulfapyridine metabolites in children with inflammatory bowel disease receiving sulfasalazine. Journal of Pediatrics 1979;95(4) 638-640.

[68] Ricart E, Taylor WR, Loftus E et al. N-acetyltransferase 1 and 2 genotypes do not predict response or toxicity to treatment with mesalamine and sulfasalazine in patients with ulcerative colitis. American Journal of Gastroenterology 2002;97(7) 1763-1768.

[69] Hausmann M, Paul G, Menzel K et al. NAT1 genotypes do not predict response to mesalamine in patients with ulcerative colitis. Zeitschrift für Gastroenterologie 2008;46(3) 259-265.

[70] Zbořil V, Pazourková M, Prokopová L et al. Imunosupresiva v léčbě idiopatických střevních zánětů. Praha: Grada Publishing; 2007.

[71] Munkholm P, Langholz E, Davidssen M et al. Frequency of glucocorticoid resistance in Crohn's disease. GUT 1994; 35(3) 360-362.

[72] Faubion WA Jr, LOFTUS EV Jr, HARMSEN WS et al. The natural history of corticosteroid therapy for inflammatory bowel disease: a population-based study. Gastroenterology 2001;121(2) 255-260.

[73] De Iudicibus S, Franca R, Martelossi S et al. Molecular mechanism of glucocorticoid resistance in inflammatory bowel disease. World Journal of Gastroenterology 2011;17(9) 1095-1108.

[74] Juliano RL, Ling V. A surface glycoprotein modulating drug permeability in Chinese hamster ovary cell mutants. Biochimica et Biophysica Acta 1976;455(1) 152-162.

[75] Cordon-Cardo C, O'Brien JP, Casals D et al. Multidrug-resistance gene (P-glycoprotein) is expressed by endothelial cells at blood-brain barrier sites. Proceedings of the National Academy of Sciences of the United States of America1989;86(2) 695-698.

[76] Farrell RJ, Murphy A, Long A et al. High multidrug resistance (P-glycoprotein 170) expression in inflammatory bowel disease patients who fail medical therapy. Gastroenterology 2000;118(2) 279-288.

[77] Farrell RJ, Kelleher D. Glucocorticoid resistance in inflammatory bowel disease. Journal of Endocrinology. 2003;178(3) 339-346.

[78] Kioka N, Tsubota J, Kakehi Y et al. P-glycoprotein gene (MDR1) cDNA from human adrenal: normal P-glycoprotein carries Gly185 with an altered pattern of multidrug resistance. Biochemical and Biophysical Research Communications 1989;162(1) 224-231.

[79] Saito S, Lida A, Sekine A et al. Three hundred twenty-six genetic variations in genes encoding nine members of ATP-binding cassette, subfamily B (ABCB/MDR/TAP), in the Japanese population. Journal of Human Genetics 2002;47(1) 38-50.

[80] Schwab M, Eichelbaum M, Fromm MF. Genetic polymorphisms of the human MDR1 drug transporter. Annual Review of Pharmacology and Toxicology 2003;43 285-307.

[81] Krupoves A, Mack D, Seidman E et al. Associations between variants in the ABCB1 (MDR1) gene and corticosteroid dependence in children with Crohn's disease. Inflammatory Bowel Diseases 2011;17(11) 2308-2317.

[82] Cascorbi I.P-glycoprotein: tissue distribution, substrates, and functional consequences of genetic variations. Handbook of Experimental Pharmacology 2011;(201) 261-283.

[83] Cascorbi I, Gerloff T, Johne A et al. Frequency of single nucleotide polymorphisms in the P-glycoprotein drug transporter MDR1 gene in white subjects. Clinical Pharmacology & Therapeutics 2001;69(3) 169-174.

[84] Ameyaw MM, Regateiro F, Li T et al. MDR1 pharmacogenetics: frequency of the C3435T mutation in exon 26 is significantly influenced by ethnicity. Pharmacogenetics 2001;11(3) 217-221.

[85] Schaeffeler E, Eichelbaum M, Brinkmann et al. Frequency of C3435T polymorphism of MDR1 gene in African people. Lancet 2001;358(9279) 383-384.

[86] Panwala CM, Jones JC, Viney JL. A novel model of inflammatory bowel disease: mice deficient for the multiple drug resistance gene, mdr1a, spontaneously develop colitis. The Journal of Immunology 1998;161(10) 5733-5744.

[87] Potocnik U, Ferkolj I, Glavac D et al. Polymorphisms in multidrug resistance 1 (MDR1) gene are associated with refractory Crohn disease and ulcerative colitis. Genes & Immunity 2004;5(7) 530-539.

[88] Honda M, Orii F, Ayabe T et al. Expression of glucocorticoid receptor beta in lymphocytes of patients with glucocorticoid-resistant ulcerative colitis. Gastroenterology 2000;118(5) 859-866.

[89] Raddatz D, Middel P, Bockemühl M et al. Glucocorticoid receptor expression in inflammatory bowel disease: evidence for a mucosal down-regulation in steroid-unresponsive ulcerative colitis. Alimentary Pharmacology & Therapeutics 2004;19(1) 47-61.

[90] Bamberger CM, Else T, Bamberger AM et al. Regulation of the human interleukin-2 gene by the alpha and beta isoforms of the glucocorticoid receptor. Molecular and Cellular Endocrinology 1997;136(1) 23-28.

[91] Kam JC, Szefler SJ, Surs W et al. Combination IL-2 and IL-4 reduces glucocorticoid receptor-binding affinity and T cell response to glucocorticoids. The Journal of Immunology 1993;151(7) 3460-3466.

[92] Bantel H, Domschke W, Schulze-Osthoff K. Molecular mechanisms of glucocorticoid resistance. Gastroenterology 2000;119(4) 1178-1179.

[93] Russcher H, Van Rossum EF, De Jong FH et al. Increased expression of the glucocorticoid receptor-A translational isoform as a result of the ER22/23EK polymorphism. Molecular Endocrinology 2005a;19(7)1687-1696.

[94] Van Rossum EF, Koper JW, Huizenga NA et al. A polymorphism in the glucocorticoid receptor gene, which decreases sensitivity to glucocorticoids in vivo, is associated with low insulin and cholesterol levels. Diabetes 2002;51(10) 3128-3134.

[95] Huizenga NA, Koper JW, De Lange P et al. A polymorphism in the glucocorticoid receptor gene may be associated with and increased sensitivity to glucocorticoids in vivo. Journal of Clinical Endocrinology & Metabolism 1998;83(1) 144-151.

[96] Russcher H, Smit P, Van Den Akker EL et al. Two polymorphisms in the glucocorticoid receptor gene directly affect glucocorticoid-regulated gene expression. Journal of Clinical Endocrinology & Metabolism 2005b;90(10) 5804-5810.

[97] De Iudicibus S, Stocco G, Martelossi S et al. Association of BclI polymorphism of the glucocorticoid receptor gene locus with response to glucocorticoids in inflammatory bowel disease. Gut 2007;56(9) 1319-1320.

[98] Hurley DM, Accili D, Stratakis CA et al. Point mutation causing a single amino acid substitution in the hormone binding domain of the glucocorticoid receptor in familial glucocorticoid resistance. Journal of Clinical Investigation 1991;87(2) 680-686.

[99] Malchoff DM, Brufsky A, Reardon G et al. A mutation of the glucocorticoid receptor in primary cortisol resistance. Journal of Clinical Investigation 1993;91(5) 1918-25.

[100] Manenschijn L, van den Akker EL, Lamberts SW et al. Clinical features associated with glucocorticoid receptor polymorphisms. An overview. Annals of the New York Academy of Sciences 2009;1179(Oct.) 179-198.

[101] Farrell R, Kelleher D. Glucocorticoid resistance in inflammatory bowel disease. Journal of Endocrinology 2003;178(3) 339-346.

[102] Roberts-Thomson C, Butler WJ. Azathioprine, 6-mercaptopurine and thiopurine S-methyltransferase. Journal of Gastroenterology and Hepatology 2005;20(6) 955-955.

[103] Colonna T, Korelitz B I. The role of leucopenia in the 6-mercaptopurie-induced remission of refractory Crohn's disease. American Journal of Gastroenterology 1994;89(3) 362-366.

[104] Krynetski E, Evans WE. Drug methylation in cancer therapy: lessons from the TPMT polymorphism. Oncogene 2003;22(47) 7403-7413.

[105] Seki T, Tanaka T, Nakamura Y Genomic structure and multiple single-nucleotide polymorphisms (SNPs) of the thiopurine S-methyltransferase (TPMT) gene. Journal of Human Genetics 2000;45(5) 299-302.

[106] Krynetski EY, Fessing MY, Yates CR, Sun D, Schuetz JD, Evans WE. Promoter and intronic sequences of the human thiopurine S-methyltransferase (TPMT) gene isolated from a human PAC1 genomic library. Pharmaceutical Research 1997;14(12) 1672-1678.

[107] Krynetski EY, Schuetz JD, Galpin AJ et al. A Single-Point Mutation Leading to Loss of Catalytic Activity in Human Thiopurine S-Methyltransferase . Proceedings of the National Academy of Sciences of the United States of America 1995;92(4) 949-953.

[108] de la Moureyre CSV, Debuysere H, Mastain B et al. Genotypic and phenotypic analysis of the polymorphic thiopurine S-methyltransferase gene (TPMT) in a European population. British Journal of Pharmacology 1998;125(4) 879-887.

[109] Tai HL, Krynetski EY, Schuetz EG et al. Enhanced proteolysis of thiopurine S-methyltransferase (TPMT) encoded by mutant alleles in humans (TPMT*3A, TPMT*2): Mechanisms for the genetic polymorphism of TPMT activity. Proceedings of the National Academy of Sciences of the United States of America 1997;94(12) 6444-6449.

[110] Sahasranaman S, Howard D, Roy S Clinical pharmacology and pharmacogenetics of thiopurines. European Journal of Clinical Pharmacology 2008;64(8) 753-767.

[111] Otterness D, Szumlanski C, Lennard L et al. Human thiopurine methyltransferase pharmacogenetics: Gene sequence polymorphisms. Clinical Pharmacology & Therapeutics 1997;62(1) 60-73.

[112] Hon YY, Fessing MY, Pui CH et al. Polymorphism of the thiopurine S-methyltransferase gene in African-Americans. Human Molecular Genetics 1999;8(2) 371-376.

[113] Schaeffeler E, Fischer C, Brockmeier D et al. Comprehensive analysis of thiopurine S-methyltransferase phenotype-genotype correlation in a large population of German-Caucasians and identification of novel TPMT variants. Pharmacogenetics 2004;14(7) 407-417.

[114] Lindqvist M, Haglund S, Almer S et al. Identification of two novel sequence variants affecting thiopurine methyltransferase enzyme activity. Pharmacogenetics 2004;14 (4) 261-265.

[115] Hamdan-Khalil R, Gala JL, Allorge D et al. Identification and functional analysis of two rare allelic variants of the thiopurine S-methyltransferase gene, TPMT*16 and TPMT*19. Biochemical Pharmacology 2005;69(3) 525-529.

[116] Yates CR, Krynetski EY, Loennechen T et al. Molecular diagnosis of thiopurine S-methyltransferase deficiency: Genetic basis for azathioprine and mercaptopurine intolerance. Annals of Internal Medicine 1997;126(8) 608-614.

[117] Collie-Duguid ESR, Pritchard SC, Powrie RH et al. The frequency and distribution of thiopurine methyltransferase alleles in Caucasian and Asian populations. Pharmacogenetics 1999;9(1) 37-42 .

[118] McLeod HL, Pritchard SC, Githang'a J et al. Ethnic differences in thiopurine methyltransferase pharmacogenetics: evidence for allele specificity in Caucasian and Kenyan individuals. Pharmacogenetics 1999;9(6) 773-776.

[119] Ganiere-Monteil C, Medard Y, Lejus C et al. Phenotype and genotype for thiopurine methyltransferase activity in the French Caucasian population: impact of age. European Journal of Clinical Pharmacology 2004;60(2) 89-96.

[120] Loennechen T, Utsi E, Hartz I et al. Detection of one single mutation predicts thiopurine S-methyltransferase activity in a population of Saami in northern Norway. Clinical Pharmacology&Therapeutics 2001;70(2) 183-188.

[121] Ameyaw MM, Collie-Duguid ESR, Powrie RH et al. Thiopurine methyltransferase alleles in British and Ghanaian populations. Human Molecular Genetics 1999;8(2) 367-370.

[122] Chang JG, Lee LS, Chen CM et al. Molecular analysis of thiopurine S-methyltransferase alleles in South-east Asian populations. Pharmacogenetics 2002;12(3) 191-195.

[123] Kumagai K, Hiyama K, Ishioka S et al. Allelotype frequency of the thiopurine methyltransferase (TPMT) gene in Japanese. Pharmacogenetics 2001;11(3) 275-278.

[124] Zhang JP, Guan YY, Xu AL et al. Gene mutation of thiopurine s-methyltransferase in uygur chinese. European Journal of Clinical Pharmacology 2004;60(1) 1-3.

[125] Arenas M, Duley J, Sumi S et al. The ITPA c.94C > A and g.IVS2+21A > C sequence variants contribute to missplicing of the ITPA gene. Biochimica et Biophysica Acta-Molecular Basis of Disease 2007;1772(1) 96-102.

[126] Lin SR, McLennan AG, Ying K et al. Cloning, Expression, and Characterization of a Human InosineTriphosphate Pyrophosphatase Encoded by the ITPA Gene Journal of Biological Chemistry 2001;276(22) 18695-18701.

[127] Bierau J, Lindhout M, Bakker JA. Pharmacogenetic significance of inosine triphosphatase. Pharmacogenomics 2007;8(9) 1221-1228.

[128] Sumi S, Marinaki AM, Arenas M et al. Genetic basis of inosine triphosphate pyrophosphohydrolase deficiency. Human Genetics 2002;111(4-5) 360-367.

[129] Herting G, Barber K, Zappala MR et al. Quantitative in vitro and in vivo characterization of the human P32T mutant ITPase. Biochimica et Biophysica Acta-Molecular Basis of Disease 2010;1802(2) 269-274.

[130] Cao HN, Hegele RA. DNA polymorphisms in ITPA including basis of inosine triphosphatase deficiency. Journal of Human Genetics 2002;47(11) 620-622.

[131] Marsh S, King CR, Ahluwalia R et al. Distribution of ITPA P32T alleles in multiple world populations. Journal of Human Genetics 2004;49(10) 579-581

[132] Shipkova M, Lorenz K, Oellerich M et al. Measurement of erythrocyte inosine triphosphate pyrophosphohydrolase (ITPA) activity by HPLC and correlation of ITPA genotype-phenotype in a caucasian population. Clinical Chemistry 2006;52(2) 240-247.

[133] Hawwa AF, Millership JS, Collier PS et al. Pharmacogenomic studies of the anticancer and immunosuppressive thiopurines mercaptopurine and azathioprine. British Journal of Clinical Pharmacology 2008;66(4) 517-528.

[134] Heller T, Oellerich M, Armstrong VW et al. Rapid detection of ITPA 94C > A and IVS2+21A > C gene mutations by real-time fluorescence PCR and in vitro demonstration of effect of ITPA IVS2+21A > C polymorphism on splicing efficiency. Clinical Chemistry 2004;50(11) 2182-2184.

[135] Marinaki AM, Ansari A, Duley JA et al. Adverse drug reactions to azathioprine therapy are associated with polymorphism in the gene encoding inosine triphosphate pyrophosphatase (ITPase). Pharmacogenetics 2004;14(3) 181-187.

[136] Zelinkova Z, Derijks LJJ, Stokkers PCF et al. Inosine triphosphate pyrophosphatase and thiopurine S-methyltransferase genotypes relationship to azathioprine-induced myelosuppression. Clinical Gastroenterology and Hepatology 2006;4(1): 44-49.

[137] Derijks LJJ, Wong DR. Pharmacogenetics of Thiopurines in Inflammatory Bowel Disease. Current Pharmaceutical Design 2010;16(2) 145-154.

[138] Zimm S, Collins JM, Oneill D et al. Inhibition of First Pass Metabolism in Cancer-Chemotherapy - Interaction of 6-Mercaptopurine and Allopurinol. Clinical Pharmacology&Therapeutics 1983;34(6) 810-817.

[139] Parks DA, Granger DN. Xanthine-Oxidase - Biochemistry, Distribution and Physiology. Acta Physiologica Scandinavica 1986;548 87-99.

[140] Guerciolini R, Szumlanski C, Weinshilboum RM Human Liver Xanthine-Oxidase - Nature and Extent of Individual Variation. Clinical Pharmacology&Therapeutics 1991;50(6) 663-672.

[141] Relling MV, Lin JS, Ayers GD et al. Racial and Gender Differences in N-Acetyltransferase, Xanthine-Oxidase, and CYP1A2 Activities. Clinical Pharmacology&Therapeutics 1992;52(6) 643-658.

[142] Sparrow MP, Hande SA, Friedman S et al. Allopurinol safely and effectively optimizes tioguanine metabolites in inflammatory bowel disease patients not responding to azathioprine and mercaptopurine. Alimentary Pharmacology& Therapeutics 2005;22(5) 441-446.

[143] Kudo M, Moteki T, Sasaki T et al. Functional characterization of human xanthine oxidase allelic variants. Pharmacogenetics and Genomics 2008;18(3) 243-251.

[144] Smith MA, Marinaki AM, Arenas M et al. Novel pharmacogenetic markers for treatment outcome in azathioprine-treated inflammatory bowel disease . Alimentary Pharmacology&Therapeutics 2009;30(4) 375-384.

[145] Agarwal A,Banerjee A, Banerjee UC. Xanthine oxidoreductase: A journey from purine metabolism to cardiovascular excitation-contraction coupling. Critical Reviews in Biotechnology 2011;31(3) 264-280.

[146] Choy EHS, Panayi GS. Mechanisms of disease: Cytokine pathways and joint inflammation in rheumatoid arthritis. New England Journal of Medicine 2001;344(12) 907-916.

[147] Horiuchi T, Mitoma H, Harashima S et al. Transmembrane TNF-alpha: structure, function and interaction with anti-TNF agents. Rheumatology 2010;49(7) 1215-1228.

[148] Tracey D, Klareskog L, Sasso EH et al. Tumor necrosis factor antagonist mechanisms of action: A comprehensive review. Pharmacology&Therapeutics 2008;117(2) 244-279.

[149] Baert F, Noman M, Vermeire S et al. Influence of immunogenicity on the long-term efficacy of infliximab in Crohn's disease. New England Journal of Medicine 2003; 348(7) 601-608.

[150] Bendtzen K, Geborek P, Svenson M et al. Individualized monitoring of drug bioavailability and immunogenicity in rheumatoid arthritis patients treated with the tumor necrosis factor alpha inhibitor infliximab. Arthritis and Rheumatism 2006;54(12) 3782-3789.

[151] Smookler DS, Mohammed FF, Kassiri Z et al. Cutting edge: Tissue inhibitor of metalloproteinase 3 regulates TNF-dependent systemic inflammation. Journal of Immunology 2006;176(2) 721-725.

[152] Hlavaty T, Pierik M, Henckaerts L et al. Polymorphisms in apoptosis genes predict response to infliximab therapy in luminal and fistulizing Crohn's disease. Alimentary Pharmacology & Therapeutics 2005;22(7) 613-626.

[153] Wu JM, Metzt C, Xu XL et al. A novel polymorphic CAAT/enhancer-binding protein beta element in the FasL gene promoter alters Fas ligand expression: A candidate background gene in African American systemic lupus erythematosus patients. Journal of Immunology 2003; 170(1) 132-138.

[154] Wu JM, Richards MH, Huang JH et al. Human FasL Gene Is a Target of beta-Catenin/T-Cell Factor Pathway and Complex FasL Haplotypes Alter Promoter Functions. Plos One 2011;6(10) 1-12.

[155] Ghavami S, Hashemi M, Ande SR et al. Apoptosis and cancer: mutations within caspase genes. Journal of Medical Genetics 2009;46(8) 497-510.

[156] Theodoropoulos GE, Gazouli M, Vaiopoulou A et al. Polymorphisms of Caspase 8 and Caspase 9 gene and colorectal cancer susceptibility and prognosis. International Journal of Colorectal Disease 2011;26(9) 1113-1118.

[157] Ferreira P, Cravo M, Guerreiro CS et al. Fat intake interacts with polymorphisms of Caspase9, FasLigand and PPARgamma apoptotic genes in modulating Crohn's disease activity. Clinical Nutrition 2010;29(6) 819-823.

[158] Ansari A, Hassan C, Duley J et al. Thiopurine methyltransferase activity and the use of azathioprine in inflammatory bowel disease. Alimentary Pharmacology&Therapeutics 2002;16(10) 1743–1750.

[159] Roberts-Thomson C, Butler WJ. Azathioprine, 6-mercaptopurine and thiopurine S-methyltransferase. Journal of Gastroenterology and Hepatology 2005;20(6) 955.

[160] Breen DP, Marinaki AM, Arenas M et al. Pharmacogenetic association with adverse drug reactions to azathioprine immunosuppressive therapy following liver transplantation.Liver Transplantation 2005;11(7) 826-33.

[161] Katsanos K, Tsiano EV. Non-TPMT determinants of azathioprine toxicity in inflammatory bowel disease. Annals of Gastroenterology 2010;23(2) 95-101.

[162] Katsanos K, Ferrante M, Henckaerts L et al. Bone marrow toxicity during azathioprine treatment in inflammatory bowel disease. Gut 2006;55 A112.

[163] Dubinsky MC, Lamothe S, Yang HY et al. Pharmacogenomics and metabolite measurement for 6-mercaptopurine therapy in inflammatory bowel disease.Gastroenterology 2000;118(4) 705-713.

[164] Colombel JF, Ferrari N, Debuysere H et al. Genotypic analysis of thiopurine S-methyltransferase in patients with Crohn's disease and severe myelosuppression during azathioprine therapy. Gastroenterology. 2000;118(6)1025–1030.

[165] Evans WE, Hon YY, Bomgaars L et al. Preponderance of thiopurine S-methyltransferase deficiency and heterozygosity among patients intolerant to mercaptopurine or azathioprine. Journal of Clinical Oncology 2001;19(8) 2293-2301.

[166] Kurzawski M, Dziewanowski K, Lener A et al. TPMT but not ITPA gene polymorphism influences the risk of azathioprine intolerance in renal transplant recipients. European journal of clinical pharmacology 2009;65(5) 533-40.

[167] Kolorz M, Bartosova L, Hosek J, Dvorackova D, et al. Importance of thiopurine S-Methyltransferase gene polymorphisms for prediction of azathioprine toxicity. Neuroendocrinology Letters 2009;30(suppl 1) 137–142.

[168] Wroblova K, Kolorz M, Batovsky M, Zboril V., Suchankova J, Bartos M, Ulicny B, Pav I, Bartosova L. Gene Polymorphisms Involved in Manifestation of Leucopenia, Digestive Intolerance, and Pancreatitis in Azathioprine-Treated Patients. Digestive diseases and sciences 2012;57(9) 2394-401.

[169] Food and Drug Administration. Table of Pharmacogenomic Biomarkers in Drug Labels http://www.fda.gov/drugs/scienceresearch/researchareas/pharmacogenetics/ucm083378.html (accessed 20 July 2012)

[170] Kaskas BA, Louis E, Hindorf U et al. Safe treatment of thiopurine S-methyltransferase deficient Crohn's disease patients with azathioprine. Gut 2003;52(1) 140-142.

[171] Relling MV, Gardner EE, Sandborn WJ et al. Clinical Pharmacogenetics Implementation Consortium Guidelines for Thiopurine Methyltransferase Genotype and Thiopurine Dosing. Clinical Pharmacology and Therapeutics 2011;89(3) 387-391

[172] Sanderson J, Ansari A, Marinaki T et al. Thiopurine methyltransferase: should it be measured before commencing thiopurine drug therapy? Annals of Clinical Biochemistry 2004;41(4) 294–302.

[173] Regueiro M, Mardini H. Determination of thiopurine methyltransferase genotype or phenotype optimizes initial dosing of azathioprine for the treatment of Crohn's disease. Journal of Clinical Gastroenterology 2002;35(3) 240–244.

[174] Gardiner SJ, Gearry RB, Begg EJ et al. Thiopurine dose in intermediate and normal metabolizers of thiopurine methyltransferase may differ three-fold. Clinical Gastroenterology and Hepatology 2008;6(6) 654–660.

[175] Kolorz M. Genové polymorfizmy ve vztahu k nežádoucím účinkům a efektivitě vytypované farmakoterapie (azathioprinem, infliximabem) u pacientů s nespecifickými střevními záněty. (English: Gene Polymorphisms and their Relationship to Adverse Drug Reactions Incidence and Effectivity of Pharmacotherapy (Azathioprine, Infliximab) on Patients with Inflammatory Bowel Disease. Dissertation. Faculty of Pharmacy, UVPS Brno, Czech republic 2012.

[176] Allorge D,Hamdan R, Broly F et al. ITPA genotyping test does not improve detection of Crohn's disease patients at risk of azathioprine/6-mercaptopurine induced myelosuppression. Gut 2005;54(4) 565-565.

[177] van Dieren JM, van Vuuren AJ, Kusters JG et al. ITPA genotyping is not predictive for the development of side effects in AZA treated inflammatory bowel disease patients. Gut 2005;54(11) 1664-1664.

[178] Gisbert JP, Gonzalez-Lama Y, Mate J. Systematic review: infliximab therapy in ulcerative colitis. Alimentary Pharmacology&Therapeutics 2007;25(1)19-37.

[179] Rutgeerts P, Sandborn WJ, Feagan BG et al. Infliximab for induction and maintenance therapy for ulcerative colitis. The New England journal of medicine 2005;353(23) 2462-2476.

[180] Alzafiri R, Holcroft CA, Malolepszy P et al. Infliximab therapy for moderately severe Crohn's disease and ulcerative colitis: a retrospective comparison over 6 years Clinical and experimental gastroenterology 2011;4 9-17.

[181] Hanauer SB, Feagan BG, Lichtenstein GR et al. Maintenance infliximab for Crohn's disease: the ACCENT I randomised trial. Lancet 2002;359(9317) 1541-1549.

[182] Sands BE, Anderson FH, Bernstein CN et al. Infliximab maintenance therapy for fistulizing Crohn's disease. New England Journal of Medicine 2004;350(9) 876-885.

[183] Kapetanovic MC, Larsson L, Truedsson L et al. Predictors of infusion reactions during infliximab treatment in patients with arthritis. Arthritis research & therapy 2006;8(4) R131.

[184] Haraoui B, Cameron L, Ouellet M et al. Anti-infliximab antibodies in patients with rheumatoid arthritis who require higher doses of infliximab to achieve or maintain a clinical response. Journal of Rheumatology 2006;33(1) 31-36.

[185] Siegel CA, Melmed GY. Predicting response to anti-TNF agents for the treatment of Crohn's disease. Therapeutic advances in gastroenterology 2009; 2(4) 245–251.

[186] Plant D, Bowes J, Potter C et al. Genome-Wide Association Study of Genetic Predictors of Anti-Tumor Necrosis Factor Treatment Efficacy in Rheumatoid Arthritis Identifies Associations With Polymorphisms at Seven Loci. Arthritis and Rheumatism 2011;63(3) 645-653.

[187] Li J, Moran T, Swanson E, Julian C et al. Regulation of IL-8 and IL-1 beta expression in Crohn's disease associated NOD2/CARD15 mutations. Human Molecular Genetics 2004;13(16) 1715-1725.

[188] Beynon V, Cotofana S, Brand S et al. NOD2/CARD15 genotype influences MDP-induced cytokine release and basal IL-12p40 levels in primary isolated peripheral blood monocytes. Inflammatory Bowel Diseases 2008;14(8) 1033-1040.

http://dx.doi.org/10.5772/53465

[189] Kullberg BJ, Ferwerda G, de Jong DJ et al. Crohn's disease patients homozygous for the 3020insC NOD2 mutation have a defective NOD2/TLR4 cross-tolerance to intestinal stimuli. Immunology 2008;123(4) 600-605.

[190] Guo QS, Xia B, Jiang Y et al. NOD2 3020insC frameshift mutation is not associated with inflammatory bowel disease in Chinese patients of Han nationality. World Journal of Gastroenterology 2004;10(7) 1069-1071.

[191] Akira S,Uematsu S,Takeuchi O. Pathogen recognition and innate immunity. Cell 2006;124(4) 783-801.

[192] Kiechl S, Lorenz E, Reindl M et al. Toll-like receptor 4 polymorphisms and atherogenesis. New England Journal of Medicine 2002;347(3) 185-192.

[193] Balistreri CR, Caruso C, Listi F et al. LPS-mediated production of pro/anti-inflammatory cytokines and eicosanoids in whole blood samples: Biological effects of +896A/G TLR4 polymorphism in a Sicilian population of healthy subjects. Mechanisms of Ageing and Development 2011;132(3) 86-92.

[194] Hajeer AH, Hutchinson IV. TNF-alpha gene polymorphism: Clinical and biological implications. Microscopy Research and Technique 2000;50(3) 216-228.

Chapter 3

The Role of the Microbiota in Gastrointestinal Health and Disease

Anne-Marie C. Overstreet, Amanda E. Ramer-Tait,
Albert E. Jergens and Michael J. Wannemuehler

Additional information is available at the end of the chapter

http://dx.doi.org/10.5772/53920

1. Introduction

Antony van Leeuwenhoek's observation of "animalcules" in the tarter of teeth in 1683 marked the beginning of humans trying to understand their relationship with microbes. Now commonly referred to as "bacteria" or the "microbiota", we share our inner and outer space with these single-celled organisms. They are present all around us in the oceans, soil, leaves, and even air [1]. One of the microbial niches that has recently garnered much attention is the human body. In this niche, we share the table with 10^{14} microbial cells, which outnumber our eukaryotic cells ten to one [1, 2]. These organisms colonize most body sites, including the skin, oral cavity, gastrointestinal, urogenital and respiratory tracts. Additionally, there is 150 times more genetic material associated with our resident bacteria when compared to our own DNA and comprise what is known as our body's "second genome," a concept recently reviewed by Zhu et al. [3]. In an effort to understand the role that these organisms have on human development, health and disease, the National Institutes of Health launched the "Human Microbiome Project" in 2007 in an effort to elucidate this host-microbe interaction [4-6].

The role of bacteria is most obvious in the gastrointestinal tract (GIT). Bacteria in this niche have the ability to break down substances that otherwise could not be digested by GIT cells; they also produce metabolites needed by the body such as vitamin K (menaquinones), folate, B12, and riboflavin [7-12]. The GIT has a surface area the size of a tennis court and is home to 10^{11}-10^{12} organisms per gram of colonic content [1, 13]. The predominant bacterial phyla present in the GIT include the Firmicutes and Bacteroidetes with low levels of Proteobacteria, Actinobacteria, Fusobacteria, and Verrucomicrobia [14-16]. It has been noted that members of the predominant factions (the Firmicutes and Bacteroidetes) belong to only three groups, *Bacteroides, Clostridium coccoides* (cluster XIVa) and *Clostridium leptum* (cluster IV) [15, 17, 18].

There are also Archaea present in the GIT and have been found to belong to one phylotype, *Methanobrevibacter smithii* [14, 19].

1.1. Initial colonization of the gastrointestinal tract

Infants are born sterile and establishment of the GI microbiota begins shortly thereafter. Studies in mice have revealed that the first organisms to colonize include lactobacilli,fFlavobacteria and Group N Streptococci [20]. These three groups were found in the stomach and the small and large intestine. When the mice were 12 days of age, the flavobacteria disappeared from all three sites. Concurrently, there was a rapid increase in the presence of enterococci and slow lactose fermenting coliform bacilli reaching 10^9 bacteria per gram of tissue in the large intestine. This spike was transient however, and as the mice aged, a shift toward a more strict anaerobic population occurred in the large intestine. This ordered colonization occurs because aerotolerant organisms are able to colonize the GIT early in the presence of oxygen. Through their metabolism, they reduce the redox potential and allow for the later colonization and replication of strict anaerobes [21].

1.2. Impact of the method of delivery on colonization

In humans, the method of delivery impacts the initial microbiota of the infant [22-24]. In a study of Venezuelan women, vaginal delivery was associated with initial colonization by *Lactobacillus, Prevotella, Atopobium,* and *Sneathia* spp.; in contrast Cesarean delivery was associated with colonization of *Staphylococcus, Propionibacterium,* and *Corynebacterium* spp. (organisms typically found on skin). It was also noted that the initial bacteria present in infants born vaginally were vertically transferred from the mother. This was not the case for those born via Cesarean. A Finnish study analyzed infant fecal samples collected between three days of age and six months of age to evaluate temporal colonization [23]. The results revealed that at three days of age, all but one infant, regardless of the delivery method, were colonized with aerobic bacteria. However, a higher percentage of vaginally delivered infants were colonized with *Bifidobacterium*-like (BLB) and *Lactobacillus*-like (LBB) bacteria as compared to Cesarean delivered infants. These differential colonization patterns were corrected by day ten for LBB and by day 30 for BLB. Additional characterization of the fecal microbiota revealed that at one month of age, infants born via Cesarean had a significant increase in *Clostridium perfringens* (25% to 56%); an increase not seen in vaginally delivered infants. This is an important observation, as *C. perfringens* has been thought to play a role in sudden infant death syndrome (SIDS) [25]. Also of note, significant differences in the levels of *Bacteroides fragilis* were observed between the two methods of delivery [23]. Specifically, this bacterium was present at statistically higher numbers in vaginally delivered infants as compared to Cesarean delivered infants at all time points throughout the six months of the study.

These differences in initial colonizers have been associated with adverse effects, as infants born via Cesarean are more susceptible to skin infections with methicillin resistant *Staphylococcus aureus* (MRSA). A 2004 report indicated that 82% of infant MRSA cases in Chicago and 64% in Los Angeles were delivered via Cesarean , all of which involved healthy, full-term infants [26]. An additional prospective cohort study indicated a link between Cesarean delivery and

Clostridium difficile infection, which was further associated with the development of wheeze, asthma, eczema, and food allergies throughout the first seven years of life [27]. Consistent with these findings, a Norwegian study documented an association between asthma and Cesarean delivered children [28]. Although the epidemiological connections between Cesarean delivery, the composition of the microbiota, and disease are still being studied, strong evidence exists that early colonization of the intestines with aerobic skin microbes is associated with health risks.

1.3. Impact of feeding method on colonization

Another factor affecting early colonization of the human gut is determined by feeding method [29]. In one study of vaginally delivered infants, the fecal microbiota of breast-fed compared to formula-fed infants within the first month of life was analyzed using fluorescence *in situ* hybridization (FISH) to evaluate 11 separate groups of organisms [29]. *Bifidobacterium* spp. were the most prominent organisms found to colonize infants fed breast milk, comprising 69% of the bacterial population, with the next most prevalent group being the *Bacteroides* and *Prevotella* spp. making up 12%. With respect to the fecal microbiota of formula-fed infants, the microbiota was actually more diverse than that found in the breast-fed babies. Formula-fed infants had *Bifidobacterium* spp. as the most predominant group, however, they only comprised 32% of the bacterial population while *Bacteroides* and *Prevotella* spp. comprised 29% of the composition. Additionally, *Atopbium* spp. were found to account for 8% of the microbiota in formula-fed infants, but only comprised 1% of the community in the breast-fed infants.

1.4. Microbial changes that occur after weaning

The next major shift in the microbial population occurs during weaning. In a study consisting of infants from five European countries, the composition of the fecal microbiota at four weeks post-weaning was analyzed via FISH using 10 different probes [30]. When considering the results from all of the infants, it was noted that the microbial communities consisted primarily of *Bifidobacterium* (37%), *C. coccoides* (14%) and *Bacteroides* (14%). When samples were obtained from infants that were separated by geographic location, differences among the groups were noticeable. Infants from Spain had significantly greater *Lactobacillus* spp. and less *Bifidobacterium* spp. as compared to infants from the UK, Sweden, Germany, and Italy. The Spanish fecal samples also had significantly greater presence of *Bacteroides* spp. and *C. leptum* compared to those from the UK, Sweden, or Italy. The numbers of *C. leptum* was highest in samples obtained from German infants. The microbiota of infants from Spain also had significantly greater amounts of enterobacteria when compared to those from the UK, Sweden, or Germany, and higher numbers of *Streptococcus* spp. compared to those from Germany. The infants with the highest amount of *Bifidobacterium* spp. were from Sweden and the UK. Further separation of the data revealed that breast-fed infants had an increased percentage of *Bifidobacterium* spp. while *Bacteroides* spp. and *C. coccoides* were reduced post-weaning. Additionally, delivery method also influenced the microbiota composition, with vaginally delivered infants having higher numbers of *Bacteroides* present.

This study also reported results from infants who provided samples before (at six weeks of age) and four weeks after weaning [30]. Switching to solid food during this time caused a significant reduction in the presence of bifidobactera, enterobacteria, and *C. difficile/C. perfringens* proportions. These reductions were accompanied by significant increases in both *C. leptum* and *C. coccoides* clusters. Again, location also played a significant role in the microbial differences at weaning. Spanish infants had the greatest increase in both *C. coccoides* and *C. leptum* post-weaning compared to the other four countries, while enterobacteria was significantly decreased in the Spanish samples compared to those from the other countries. The samples from Spanish infants also had significant increases in *Atopobium* spp. compared to those from Sweden and Germany and *Streptococcus* spp. compared to Germany and Italy. The authors also report significant decreases post-weaning in the enterobacteria present in the Italian infant samples as compared to samples from Sweden and the UK. As mentioned previously, feeding and delivery method alter the composition of the microbiota at birth; this is also true after weaning. Formula-fed infants had higher proportions of *C. leptum* in their feces compared to breast-fed infants post-weaning. Infants born via Cesarean section possessed increased levels of *Bacteroides* spp. after weaning, whereas there was no change in the abundance of this group in vaginally delivered infants. Additionally, *Atopobium* spp. decreased in vaginally delivered children but increased in Cesarean delivered children post-weaning [30].

Studies describing development or maturation of the human microbiota reveal that as an individual ages, the microbiota shifts from predominantly facultative anaerobes to strict anaerobes, just as previously observed in rodents [20]. Notably, variations in initial colonization associated with different delivery and feeding methods seems to profoundly impact the microbial community post-weaning. Additionally, geographic location plays an important role in the initial colonization of the (GIT). In spite of all these variables, several themes for colonization can be described. Initially, *Bifidobacterium* spp. are the primary colonizers of the infant GIT along with other species such as *Bacteroides, Lactobacillus, Prevotella,* and *Atopobium.* As the infant matures, the oxygen presence in the gut is reduced and the infant begins eating solid food, which promotes a transition towards the growth and maintenance of the anaerobes found in the *C. coccoides* and *C. leptum* clusters.

1.5. The microbiota and gastrointestinal homeostasis

The commensal microbiota has a tremendous influence on the development and functional capabilities of the GIT of its host. Numerous studies have documented the effects that the microbiota has on GIT development in mice. Specifically, the morphology of the intestines differs significantly in animals devoid of microbes (i.e., germfree) compared to conventionally-reared (CONVR) mice [31]. The mucus layer is thinner and epithelial cells have a slower rate of turnover compared to those from conventional animals, primarily because of extended time in the S and G_1 phases of the cell cycle [32]. This can be corrected by bacterial colonization. In Figure 1, panel A shows intestinal tissue from germfree (GF) mice and panel B shows tissue from a mouse colonized with *Brachyspira hyodysenteriae.* Colonization with *B. hyodysenteriae* elicits the production of goblet cells and increases the heights of the mucosa, resembling what is seen in CONVR mice.

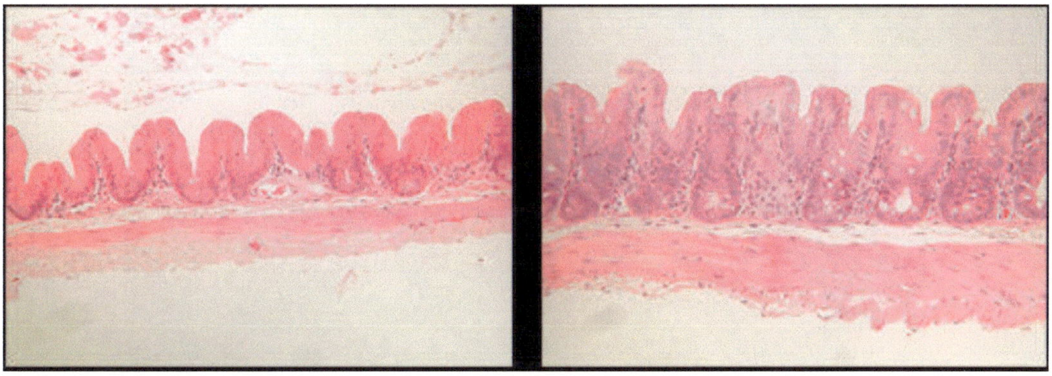

(a) (b)

Figure 1. Photomicrographs of cecal tissue from a) a germfree mouse and b) a mouse monoassociated with *Brachyspira hyodysenteriae.* Note the changes in the cellularity, presence of goblet cells, and height of the mucosa in the ceca from the monoassociated mouse 28 days after colonization with *B. hyodysenteriae*.

In the small intestine, this change in epithelial cell transit time is doubled, going from 53 hours in a CONVR mouse to 115 hours in a GF mouse [33]. The most noticeable gross change in GF mice is the enlargement of the cecum, which can comprise up to 19% of the mouse's body weight [34]. The cecum of a GF mouse can assume a more normal size (4.5% body weight) following colonization with a mixture of *Lactobacillus* spp., Group N streptococci , *Bacteroides* spp., enterococci and coliform bacilli recovered from CONVR mice [34]. As shown in Figure 2, monoassociation with *B. hyodysenteriae* also returns the cecum to a more normal size.

Of interest, not all bacteria tested were able to return the cecum to a normal size. It was noted that colonizing mice with *Lactobacillus* spp. and Group N streptococci only was not sufficient to change the morphology of the cecum. However, when *Bacteroides* spp. colonized the mice, the morphology assumed a more normal size. Other differences between GF and CONVR mice include the consistency of the cecal contents, with the contents from a GF mouse being more liquid, hypotonic and alkaline than in a CONVR mouse [35]. Additionally, GI transit time is slower in GF mice, which are also prone to vitamin deficiency due to a lack of bacterial metabolism [36-38]. In GF rats, monoassociation with either a rat-derived *Escherichia coli* strain or a sarcina-like micrococcus was able to reverse the vitamin K deficiency. Research identifying the response to *Salmonella enteritis* serovar Typhimurium challenge indicated that there was a 50-fold greater translocation of bacteria to the mesenteric lymph node, and organisms were present in the blood of GF mice, something not seen in CONVR mice [37]. This phenomenon occurred due to the decreased transit time in the small intestine of GF mice, thereby allowing the *Salmonella* to multiply in the host and translocate to other tissue sites.

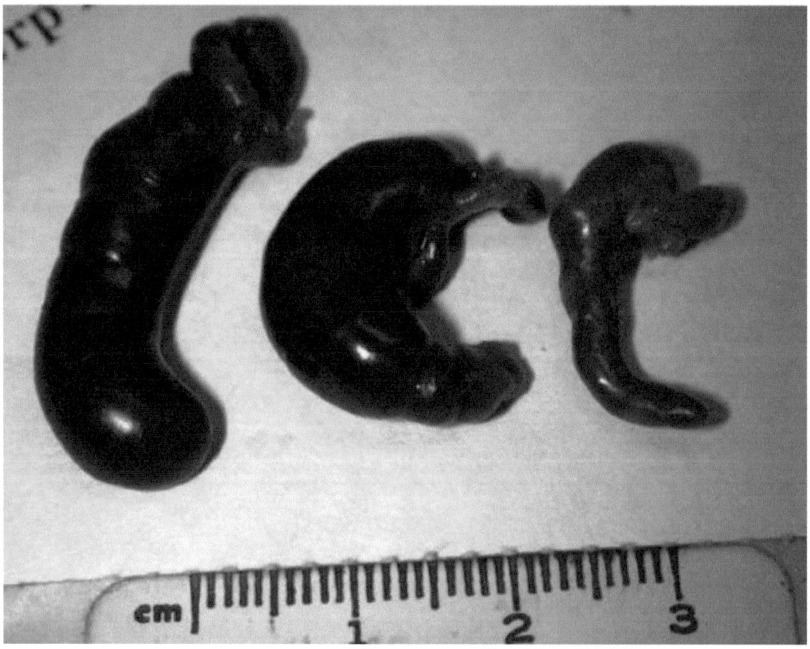

Figure 2. Physical and morphological changes associated with microbial colonization. Shown here are ceca from a germfree mouse (left), monoassociated mouse (center), and conventional microbiota mouse (right). Note the increased size of the cecum from the GF mouse. The distal end of the cecum (appendix) of the monoassociated mouse has begun to undergo morphological changes, including the development of a lymphoid tissue known as a cecal tonsil.

1.6. Effect of bacterial colonization on immune development

In addition to its importance in maintaining gut homeostasis, the GI microbiota is also critical for normal priming and development of the immune system [39-41]. GF mice have reduced numbers of immune cells present in the lamina propria and have smaller Peyer's patches compared to CONVR mice. They also have a diminished capacity for antibody production, fewer plasma cells, smaller mesenteric lymph nodes, and reduced numbers of germinal centers compared to CONVR mice [39]. However, this underdeveloped immune system is fully capable of mounting a response comparable to that of a CONVR mouse when stimulated with bacterial antigen or protein [40, 41]. Macrophages from CONVR mice process antigen faster than those from GF mice, likely because the continued exposure of CONVR macrophages to bacterial antigen allows them to be "primed" for antigen degradation; a phenomenon that does not occur in GF mice [41]. The presence of bacteria in the GIT promotes decreased immunoreactivity towards commensal organisms. The barrier between the gut microbiota and the underlying gastrointestinal associated lymphoid tissue consists of a single layer of epithelial cells covered by two layers of mucus [42, 43]. The inner layer of mucus is approximately 100 µm thick while the outer layer is approximately 700 µm in the rat colon [43]. The inner layer is firmly attached to the epithelial cells and devoid of bacteria, while the outer layer is "loose"and contains commensal organisms [44]. The major constituent of these layers is a protein known as Muc2 [42]. The importance of Muc2 has been highlighted by the development of Muc2$^{-/-}$ mice. These mice fail to gain weight, have diarrhea by seven weeks of age, occult blood present in their feces by eight weeks of age, and the majority of mice had gross bleeding and reversible rectal prolapse by nine weeks of age [45]. These mice also develop microscopic evidence of colitis as early as five weeks of age.

Underneath the mucus layers lay the intestinal epithelial cells, which are held together by tight junction proteins such as occludins, claudins, and junctional adhesion molecules [46]. These proteins seal the paracellular junction between the cells and regulate the entry of nutrients, ions and water. They also act as a barrier against bacterial entry. Loss of epithelial barrier function promotes a break in immunological tolerance and facilitates immunoreactivity towards the normal commensal microbiota (Figure 3). This phenomenon has been demonstrated in mouse studies employing 2,4,6 trinitrobenzensulfonic acid (TNBS), a chemical that disrupts the epithelial barrier to allow translocation of bacteria, resulting in the induction of both innate inflammatory responses and antigen-specific immune responses [47]. Subsequent to the loss of epithelial barrier function, these mice develop severe gastrointestinal inflammation, which can be ameliorated by pretreating with antibiotics to reduce the microbial load [47].

The role of the commensal bacteria in regulating the immune response was elegantly demonstrated in a study by Wlodarska et al. [48]. Mice administered metronidazole were more susceptible to subsequent infection with the pathogen, *Citrobacter rodentium*. Metronidazole-treated mice had increased submucosal edema, ulcerations, mucosal hyperplasia and decreased numbers of goblet cells. The author also noted enhanced expression of *IL-25* and *Reg3γ* mRNA and an increased presence of NK cells and macrophages in the lamina propria of these mice, indicating an increase in microbial stimulation. The inner mucous layer of metronidazole-treated mice was significantly thinner and mRNA expression of genes encoding for the goblet-cell specific proteins Muc2, TFF3, and RelmB was also decreased in these mice [49, 50]. The thinning of the inner mucous layer following metronidazole treatment allowed for *C. rodentium* to more closely associate with the epithelium and promote production of the pro-inflammatory cytokines and chemokines TNF-α, IFN-γ, and MCP-1. This study highlights the contribution of the commensal microbiota in the production of the mucus barrier and subsequently in maintaining mucosal homeostasis [48].

It has also been noted that specific members of the resident microbiota are able to illicit specific immune functions. Colonization with *Bacteroides fragilis* expressing polysaccharide A (PSA) suppressed development of T helper 17 (T_h17) $CD4^+$ T cells by promoting the development of $Foxp3^+$ T regulatory (T_{reg}) $CD4^+$ T cells and inducing IL-10 expression via TLR2 signaling [51]. Additional studies have demonstrated that purified PSA is sufficient to expand the numbers of $Foxp3^+$ T_{reg} cells [52]. *B. fragilis* inhabits colonic crypts. This niche puts the organism in close contact with the immune system but its production of PSA ensures that no inflammatory response is induced. Both prophylactic and therapeutic treatment of mice with PSA has been shown to ameliorate TNBS-induced colitis in mice [52]. More recently, work from Atarashi et al., eloquently demonstrated a role for indigenous *Clostridium* species in the induction of colonic T_{reg} cells [53]. Colonization of GF mice with a cocktail of 46 *Clostridium* strains enriched for clusters IV and XIVa promoted TGF-β production from intestinal epithelial cells and increased the number of Foxp3⁺ T_{reg} cells in the colon. Furthermore, inoculation of young CONVR mice with *Clostridium* species facilitated resistance to both dextran sodium sulfate (DSS)- and oxazolone-induced colitis as well as increased systemic Immunoglobuin E (IgE) production as adults.

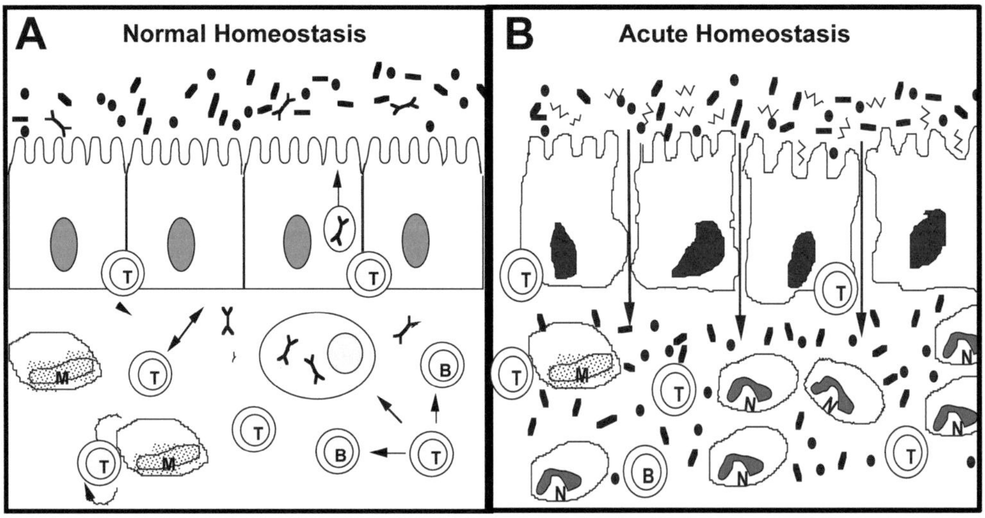

Figure 3. Panel A shows normal mucosal homeostasis. The epithelial cells provide a barrier between the commensal bacteria and the underlying immune cells. Panel B depicts acute inflammation. The epithelial cell barrier has been breached, allowing bacteria to be readily detected by the immune system and promote a pro-inflammatory immune response.

The segmented filamentous bacteria (SFB) is another microorganism of interest that has been implicated in the induction of T_h17 responses [54]. Ivanov et al. found that C57BL/6 mice purchased from the Jackson Laboratory had significantly less IL-17-producing $CD4^+$ T cells in the small intestine compared to those from Taconic Farms. This discrepancy could be corrected via intragastric gavage of the Jackson mice with contents from the small intestines of the Taconic mice. Using a 16S ribosomal RNA PhyloChip analysis, SFB were identified in the microbiota of mice from Taconic Farms but not in those from the Jackson Laboratory. Monoassociation of mice with SFB induced the production of T_h17 cells and up-regulated genes encoding antimicrobial peptides and serum amyloid A (SAA). SAA co-cultured with naive $CD4^+$ T cells and lamina propria derived dendritic cells induced T_h17 cell differentiation *in vitro*. The authors concluded that SFB, which tightly adheres to and imbeds itself among the microvilli on the epithelial cell surface, induces the production of SAA by intestinal epithelial cells. In turn, the SAA acts on lamina propria dendritic cells to stimulate the induction of T_h17 cells. Colonization with SFB has also been shown to protect against *C. rodentium* infection. Th17 cytokines such as

IL-22 likely stimulate intestinal epithelial cells to secrete antimicrobial peptides to limit the growth of the pathogen and its infiltration into the colonic wall [54].

1.7. Effect of bacterial colonization on other aspects of the body

In addition to promoting immune maturation, the commensal microbiota also helps to regulate fat storage. GF mice eat 29% more food than conventional mice yet have 42% less body fat and a decreased metabolic rate [55]. Colonization of GF mice with cecal contents from conventional mice for 14 days caused a 57% increase in total body fat with a concomitant 27% reduction in food intake. These "conventionalized" mice also had increases in leptin, fasting glucose, and insulin levels compared to GF mice; they also developed insulin resistance. Levels of mRNA specific for the transcription factors, SREBP-1 and ChREBP, were also elevated leading to increased production of lipogenic enzymes. Fat formation is aided by the regulator lipoprotein lipase (LPL) and is inhibited by the *fiaf* gene product whose expression is suppressed in microbiota-bearing conventional mice. The authors suggest that the bacteria in the gut breakdown dietary polysaccharide into monosaccharaides that are then transported to the liver to activate lipogenic enzymes. This process promotes fat formation in the peripheral tissues due to the suppression of *fiaf*. In addition to the production of white adipose tissue, the microbiota may also play a role in eye health [56]. A recent study revealed differences in the lipid profiles in the lens and retinas of GF mice as compared to CONVR mice. The CONVR mice had reduced concentrations of multiple phosphatidylcholines and an overall reduced presence of phospholipids in the lens. The authors postulate these changes may be due to the increased exposure of the CONVR mice to more oxidative stress than their GF counterparts [56]. Together, these studies help us realize the effects that the gut microbiota may have on host systems that, at the surface, seem to have limited or no connection to the GIT.

1.8. Bacterial production of short chain fatty acids

Another health benefit that the microbiota provides its host revolves around the production of short-chain fatty acids (SCFA) such as acetate, propionate, and butyrate as end products of anaerobic fermentation [57]. These SCFA (predominantly butyrate) can be utilized as energy sources by eukaryotic cells. Members of the *Clostridium* clusters IV (e.g., *Faecalibacterium prausnitzii)* and XIVa (e.g., *Roseburia* spp. and *Eubacterium rectale*) are the primary butyrate producers in the GIT, and they comprise approximately 2-15% of the total gut microbiota [14, 58-61]. Butyrate, a four-carbon fatty acid, is produced by bacteria via one of two metabolic pathways. The first pathway utilizes the enzymes phosphotransbutyrylase and butyrate kinase to form butyrate from butyryl-CoA to yield one ATP per one molecule of butyrate produced [62, 63]. The second pathway, which is utilized by most organisms in the gut, uses butyryl-CoA acetate CoA transferase to form butyrate and acetyl-CoA from butyryl-CoA [64, 65].

Once produced, butyrate has multiple effects on gut health. A primary use is as a preferred energy source for colonocytes, and the mechanisms by which butyrate is utilized in the GIT is summarized in Figure 4 [66-69]. Two biomarkers of energy homeostasis, ATP and NADH/NAD$^+$ levels, are both significantly reduced in only the colonic tissues of GF mice as compared to CONVR mice [70]. This observation indicates that GF mice have a reduction in TCA cycle activity, and subsequently less ATP is generated for cellular energy. Moreover, this reduction in ATP was correlated with increased signs of energetic stress in colonocytes, including increased expression of 5′-adenosine monophosphate-activated protein kinase (AMPK). Consistent with previous reports describing a role for AMPK in inducing autophagy [71], GF coloncytes also expressed elevated levels of the autophagosome marker LC3-11. Transmission election microscopic analysis revealed that significantly more GF colonocytes were undergoing autophagy than colonocytes from CONVR mice. Colonizing GF mice with a conventional microbiota reversed these effects, as did incubation of isolated colonocytes with butyrate. Additional experiments employing the fatty-acid oxidation blocker, etomoxir, demonstrated that colonocytes consume butyrate as an energy source and not as a histone deacetylase (HDAC) inhibitor, another known function of butyrate [72, 73].

Butyrate functions as an HDAC inhibitor by blocking cellular deacetylase activity and allowing histone acetylation [72, 73]. Histone modification causes changes in cellular gene expression patterns; compounds and molecules that can elicit these modifications are being studied as potential anti-cancer therapeutics [74]. A comparative study of gene expression patterns in HT-29 cells (a colon carcinoma-derived cell line), treated with either butyrate or trichostain A (a known HDAC inhibitor) revealed that both substances had similar effects on gene expression [75]. Upregulated genes (21 total) were found to regulate the cell cycle, signal transduction, DNA repair and genome transcription. Only two genes were down-regulated—lactoferrinδ and MAPKAP kinase. It is also important to note that both butyrate and trichostain A inhibited the growth of HT-29 cells by creating an arrest in the G_1 phase of the cell cycle [76]. Butyrate may also down-regulate pro-inflammatory responses via its HDAC activity, as incubation of butyrate with inflamed biopsy samples or LPS-induced peripheral blood mononuclear cells (PBMCs) reduced the mRNA expression of IL-6, TNF-α, TNF-β, and IL-1β [77]. Additionally, in murine studies of TNBS- and DSS-induced colitis, and in ulcerative colitis (UC) patients, administration of butyrate enemas ameliorates disease activity via NFκB inhibition [77-79]. Butyrate has been shown to decrease both COX-2 and PGE_2 expression in HT-29 cells stimulated with TNF-α [80].

The information presented in this section clearly defines a central role for the gut microbiota in many physiological processes; the microbiota even has a tremendous impact on the host's health status. Causal links likely exist between the methods by which infants are delivered, their gut microbial colonization patterns and subsequent health concerns, including asthma, eczema and, food allergies. Associations between gut bacterial communities and obesity, diabetes, and cardiovascular disease have also been documented [81-83]. A significant body of literature also links changes in the composition of the gut microbiota with inflammatory bowel disease (IBD), which is discussed in detail in the following section [84-89].

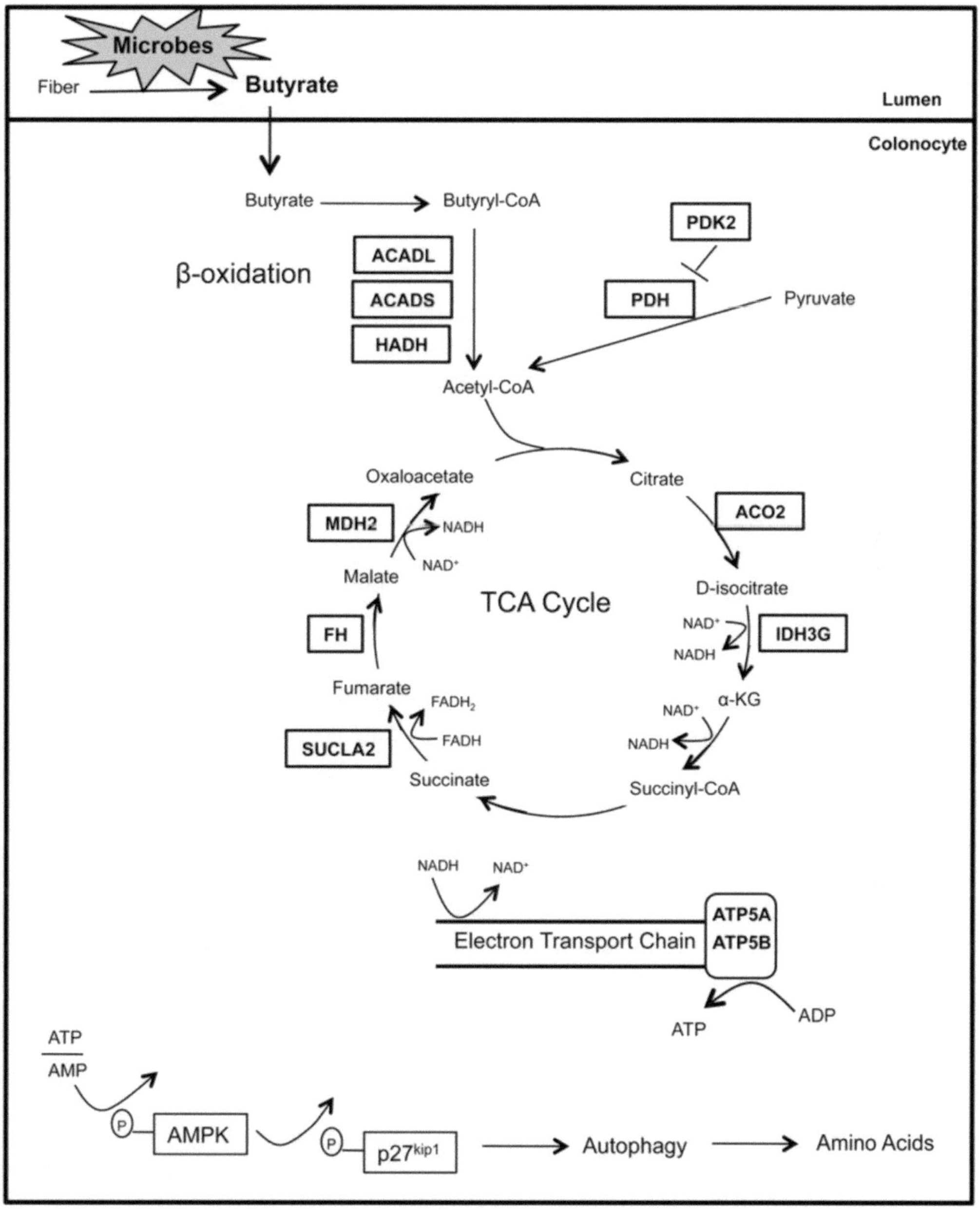

Figure 4. Microbial regulation of colonocyte metabolism. Schematic depicting how dietary fiber is fermented by microbes into butyrate in the lumen of the colon, which is then transported into the colonocyte. In the colonocyte, butyrate promotes oxidative metabolism and inhibits autophagy. Based on transcriptome and proteome experiments, enzymes regulated by microbes are shown in boxes. In all cases, boxed enzymes that function in β-oxidation and the TCA cycle are downregulated in GF colonocytes, revealing that microbes positively regulate their expression. Diminished ATP results in phosphorylation of AMPK and p27, which culminates in autophagy. (Cell Metab. 2011 May 4;13(5): 517-5) Reprinted with permission from the publisher license number 2977121495018

2. Introduction to inflammatory bowel disease

In 1932, three physicians, Burrill Crohn, Leon Ginzburg, and Gordon Oppenheimer described a disease of unknown etiology in the terminal ileum of young adults [90]. The disease was characterized as being similar to UC (fever, diarrhea and weight loss) and having ulcerations of the mucosa that would eventually lead to stenosis of the lumen and formation of multiple fistulas. Eventually, surgical intervention was used to resect the affected portion of the intestinal tract and patients recovered with little signs of the disease persisting. In their 1932 report, Crohn and colleagues discuss observations from other physicians regarding observations of granulomas in the small and large intestine of unknown etiology being classified under the umbrella term "benign granulomas". Still today Crohn's disease (CD) and UC are both included under the umbrella term "inflammatory bowel disease." Crohn and colleagues described the disease as beginning at the ileocecal junction with lesions separated by normal mucosa [90]. They described inflammation of the submucosa and the muscularis resulting in a markedly thickened bowel wall. The presence of "giant cells" was also noted, which they attributed to vegetable matter becoming entrapped in the ulcers and become encapsulated during healing. The authors concluded that the presence of these giant cells in the granulomatous lesion led others to believe that the inflammation was due to an unusual form of tuberculosis. However, the authors could not find any evidence of tuberculosis in their 14 patients.

Clinically, the patients with IBD were characterized as young adults with fever, diarrhea, dull abdominal pain, and vomiting; they were also weak, anemic and had poor appetite. Upon physical examination, the author noted five commonalties: 1) a mass in the right iliac region, 2) evidence of fistula formation, 3) emaciation and anemia, 4) approximately half of the subjects had undergone an appendectomy, and 5) evidence of intestinal obstruction. Treatment was supportive and surgical resection of the affected portion of the intestinal tract was recommended; 13 of their 14 patients had no symptoms post-operatively. For the one patient that developed recurrent symptoms, it was later determined that not all of the affected intestinal tissue had been resected during the first surgery.

Eighty years after the first published article of what would become known as "Crohn's disease," there is still no cure for this disease nor do we fully understand its etiology. Unfortunately, the number of people being diagnosed with IBD is increasing yearly [91]. There is not one specific, causative agent of IBD; instead the etiology is thought to be multifactorial in nature, with host genetics, environmental factors, the induction of aberrant immune responses, and the gastrointestinal microbiota all contributing to disease pathogenesis.

2.1. Genetic factors affecting IBD

As of 2011, genome-wide meta-analyses had identified 71 susceptibility loci associated with CD, 47 with UC and 28 associated with both, some of which are shown in Figure 5 [92-95]. Here, we focus on genetic variants within specific genes involved in mediating host responses to microbial components.

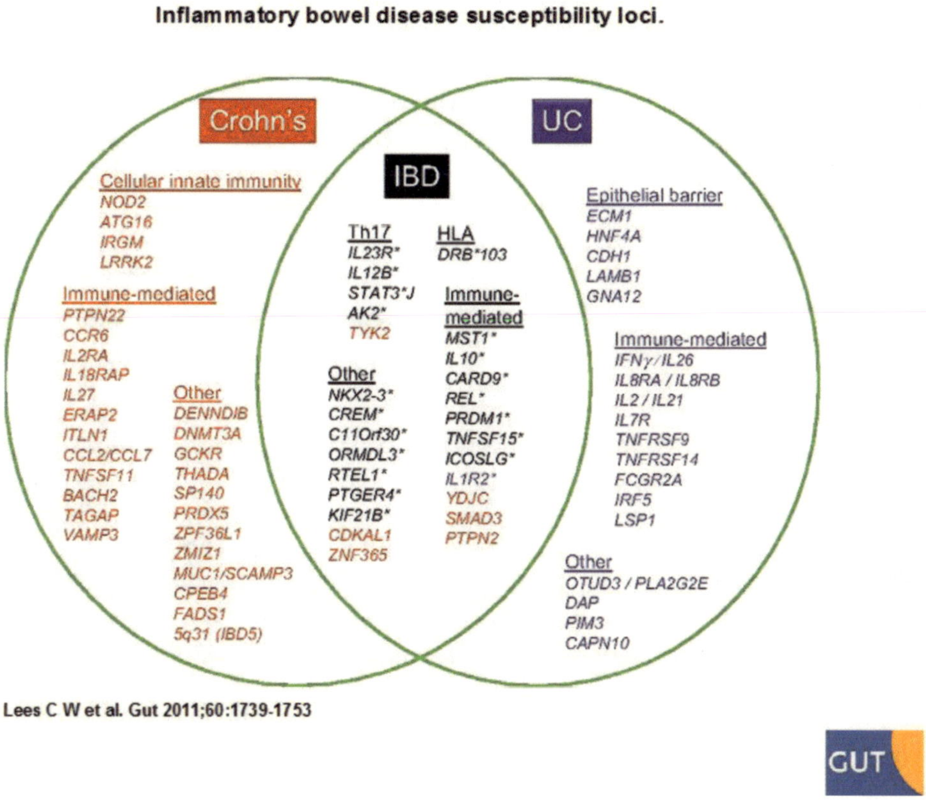

Figure 5. Inflammatory bowel disease susceptibility loci. The loci (depicted by lead gene name) attaining genome wide significance ($p < 5x10^{-8}$) are shown for Crohn's disease (CD, red), ulcerative colitis (UC, blue) and IBD (black where $p < 5x10^{-8}$ in CD and UC; red were $p < 5x10^{-8}$ in CD and $p < 5x10^{-4}$ in UC; blue where $p < 5x10^{-8}$ in UC and $p < 5x10^{-4}$ in CD. Reprinted with permission from the publisher license number: 2977121069437

2.1.1. *Nod2*

One of the first candidate genes linked to IBD susceptibility was *Nod2*. Located on chromosome 16, the defective allele affects the activation of the transcription factor NF-κB. NOD2 is expressed in antigen-presenting cells, macrophages, lymphocytes, ileal Paneth cells, and intestinal epithelial cells and functions as an intracellular microbial recognition molecule [96-100]. NOD2 senses muramyl dipeptide (MDP), a minimally bioactive motif of peptidoglycan from both Gram-negative and Gram-positive bacteria. Once activated by its ligand, NOD2 undergoes a conformational change to expose its CARD domains and recruits the kinase RIP2 to the complex which associates with NOD2 via homophillic CARD-CARD interactions [97]. This process leads to the activation of IKK and the subsequent degradation of IκB and ultimately results in the translocation of NF-κB to the nucleus [96, 101].

Petnicki-Ocwieja et al. demonstrated that MDP stimulation of ileal crypts induced bactericidal secretions capable of killing *E. coli* [102]. Moreover, the same authors showed that NOD2 was required for the bactericidal activity of crypt secretions of the terminal ileum. The composition of the ileal microbiota of the NOD2$^{-/-}$ mice was significantly altered in comparison to their WT counterparts. Specifically, NOD2$^{-/-}$ mice had increased numbers of Firmicutes, specifically *Bacillus* species and *Bacteroides* species. Wild-type mice were able to clear an infection of *Helicobacter hepaticus*, an opportunistic mouse pathogen, within seven days while NOD2$^{-/-}$ mice remained colonized with *H. hepaticus* for at least 14 days post-infection [102]. Also of note, the presence of a gut microbiota was required for the expression of NOD2. GF mice possessed decreased levels of NOD2—a phenotype that could be reversed following monoassociation with either Gram-negative or Gram-positive organisms. Together, these results outline a reciprocal regulatory relationship between NOD2 expression and the gut microbiota.

2.1.2. ATG16L1

Another gene implicated in the pathogenesis of IBD that regulates cellular autophagy is *ATG16L1* [95, 103]. Autophagy is a process utilized by cells to recycle cellular components. This process may also be utilized by cells as a non-apoptotic method of programmed cell death [104]. *ATG16L1* is expressed by CD4$^+$ and CD8$^+$ T cells, CD19$^+$ B cells, epithelial cells, and macrophages [105, 106]. Studies by Caldwell et al. utilizing mice engineered to express low or hypomorphic levels of *ATG16L1* revealed that this gene is indeed an autophagy-related protein. Elevated levels of cytosolic proteins normally degraded by a rapamycin-induced degradation pathway were found in the cells of the *ATG16L1* hypomorphic (ATG16L1^{HM}) mice [95]. Additionally, cells from ATG16L1^{HM} mice possessed fewer autophagosomes following rapamycin treatment or nutrient deprivation. The small intestines and colons of ATG16L1^{HM} mice had no morphological defects in crypt height or villus length but did possess abnormalities found in their Paneth cells. Specifically, lysozyme within Paneth cells was found to be either depleted/absent or diffuse, which is in contrast to the normal and orderly packaging of lysozyme within granules. Decreased levels of lysozyme were also observed in the ileal mucus layer of ATG16L1^{HM} mice. However, there were intact granules observed in the crypt lumen, indicating a potential role of *ATG16L1* in the maintenance of the Paneth cell granule exocytosis pathway. The authors observed no differences between WT and ATG16L1^{HM} mice in terms of resistance to a challenge with *Listeria monocytogenes*. However, others have reported a reduction in intracellular bacteria targeted to autophagic vacuoles following in vitro infections of HeLa or Caco-2 cells with *S. typhimurium* in conjunction with siRNA to reduce the expression of *ATG16L1* [105, 107]. Additional work by Caldwell et al. revealed that 100 % of ileocolic resection specimens obtained from humans with the *ATG16L1* risk allele had abnormal Paneth cells that looked similar to those found in the ATG16L1^{HM} mice [95].

Using siRNA to reduce *ATG16L1* expression in THP-1 macrophages revealed an increase in intracellular adherent and invasive *E. coli* (AIEC) as compared to normal THP-1 infected macrophages [106]. AIEC promote enhanced production of TNF-α and IL-6 from macrophages. Silencing of *ATG16L1* expression resulted in significant increases in both cytokines. The authors postulate that bacterial clearance is less efficient in individuals with the risk alleles for

ATG16L1. When AIEC are present, this reduction in bacterial clearance likely leads to increased production of pro-inflammatory cytokines, which could tip the immune balance to an inflammatory state. Thus, it appears that the presence of bacterial provocateurs (e.g., AIEC) in the microbiota increases the risk of developing IBD in individuals possessing polymorphisms in genes such as *ATG16L* or *NOD2*.

2.2. The immune response and IBD

The mucosal immune system is charged with the monumental task of balancing responsiveness and tolerance to a tremendous number of environmental antigens, including those from both food and bacteria. Although the exact cause of IBD remains elusive, significant evidence supports the hypothesis that GIT inflammation is initiated and perpetuated by a dysregulated immune response directed against the gut microbiota resulting in deleterious responses in genetically susceptible individuals following an environmental trigger. The host with a genetic predisposition for IBD may possess defects in epithelial permeability and/or altered regulation (i.e., NOD2 deficiency) of commensal bacteria. Potential environmental triggers may include smoking, certain medications, or a gastrointestinal illness that induces a break in homeostasis. Regardless of the specific genetic or environmental trigger, what ensues is an exaggerated, inappropriate mucosal immune response characterized by chronic activation of T cells and the production of cytokines and other inflammatory mediators.

The success of cytokine-targeted immunotherapies for a subset of IBD patients supports the idea that these chemical messengers of the immune system play an important role in disease pathogenesis. However, the nature of the immune phenotypes observed in CD and UC patients do differ [108]. The immune response of CD is typically associated with a T helper 1 (Th1) phenotype while UC is characterized by a T helper 2 (Th2) phenotype [108]. Isolated lamina propria (LP) $CD4^+$ T cells from CD patients produce IFN-γ when stimulated via the CD2/CD28 pathway; in contrast, LP $CD4^+$ T cells from UC patients secreted mostly IL-5 [109]. Another cytokine with a strong link to CD is IL-12 [110]. Messenger RNA for IL-12p40 in LP mononuclear cells (LPMC) was found in 85 % of CD patients, a percentage significantly higher than that found in healthy and UC GIT tissue samples. Similarly, IL-12p35 mRNA was detectable in the LPMC of 92 % of CD patients; expression was again significantly higher than for healthy and UC patients. Elevated levels of IL-12 were also detectable in the serum of CD patients [110], and this potent Th1-promoting cytokine is able to induce IFN-γ production from LP lymphocytes (LPL) isolated from CD patients [111]. Additionally, studies employing a murine model of TNBS-induced colitis have revealed that administration of anti-IL-12 antibodies ameliorated disease severity, presumably by decreasing IFN-γ secretion from LP $CD4^+$ T cells [112].

In UC, production of the cytokines IL-5 and IL-13 appear to mediate the disease process. Using LPMC from IBD patients, those with UC had increased production of IL-13 and IL-5 upon *in vitro* restimulation as compared to LPMCs recovered from either CD patients or healthy individuals [113]. Levels of IFN-γ produced by LPMC from UC patients were similar to those produced by cells from healthy controls. The authors specifically identified that $CD4^+$ $CD161^+$

NK T cells were the primary source of IL-13 in UC patients, as these cells produced 30-fold more IL-13 than NK T cells from CD patients following *in vitro* restimulation.

More recent work has implicated the T helper 17 (Th17) lineage of $CD4^+$ T cells in the chronic inflammation observed in IBD [114, 115]. The development of Th17 T cells is dependent upon the presence of both IL-6 and TGF-β [115]. Colonic biopsies from UC and CD patients expressed higher levels of IL-17A mRNA as compared to those from healthy controls [115-117]. Immunohistochemical analysis of these tissues identified increased numbers of IL-$17A^+$ cells in both the LP and the epithelium of UC and CD patients as compared to controls [116]. Additional work also noted the presence of IL-17^+ cells in patients with active IBD [114]. However, the IL-17^+ cells were found predominantly in the LP of UC patients but in the submucosa and muscularis propria of CD patients [114]. These different locations of IL-17^+ cells complements prior observations that CD lesions often present as transmural while those in UC are superficial. Also of note, a comparison of biopsies from patients with active versus inactive disease revealed that IL-17^+ cells were only increased in numbers during active disease. The authors also determined that both T cells and monocytes/macrophages are a source of IL-17, and that IBD patients have elevated levels of IL-17 in their sera as compared to undetectable levels of this cytokine in the sera of healthy individuals.

The maintenance of Th17 T cells requires the presence of IL-23 [115]. Of interest, a gene variant significantly associated with CD encodes for the IL-23R, which, along with IL-12Rβ1, comprises the IL-23 receptor complex [118, 119]. This receptor complex interacts with IL-23 (a heterodimer of IL-12p40 and IL-23p19) to direct the production of a T_H17 immune response [120-122]. Anti-IL-23 antibodies have been shown to both prevent and ameliorate established disease in a T-cell transfer model of murine colitis [123]. Studies of human tissues demonstrate that IL-23R expression is upregulated not only on IL-17 producing $CD4^+$ T cells, but also on IFN-γ^+ T cells in both UC and CD patients [115]. Stimulation of LP $CD4^+$ T cells from UC patients with IL-23 significantly increased IL-17 production; in contrast, IL-23 stimulation of LP $CD4^+$ T cells from CD patients resulted in enhanced IFN-γ secretion [115]. In addition to promoting the production of T_H17 cells, IL-23 also inhibits the production of $Foxp3^+$ T_{reg} cells [124] and suppresses production of IL-10, a key regulatory cytokine [125].

Another important hallmark of the immune response observed in IBD is the production of IgG antibodies against the normal commensal microbiota [126]. Increased intestinal permeability, be it through genetic predisposition or environmental trigger, promotes enhanced immunoreactivity to bacterial antigens. The mucosal immunoglobulin profile of healthy adults consists predominantly of IgA with only a small amount of IgG. In contrast, patients with active IBD presented with significantly higher amounts of IgG in their mucosal secretions with no difference in amounts of IgA as compared to controls. The IgG antibodies present in IBD patients were identified as binding to non-pathogenic bacterial commensals, including *E. coli, B. fragilis, C. perfringens, Klebsiella aerogenes, and Enterobacter faecalis.* Patients with CD had significantly higher titers than UC patients, while antibody titers to these commensal bacteria were at or below the limit of detection in serum samples from healthy controls. Notable differences were also observed in the isotypes of IgG present in UC versus CD patients. Specifically, UC patients produced predominantly IgG_1 and IgG_3 antibodies to bacterial antigens, while IgG_1, IgG_2, IgG_3 were the predominant isotypes reacting with the bacterial antigens in serum samples from CD patients [126]. Conversely, other reports have described an increase in IgG_1 antibodies in UC patients and an increased in IgG_2 antibodies in CD patients [127-130]. Additional analyses have determined that IgG antibodies in CD patients are primarily directed towards bacterial cytoplasmic proteins rather than membrane associated proteins [126]. Despite the presence of many types of antibodies in both the mucosal secretions and serum of IBD patients, no direct evidence for their involvement in IBD immunopathogenesis has been reported, indicating that they may simply be a marker for immune responsiveness and/or dysregulation [131].

2.3. Environmental factors affecting IBD

Although there are allelic differences in many people with IBD, genetics alone cannot completely account for the development of IBD nor the increase in the incidence of IBD worldwide. Studies of monozygotic twins best highlight this concept, as there are disease concordance rates of only 50 % for CD and only 20 % for UC [132, 133]. Of interest, a British study assessing discordant twins with CD found an association with mumps infection, smoking, and oral contraceptive usage with the development of CD [134]. Additionally, the twin(s) with CD had suffered both a medical illness, more episodes of gastroenteritis, and spent more time with animals. Smoking is one confounding environmental factor that is of special interest, because it appears to have a protective effect on UC, but increases the risk of CD [132, 135-137]. Another factor that appears to be protective for UC is an appendectomy; its effect on CD is not as evident [138-140]. The equivalent procedure performed in mice has been shown to ameliorate colitis in both chemically-induced and genetically-engineered murine colitis models [141, 142]. Modest associations between oral contraceptive use and IBD have been documented, while others have found breast-feeding to be protective against both UC and CD [143, 144]. A meta-analysis performed by investigators in New Zealand identified other potential environmental factors, including being an only child, using antibiotics prior to and during adolescence (four or more courses in year), and having a pet in the house during childhood [145]. IBD also tends to occur in extended families as first and second degree relatives of IBD patients reported the occurrence of disease with a significantly higher frequency than the general population [146]. These finding strengthen the interconnection between genetics, environmental factors, and the incidence of IBD.

2.3.1. Antibiotic usage

Antibiotics are used in the treatment of IBD to reduce microbial load and dampen inflammatory immune responses. However, their use prior to disease diagnosis is now being identified as a risk factor for developing IBD. A Danish study of IBD patients revealed that antibiotic users were 1.84 times more likely to develop IBD, which correlated to a 12 % increase in disease risk for each course of antibiotics taken [147]. Further analysis revealed that antibiotic users were 3.41 times more likely to develop CD than UC, which correlated to an increased risk of 18 % per course of antibiotics used. Specifically, usage of penicillin V and extended spectrum penicillins were associated with the greatest disease risks. A Swedish study focused on the use of antibiotics from birth to age 5, a time when the microbiota and immune response are still developing and/or maturing, as a risk factor for IBD. They reported an association between a diagnosis of pneumonia, subsequent antibiotic treatment and the onset of both pediatric and adult CD [148]. Another study by Card et al. revealed a statistically significant association between antibiotic usage 2 to 5 years prior to diagnosis of CD in patients from the United Kingdom [149]. This finding was confirmed in a Canadian study, which reported that the more antibiotics taken within 2 to 5 years of diagnosis, the greater the risk of developing IBD [150]. That same study found that disease risk was weakly associated with penicillin use and greatly associated with metronidazole use, which was prescribed primarily for "non-infectious gastroenteritis." This association with antibiotic usage may be explained by the failure of the gut microbiota to reestablish its normal community structure and function following a course of antibiotics [151]. This alteration in the microbiota or dysbiosis may be a predisposing factor to the onset of IBD in a susceptible individual.

2.3.2. MAP

Another potential environmental risk factor for the development of IBD is a chronic pathogenic infection in the GIT. To date, no one particular organism has been found to be the causative agent of IBD. Although many microbial pathogens have been implicated as causative, only two have been significantly investigated. The first organism hypothesized to be associated with IBD was *Mycobacterium avium* subsp. *paratuberculosis,* which causes Johne's disease in cattle [152, 153]. The granulomatous inflammation observed in CD patients led many early researchers to investigate various types of *Mycobacterial* spp. in CD pathogenesis but confirmation was never achieved (reviewed in [154]). The first report of *M. paratuberculosis*-like organisms isolated from patients with CD in was published 1984. Now known as *M. avium* subsp. *paratuberculosis* (MAP), there is still no consensus as to whether or not it plays a role in the onset of IBD in a subset of genetically susceptible patients [155]. Using PCR to amplify the DNA insertion element IS*900,* which is specific to MAP, in biopsy sections, Sanderson et al. reported that 65 % of adult CD patients examined were PCR positive [156]. Dell'Isola et al. reported that 72 % of pediatric CD patients examined were PCR positive for the presence of MAP [156, 157]. While many studies have reported the presence of MAP DNA in CD patients, just as many have found MAP DNA in samples from healthy individuals and UC patients [156-162]. Moreover, multiple studies have failed to detect MAP-specific DNA in any CD patient sample examined [163-169]. The ability to detect MAP in some tissue samples and not others may be due, in part, to the organism's fastidiousness, slow growth, and/or the presence of PCR inhibitors in fecal/tissue samples that inhibit the detection of IS900. Serological evidence also fails to provide definitive answers for the involvement of MAP in the pathogenesis of IBD. Some studies assessing the presence of serum antibody titers against MAP-derived antigens find an association with IBD [170-176] while others do not [177-182]. More recent work has identified a possible link between variants in the *Nod2* gene and the presence of MAP [183]. In this study, 68 % of CD patients were positive for MAP DNA based on PCR analysis as compared to 21 % of the healthy individuals. Fifty-one percent of the CD patients were carriers of NOD2 polymorphisms as compared to 21 % of healthy individuals, and 74 % of the CD patients possessing one of the mutated NOD2 alleles were positive for MAP DNA. Even with of all of the data collected, the debate continues as to whether or not MAP plays an important role in the pathogenesis of CD [184, 185].

2.3.3. *Adherent-invasive Escherichia coli*

Another organism implicated in IBD pathogenesis is adherent-invasive *Escherichia coli* (AIEC). First described in 1998, AIEC isolates were recovered from the ileal mucosa of CD patients [186]. These organisms are found in higher numbers in CD patients (22 %) as compared to healthy controls (6 %) [187]. These isolates were able to adhere to Caco-2 cells and did not posses any of the virulence genes associated with known *E. coli* pathotypes (e.g., ETEC, EHEC) [186]. A characterization of expressed adhesions in AIEC strains revealed the *Pap* and *Sfa* adhesion or colonization factors, both of which are found in uropathogenic *E. coli* strains; however many of the AIEC strains did not possess any of the known adhesions associated with pathogenic *E. coli* (e.g., intimin). Some of the cytotoxic strains were found to express the *hly* operon, and it was subsequently demonstrated that these organisms express a type 1 pili similar in sequence to an *E. coli* strain associated with avian colisepticemia and meningitis [188]. Type 1 pili are involved in both the adherence and internalization of *E. coli* into host cells. They specifically bind to the CEACAM6 receptor on ileal enterocytes, which is expressed at significantly higher levels in the inflamed small intestinal epithelium of CD patients as compared to healthy controls [189].

Further research involving the prototypic AIEC strain, LF82, has shown that this pathogenic group of *E. coli* invades epithelial cells via engagement of actin microtubules and microfilaments and replicates intracellularly even without possessing any of the known invasive determinants found in other invasive *E. coli* strains [190]. AIEC strains are also able to survive and replicate within macrophages without causing apoptosis; they also induce production of the pro-inflammatory cytokine TNF-α [191]. LF82 is also able to induce *in vitro* aggregation of peripheral blood mononuclear cells (PBMCs), an observation reminiscent of the granulomas observed in the colonic tissue of CD patients [192].

In addition to being detected with increased frequency in human IBD patients, AIEC strains have also been isolated from Boxer dogs with granulomatous colitis. These *E. coli* isolates were found to have the same adherent-invasive phenotype as human AIEC strains. The Boxer dog isolates were also of the same phylotype (B2 and D) and possessed similar virulence gene profiles as LF82. In contrast to the human AIEC strains, however, the canine AIEC strains were only isolated from diseased dogs and not healthy controls. Simpson and colleagues also demonstrated that remission of colitis in Boxer dogs could be achieved by treatment with enrofloxacin, the use of which resulted in the eradication of AIEC *E. coli* [193].

2.4. The microbiota and IBD

Although no single organism has been implicated in the induction of IBD, a preponderance of studies indicates that the GI microbial community of IBD patients is different from that of healthy individuals. This imbalance is known as "dysbiosis". Characteristics of a dysbiotic community in IBD include a reduction in members of the *C. leptum* and *C. cocciodes* clusters (members of the Firmicutes phyla and major butyrate producers) and an increase in *Enterobacteriaceae* and members of the Bacteroidetes, thereby leading to a reduction in the microbial diversity of the gut. Another notable difference is the greater concentration of mucosally-associated bacteria in IBD patients as compared to healthy individuals [194-197]. Using fluorescence *in situ* hybridization (FISH), patients with CD were found to have predominantly *Enterobacteriaceae, γ-Proteobacteria,* or *Bacteroides/Prevotella* adherent to their mucosa and present in their submucosa [195]. Another FISH-based analysis revealed that *Bacteroides* spp. were the dominant gut bacteria, representing up to 80 % of the total mucosally-adherent bacterial population in some samples. Of interest was the authors' additional finding that treatment of IBD patients with mesalamine (an anti-inflammatory therapeutic drug) significantly reduced the numbers of mucosally-adherent bacteria [198].

Sample origin is an important factor to consider when interpreting data for microbial analyses. Although stool samples are easy to obtain, it may not accurately reflect the microbial community in the cecum and proximal colon of patients [14]. In a comparative study of the microbial populations detected in cecal versus fecal samples, more anaerobes and *Bifidobacterium* spp. were detected in fecal samples using culture-based methods [199]. Molecular probe hybridization revealed that facultative anaerobes represented by *Lactobacillus, Enterococcus,* and *E. coli* were higher in numbers in cecal contents, yet the number of strict anaerobes represented by the *Bacteroides, C. leptum,* and *C. coccoides* groups were significantly lower in the cecal contents. Differences in microbial composition have also been observed when comparing colonic biopsies versus feces [200]. Analysis of feces from Japanese IBD patients showed that *Faecalibacterium* spp. were significantly decreased in CD patients, while *Bacteroides* spp. were significantly increased only in patients with active IBD [201]. Based on the Shannon diversity index, this study demonstrated that microbial diversity was significantly reduced in CD patients both during active disease and remission as compared to healthy individuals.

Several studies have noted a specific decrease in the numbers of *C. leptum* and *C. coccoides* clusters present in colonic contents or feces in IBD patients [18, 197, 202-206]. A reduction in the *C. coccoides* group in UC patients and *C. leptum* in CD patients has been shown using FISH probes on patient feces [202]. Another study employing a combination of PCR and FISH analysis of fecal samples found a reduced presence of both *C. leptum* and *C. coccoides* clusters in IBD patients [197]. Additional analyses revealed significant decreases in the concentrations of the SCFAs (e.g., butyric and propionic acid) in the feces of IBD patients [197]. In other work, high throughput sequencing demonstrated reduced numbers of *Faecalibacterium, Ruminococcaceae, Alistipes, Collinsella,* and *Roseburia* and increased numbers of *Enterobacteriaceae* in a twin with ileal CD as compared to the healthy twin [204]. This latter study again emphasizes the involvement of the microbiota in the development of IBD in a genetically susceptible host, as only one of the twins developed disease.

One specific member of the *C. leptum* cluster, *Faecalibacterium prausnitzii*, has recently been the subject of many published studies. This organism is a major butyrate producer that also possesses some anti-inflammatory properties [59, 207]. A study by Sokol et al. described a reduction of both *C. leptum* and *C. coccoides* clusters in the stool of patients with active IBD along with a skewed Firmicutes/Bacteroidetes ratio [203]. The authors specifically identified a reduction in *F. prausnitzii* in IBD patients, confirming results obtained using biopsy samples from twins analyzed via qPCR [205]. In other work, denaturing gradient gel electrophoresis (DGGE) analysis of biopsy samples also demonstrated a significant decrease in *Faecalibacterium* spp. along with increased levels of *E. coli* and *Clostridium* spp. in CD patients as compared to healthy individuals [208]. Using fecal cylinders and 11 different FISH probes to analyze sections GIT tissue specimens, Swidsinski and colleagues found the presence of *F. prausnitzii* to be significantly reduced in CD patients [209]. Of special note, analysis of samples from IBD patients given high-dose cortisol or infliximab to reduce inflammation revealed a dramatic increase (>14 $x10^9$) in the levels of *F. prausnitzii* within days of initiating treatment. This increase was short-lived, however, as levels of *F. prausnitzii* decreased when the cortisol dose was reduced or the time between infliximab infusions was increased. Together, these data indicate that inflammation plays a major role in shaping the intestinal microbiota.

Work in murine models of colitis also demonstrates that inflammation in the gut, be it chemically or bacterially induced, causes an increase in *Enterobacteriaceae* [210]. Colonization of mice with *Citrobacter rodentium* resulted in a reduction of the total number of bacteria in the colon at 7 and 14 days post-infection; this decrease coincided with the highest levels of both *C. rodentium* and intestinal inflammation [211]. Further analysis specifically determined that members of the Cytophaga-Flavobacter-Bacteroides phylum were decreased. Infection with *C. rodentium* infection is self-limiting, and the total bacterial levels returned to normal following pathogen clearance. These changes in the bacterial load were not simply associated with colonization of a new organism to the microbial community, such as *Campylobacter jejuni*, an organism that does not cause intestinal inflammation in immunocompetent CONVR mice [212], induced no detectable changes in microbial load.

The induction of GIT inflammation in mice via administration of dextran sulfate sodium (DSS) in the drinking water for seven days was associated with increased numbers of aerobic bacteria, specifically *Entercococcus faecalis* [210]. Bacteroidetes were eliminated from the community and the total number of bacteria was also decreased. A dramatic increase in the numbers of a non-pathogenic *E. coli* following DSS treatment was also observed. The authors subsequently colonized IL-$10^{-/-}$ mice, which spontaneously develop colitis [213], with this non-pathogenic *E. coli*. Upon the development of GIT inflammation, the *E. coli* was able to proliferate to the same level observed in DSS treated mice, but displacing the Firmicutes phylum instead of the Bacteroidetes. These results indicate that regardless of the source, GIT inflammation creates a niche that favors the colonization and expansion of *Enterobacteriaceae*. Collectively, these data suggest that the induction of inflammation following the colonization of the GIT by a bacterial provocateur along with perturbations of the microbiota together have a deleterious impact on the microbiota and mucosal homeostasis.

2.5. Canine IBD

In addition to affecting humans, IBD can also occur in dogs as well [214]. As in human IBD, the interactions between genetics, the mucosal immune system, inflammation, and environmental factors (ie, diet and imbalances in the intestinal microbiome) all contribute to the pathogenesis of canine IBD (Figure 6) [215-217].

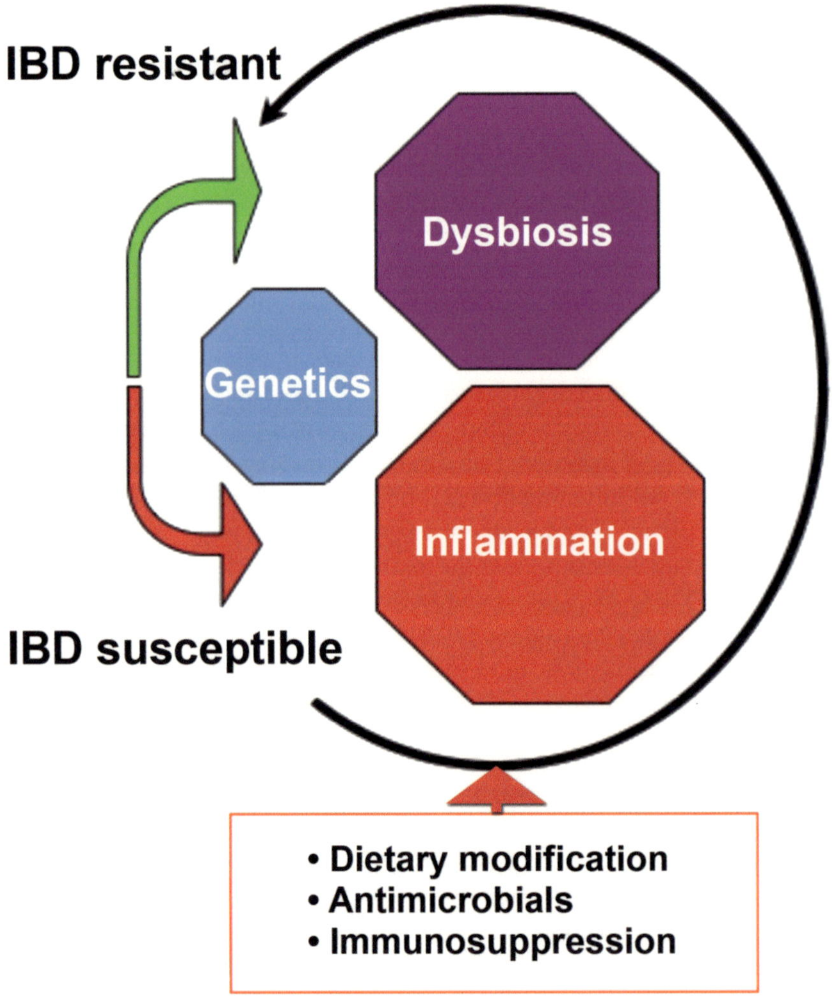

Figure 6. The etiology for canine IBD involves complex interactions between host genetics, mucosal immunity, and the enteric microbiota. Therapeutic intervention with diet, antibiotics and immunosuppressive drugs is aimed at reducing inflammation and dysbiosis.

http://dx.doi.org/10.5772/53920

Mutations in innate immune receptors in German shepherd dogs (TLR5, NOD2) have been linked to IBD susceptibility which in the presence of an inappropriate enteric microbiota may lead to upregulated pro-inflammatory cytokine production (e.g., IL-17, IL-22, TNF-α) and reduced bacterial clearance, thereby promoting chronic intestinal inflammation [218, 219]. Commensal bacterial antigens are likely to be important in disease pathogenesis because it has been observed that boxer dogs with granulomatous colitis (GC) show clinical remission following the eradication of mucosally associated AIEC that share a novel adherent and invasive pathotype which bears phylogenetic similarity with AIEC strains recovered from patients with ileal Crohn's disease [193, 220, 221]. Moreover, genome-wide analysis in affected boxer dogs has identified disease-associated single nucleotide polymorphisms (SNPs) in a gene (*NCF2*) involved with killing intracellular bacteria [222]. Still others have shown that $CD11c^{+}$ cells are significantly decreased in the intestines of dogs with IBD suggesting that chronic mucosal inflammation may involve an imbalance in the intestinal dendritic cell population leading to aberrant immune activation [223]. Molecular analysis of the intestinal microbiome in different breeds of dogs with IBD have consistently shown that diseased tissues are enriched with members of the families *Enterobacteriaceae* and *Clostridiaceae* [224, 225]. These bacteria are believed to contribute to the pathogenesis of GIT inflammatory disease in dogs as in humans [187, 226]. A recent trial using high throughput 16S rDNA sequencing methods (ie, 454 pyrosequencing) on intestinal biopsies of IBD dogs revealed a dysbiosis in the mucosally-adherent microbiota with an increase in sequences belonging to Proteobacteria and a decrease in Bacteroidetes, Fusobacteria, and the Clostridiales [227]. Taken together, these studies suggest that chronic intestinal inflammation of canine IBD may be due to overly aggressive adaptive immune responses to enteric bacteria (or fungi) [225] in hosts with genetic defects that fail to properly regulate microbial killing, mucosal barrier function, or immune responses. As in human IBD, environmental factors (diet, microbiota imbalances) likely govern the onset of inflammation or reactivation and modulate genetic susceptibility to disease.

2.5.1. Clinical and diagnostic features

The clinical manifestations of IBD are diverse and are influenced by the organ(s) involved, presence of active versus inactive disease, and physiologic complications seen with enteric plasma protein loss and/or micronutrient (cobalamin) deficiency [215, 216, 228, 229]. Canine IBD is a disease that predominantly affects middle-aged animals. Vomiting and diarrhea are most commonly observed and are often accompanied by decreased appetite and weight loss. Gastric and duodenal inflammation is associated with vomiting and small bowel diarrhea while colonic involvement causes large bowel diarrhea with blood, mucus, and straining. The clinical course of IBD is generally cyclical and is characterized by spontaneous exacerbations and remissions. Importantly, the clinical signs of IBD are not disease specific and share numerous over-lapping features with other canine disorders. A diagnosis of IBD is one of exclusion and requires careful elimination of IBD mimics [230]. The possible causes for chronic intestinal inflammation may be excluded through the integration of history, physical findings, clinicopathological testing, diagnostic imaging, and histopathology of intestinal biopsies. A baseline CBC, biochemistry profile, urinalysis, and diagnostic imaging are useful in eliminating the most common systemic and metabolic disorders (e.g., renal disease, hepatopathy, hypoadrenocorticism) causing chronic GI signs in dogs. The measure of clinical disease activity by means of quantifiable indices is well established in human IBD [231-233].

A canine IBD activity index (CIBDAI) used for assessment of inflammatory activity in dogs has been recently designed [234]. Similar to other indices, the magnitude of the numerical score is proportional to the degree of inflammatory activity. This index serves as the principal measure of response to a therapeutic regimen and may be used to tailor medical therapy for an individual patient's needs [235]. Intestinal biopsies are required to confirm histopathological inflammation and to determine the extent of mucosal disease. Diagnostic endoscopy is preferred since this technique allows for direct assessment of mucosal abnormalities and the acquisition of targeted biopsy specimens. The microscopic findings in canine IBD consist of minimal to pronounced inflammatory cell (lymphoplasmacytic) infiltration of the intestinal lamina propria accompanied by varying degrees of mucosal architectural disruption similar to that observed in tissue from human IBD patients (Figure 7).

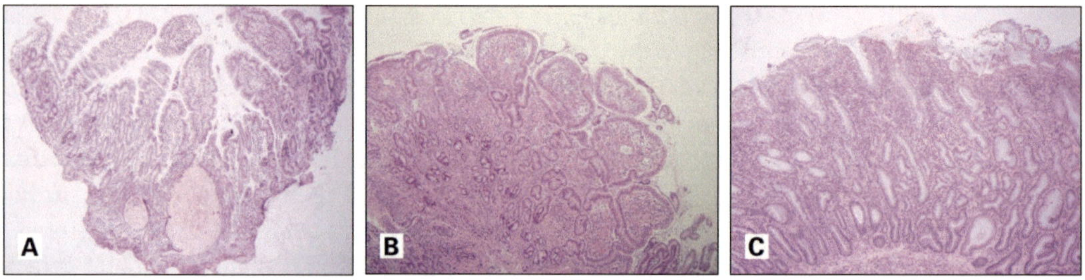

Figure 7. Histopathological lesions of (A) crypt distortion with abscessation, (B) diffuse villous atrophy, and (C) mucosal ulceration seen in duodenal biopsies of dogs with IBD.

Unfortunately, biopsy interpretation is notoriously subjective and suffers from extensive intra-observer variability and the technical constraints of procurement/processing artifacts inherent in evaluation of endoscopic specimens [236]. Although several histopathological scoring schemes have been proposed there are no uniform grading criteria that pathologists can universally agree on. One small study has resulted in development of a 'simplified model system' for defining intestinal inflammation of IBD that is presently being tested in a separate clinical trial.

2.5.2. Therapeutic approach

Treatment principles for canine IBD are empirical and consist of combination therapy using both dietary and pharmacologic interventions. As compared to clinical trials evaluating the efficacy of therapy for CD and UC, only one randomized, controlled drug trial for canine IBD has been reported [235]. There are, however, abundant evidence-based observations that feeding elimination diets and administering corticosteroids, immunosuppressive drugs, and/or select antibiotics are useful in the clinical management of canine IBD. Some clinicians prefer a sequential approach to nutritional and drug therapy for IBD. The optimal drug or drug combinations as well as duration of therapy for induction and maintenance of remission of clinical signs have not been determined for most protocols [216, 230]. In general, the administration of corticosteroids (i.e., prednisone, prednisolone or budesonide), antimicrobials (i.e., metronidazole or tylosin), and immunosuppressive drugs (i.e., cyclosporine, chlorambucil, azathioprine) used alone or in some combination are effective in inducing clinical remission in most animals. Some dogs will require intermittent or life-long drug therapy.

The rationale for nutritional therapy of IBD is that restricting exposure to antigens (i.e., dietary proteins) known to evoke sensitivity will reduce exaggerated host responses and attenuate intestinal inflammation. Other indications for specialized nutrition include the presence of decreased appetite, impaired nutrient absorption, or enteric plasma protein loss seen with moderate-to-severe mucosal inflammation. While evidence-based observations indicate that most dogs respond favorably to dietary intervention, the superiority of one novel protein source versus another or the advantage in feeding an intact protein elimination diet versus a hydrolyzed protein elimination diet has not been shown to date. Modifying the dietary n3:n6 fatty-acid ratio may also modulate inflammatory responses by reducing production of pro-inflammatory metabolites [237]. There is relatively sparse clinical data investigating prebiotic or probiotic therapy for canine IBD (see subsequent section on probiotics).

2.5.3. Future directions in canine IBD

Canine IBD represents a common and frustrating GI disorder in veterinary medicine. More research is needed to unravel the mechanisms responsible for disease development and to translate these findings directly to human IBD. The primary features of IBD in humans and animals are remarkably similar (Table 1).

Feature	Human IBD	Canine IBD
Genetic basis	Yes	Likely
Etiology	Unknown but multifactorial	Unknown but multifactorial
Involves the microbiota	Yes	Yes
Hematochezia	Yes	Yes
Diarrhea	Yes	Yes
Definitive Diagnosis	GI biopsy	GI biopsy
Disease activity assessment	Clinical indices, biomarkers (ASCA, pANCA, CRP, calprotectin)	Clinical indices, biomarkers (pANCA, CRP, calprotectin ?)
Responsive to anti-inflammatory drugs	Yes	Yes
Responsive to antibiotics	Yes	Yes
Spontaneous GI flares	Yes	Yes

Table 1. Comparative features of IBD in humans and dogs.

Recent advances in clinical indices, histopathological standards, and the development of species-specific immunologic reagents and innovative molecular tools have made the dog an excellent 'spontaneous' animal model to study chronic immunologically-mediated intestinal inflammation. In addition, the dog has higher genomic sequence similarity to that of humans than do mice, a species traditionally used for comparative disease genetics [238]. However, clinical manifestations of complex disease in the mouse do not compare to the human form as closely as they do in the dog. Furthermore, the lifespan of the dog is much shorter than that of a human; thus, clinical trials aimed at treatment of IBD can be carried out much quicker and yield results that should have relevant application to human trials [230, 235, 239].

2.6. Treatment for human IBD

Treatments for human IBD patients typically involve the use of anti-inflammatory drugs, antibiotics, and there is a growing trend of probiotics and prebiotics being studied to determine their effects on disease activity. When patients fail to respond to treatment, the last and most drastic treatment option is surgery to resect sections of the inflamed bowel [240]. Most treatment options are primarily focused on reducing the inflammation associated with IBD. Some of these drugs also impact the microbiota and those will be discussed below.

2.6.1. Antibiotics

Given the importance of the microbiota in the pathogenesis of IBD, antibiotic therapy may seem an obvious treatment option. A meta-analysis by Khan et al. in 2011 reviewed randomized controlled trials utilizing antibiotics in the treatment of IBD [241]. Rifamycin derivatives, ciprofloxacin, and clofazamine all induced remission in CD patients. Rifaximin (a rifamycin derivative) is effective against both Gram-negative and Gram-positive anaerobes and aerobes; it is also poorly absorbed after oral administration, resulting in little to no systemic side effects [242, 243]. Analysis of the effect of the drug using an *in vitro* continuous culture method with fecal samples from CD patients revealed increases in beneficial bacteria post-rifaximin administration [244]. Significant increases in *Bifidobacterium* spp., the *Atopobium* cluster, and *F. prausnitzii* were noted, as were increases in levels of lactate, acetate, and propionate as determined by ^{1}H-NMR spectroscopy [244].

Ciprofloxacin is a fluoroquinolone with broad-spectrum antibiotic activity [245]. In addition to having anti-bacterial properties, this drug has also been shown to have immunomodulatory properties as well [246]. In a TNBS mouse model of colitis, administration of ciprofloxacin ameliorated disease as compared to mice given ceftazidime (an antibacterial with a similar spectrum of activity compared to ciprofloxacin) [245]. Clinically, mice treated with ciprofloxacin did not lose weight and had reduced histopathological inflammatory scores associated with their colons. Ciprofloxacin treated mice also had reduced expression of IL-1β, IL-8, and TNF-α as measured from colonic homogenates as well as reduced expression of NF-κB. Since ceftazidime was less effective in ameliorating GIT inflammation, there appears to be additional benefits (i.e., anti-inflammatory) to the use of ciprofloxacin in addition to its spectrum of antimicrobial activity.

Clofazamine has also been documented to significantly affect the rate of remission in CD patients [241]. This drug, used to treat leprosy, is similar to ciprofloxacin, in that it has both anti-bacterial and anti-inflammatory properties [247-249]. It is only effective against Gram-positive organisms, and its effectiveness increases in anaerobic environments [250]. Its effects on the immune system include increasing the presence of lysosomal enzymes in macrophages [251] and increasing phagocytosis by macrophages resulting in enhanced uptake and digestion of immune complexes [252]. Clofazamine has also been shown to inhibit TCR-mediated IL-2 production by T cells, thereby limiting T cell activation, a component of the pathogenesis of IBD [253].

2.6.2. Corticosteroids

The most commonly used corticosteroids used are prednisolone, methylprednisolone, and budesonide [254]. These drugs are very effective at inducing remission, however, they are not without side effects. In a study comparing prednisolone and budesonide, both were found to be effective at inducing remission [255]. However, patients on budesonide had reduced evidence of adrenal axis suppression and peripheral leucocyte counts compared to those treated with prednisolone. These results indicate that budesonide is a safer choice yet it is still as effective as prednisolone. Corticosteroids are able to prevent NFκB activation [256] as well as block infiltration of neutrophils, prevent vasodilation and enhanced vascular permeability and downregulate the production of pro-inflammatory cytokines [254]. Although it is well established that these corticosteroids have an anti-inflammatory effect, little research has been conducted on the effects they have on the gut microbiota. A study by Swidsinski et al., mentioned previously, indicated that administration of cortisol increased the population of *F. prausnitzii* in a dose dependent manner [209].

2.6.3. Immunosuppressive therapy

Drugs such as methotrexate, 6-mercaptopurine (6-MP) and azathioprine (the prodrug of 6-MP) work by inhibiting the proliferation and activation of lymphocytes and decreasing the production of pro-inflammatory cytokines [254]. 6-mercaptopurine (6-MP) and azathioprine are purine antagonists and inhibit cellular metabolism by interfering with DNA replication [257, 258]. Methotrexate is a folic acid analog that inhibits DNA synthesis and, therefore, has an anti-proliferative effect [259]. Antibacterial effects, including growth inhibition of MAP, have also been demonstrated for methotrexate and 6-MP [258].

2.6.4. 5-aminosalicyclic acid (5-ASA)

Sulfasalazine was the first 5-ASA-type drug developed and is a combination of sulfapyridine (an antimicrobial) and salicyclic acid (an anti-inflammatory) to form a pro-drug. Upon entering the colon, this pro-drug is cleaved by colonic bacteria into the two separate molecules [260, 261]. Unfortunately, the frequency of gastrointestinal side effects was quite high due to the sulfapyridine moiety [262, 263]. It was later determined that the active moiety is 5-aminosalicyclic acid (5-ASA, mesalazine) [264]. More recently formulations of this pro-drug have eliminated the sulfapyridine moiety and replaced it with either a second salicyclic acid moiety (disodium azodisalicylate [265]) or an inert carrier (balsalazide [266]) thereby reducing the side effects.

In addition to being an anti-inflammatory agent [267-270], 5-ASA also affects the gut microbiota. As mentioned previously, patients taking mesalamine had a reduction in mucosa-adherent bacteria [198, 271]. 5-ASA has also been shown to inhibit the growth of MAP [272] and *Bacteroides* spp. [273] and moderately inhibit the growth of *C. difficile* and *C. perfringens* in culture [273]. This drug also effects bacterial gene expression, as *Salmonella enterica* serovar Typhimurium incubated with 5-ASA had no change in growth but differentially expressed 110 genes [274]. Those genes characterized were found to be involved in invasion, metabolism, and antibiotic and stress resistance. *In vitro* assays revealed attenuation in the invasiveness of *S. enterica* serovar Typhimurium towards HeLa cells when pretreated with 5-ASA. These results indicate that in addition to inhibiting host-mediated inflammation, 5-ASA also has the potential to affect the intestinal microbiota.

2.6.5. Anti-TNF monoclonal antibodies

The induction of TNF-α is most often a downstream event following the interaction of phlogistic microbial components with toll-like receptors (TLRs) on host cells. The interest in TNF-α as a therapeutic target for IBD treatment began when the expression and secretion of this cytokine was found to be increased in IBD patients [275, 276]. For example, pediatric patients with either active UC or CD present with elevated levels of TNF-α in their stool [275]. Additionally, the incubation of GIT tissue sections in culture medium has demonstrated that significantly elevated levels of TNF-α are spontaneously secreted from inflamed tissue of both UC and CD patients when compared to the amounts produced by non-inflamed tissue and tissue from otherwise healthy individuals [276]. The predominant cell type producing the TNF-α has been shown to be the macrophage [276]. Based on the central role TNF-α appears to play in the pathogenesis of IBD, there was interest in developing a therapeutic approach to control the harmful effects of this cytokine.

Clinically, the use of monoclonal antibodies to treat IBD patients began with Infliximab, an IgG1 murine-human chimeric monoclonal antibody specific for TNF-α, which was approved for human use in 1998 for CD [277, 278]. This monoclonal antibody consists of human constant regions and murine antigen binding regions [277]. These chimeric antibodies reduce the risk of immunoreactivity that occurs when murine antibodies are used. In addition to being less immunoreactive, this chimeric antibody had improved binding and neutralization characteristics for TNF-α than that of the original murine antibody [277]. Another monoclonal anti-TNF antibody, Adalimumab, is a fully humanized IgG1 antibody that avoids the induction of anti-species IgG that neutralize the effectiveness of the anti-TNF-α reagent [278, 279]. Lastly, Certolizumab is a monoclonal antibody fragment with a polyethylene glycol moiety (PEGylated) [278]. Certolizumab lacks the crystallizable fragment (Fc) portion of the immunoglobulin molecule and is an IgG4 isotype unlike Infliximab and Adalimumab, which are IgG1 antibodies [278, 280, 281]. In addition, the PEGylation increases the half-life of the antibody thereby reducing the frequency of administration.

Anti-TNF-α therapy works via multi-factorial mechanisms. First, it neutralizes TNF-α by blocking its ability to bind to TNF receptors, thus, inhibiting the pro-inflammatory response. Second, Anti-TNF-α binds to cell surface bound TNF-α on $CD4^+$ T cells and macrophages, resulting in both complement- and antibody-dependent cell-mediated cytotoxicity [282]. All three monoclonal antibodies bind to and neutralize both soluble and membrane forms of TNF-α [281]. Infliximab and Adalimumab both mediate complement- and antibody-dependent cell-mediated cytotoxicity; however, Certolizumab only mediates complement-dependent cellular cytotoxicity as it lacks of an Fc region. Furthermore, Infliximab and Adalimumab induce apoptosis in peripheral blood lymphocytes and monocytes, as well as cause degranulation and loss of membrane integrity of PMNs. These activities were not induced with Certolizumab. Lastly, all three monoclonal antibodies inhibit the production of IL-1β after LPS stimulation in vitro, suggesting that there is a sequential production of pro-inflammatory cytokines induced by microbial components. Infliximab and Adalimumab both inhibit T cell proliferation in mixed lymphocyte reactions in vitro, again suggesting that anti-TNF-α monoclonal antibodies ameliorate the inflammation associated with IBD via more than one mode of action [283]. The impact of these therapies on the microbiota, however, is not well studied. As previously mentioned, treatment with Infliximab resulted in increased levels of *F. prausnitzii* after administration [209]. As mentioned above, it is clear that the host inflammatory response often negatively impacts (i.e., shapes) the composition of the GIT microbiota, and that controlling mucosal inflammation benefits the health of the microbiota as well. Otherwise, there have been no specific studies performed to directly evaluate the role of anti-TNF-α therapies on the gut microbiota.

2.6.6. Complementary and alternative therapies

An estimated 70 % of IBD patients have reported using complementary and alternative medicine (CAM) products at some time to treat their symptoms In a Canadian study of IBD patients, some of the most commonly used CAM treatments included massage therapy, chiropractic visits, probiotics, herbs, and fish oils [284]. A systematic review of the literature on the use of herbal medicines reveals some anti-inflammatory benefits associated with the administration of these herbs to both animals and humans [285]. It should be stressed that prior to utilizing any herbal remedy, which are potentially biologically active, patients need to consult their physician. This is especially important because the number two reason patients using CAM gave as to why they sought these products was that "natural therapy is safe"[286]. Some of the biological properties associated with CAM products include the reduction of pro-inflammatory cytokines, increased antioxidant production, inhibition of leukotriene B4, decreased NF-κB activation, and inhibition of platelet activation [285].

Increasing evidence supports a potential therapeutic role for prebiotic and probiotic therapy in human IBD [287, 288]. If IBD in dogs is indeed driven by loss of tolerance to components of the intestinal microbiota as it is in humans, then prebiotics and probiotics may also prove beneficial as primary or adjunct therapies with diet and drugs. *Probiotics* are living microorganisms that, upon ingestion in sufficient numbers, impart health benefits beyond those of inherent basic nutrition [289]. Lactobacilli and Bifidobacterium have been the most commonly used human probiotics, but multi-strain cocktails (e.g., VSL#3), *E. coli* Nissle 1917, and nonbacterial *Saccharomyces boulardii* have also been used as probiotics [226]. Probiotic bacteria have measurable host benefits, including the ability to improve epithelial barrier function, modulate the mucosal immune system, and alter the intestinal flora [290]. *Prebiotics* are non-digestible dietary carbohydrates, such as lactosucrose, fructo-oligosaccharides (FOS), psyllium, bran, which beneficially stimulate the growth and metabolism of endogenous enteric bacteria upon consumption [291]. Beneficial effects of prebiotics are also associated with the production of short chain fatty acids (SCFA) due to fermentation by colonic bacteria. *Synbiotics* are combinations of probiotics and prebiotics that are an emerging therapeutic modality. Increasing evidence supports a therapeutic role for probiotics, prebiotics, and synbiotics in treating gastrointestinal diseases of humans, including infectious diarrhea, *H. pylori* infection, irritable bowel syndrome, lactase deficiency, and IBD [84]. A comparison of prebiotic and probiotic preparations is outlined in Table 2.

2.6.7. Probiotics

VSL#3 is one of the most commonly used probiotic cocktails and contains a very high bacterial concentration per gram of product characterized by greater number of different bacterial species as compared to traditional probiotic preparations [292]. This commercially prepared formulation consists of 450 billion bacteria/g of viable lyophilized bacteria comprised of eight bacterial strains (*Lactobacillus casei, L plantarum, L. bulgaricus, L. acidolphilus, Bifidobacterium longum, B. breve, B. infantis* and *Streptococcus thermophiles*). While the exact mechanism of action of VSL#3 is unknown, several studies have demonstrated the effects of VSL#3 on epithelial barrier function and down regulation of cytokine secretion from immune cells. For example, Madsen [293] has shown in *in vitro* studies that epithelial barrier function could be enhanced by exposure to a soluble factor secreted by VSL#3 bacteria. Moreover, this same study demonstrated that VSL#3 did not alter the ability of the epithelial cell to activate a mucosal inflammatory response to a bacterial invasion. Studies with VSL#3 formulations have also been conducted in several animal models of colitis, inflammatory liver disease, sepsis, and irritable bowel syndrome (IBS). In models of experimentally-induced colitis, these studies demonstrated that VSL#3 normalized gut permeability and barrier function, and that VSL#3 modulated inflammatory and immune responses [226, 294]. Animal models of sepsis have also demonstrated that VSL#3 administration reduced bacterial translocation and significantly attenuated damage to the liver and intestinal mucosa [295]. The use of VSL#3 as an innovative probiotic preparation, developed specifically to balance the intestinal microbiota, is supported by studies in humans with IBD (ulcerative colitis [296], pouchitis) and in other patients with diverse gastrointestinal disorders, such as IBS [297, 298].

Studies have shown VSL#3 to induce remission of inflammation in 77 % of adult UC patients with no adverse effects [298] and 56 % of pediatric UC patients [299]. These same pediatric UC patients had a reduction in disease activity index and sigmoidoscopy scores following VSL#3 treatment. They also had reduced levels of the pro-inflammatory cytokines TNF-α and IFN-γ following therapy [299]. *In vitro* analysis of the effects of VSL#3 on Mode-K epithelial cells revealed that only one of the eight organisms, *L. casei*, inhibited TNF-induced secretion of the pro-inflammatory chemokine IP-10 [300]. The most recent studies with VSL#3 treatment of UC show increased fecal concentrations of beneficial bacterial species, improved clinical, endoscopic and histopathological scores in most patients, and higher rates of remission compared to placebo [298]. The most recent studies with VSL#3 treatment of UC show increased fecal concentrations of beneficial bacterial species, improved clinical, endoscopic and histopathological scores in most patients, and higher rates of remission compared to placebo [298]. VSL#3 is available without prescription and can be ordered via the internet or obtained locally at the pharmacy in the U.S. [301].

	Probiotics	Prebiotics
Definition	Live microorganisms which, given in adequate amounts confer health benefits to the host	Non-digestible carbohydrate which stimulate replication of protective enteric bacteria when consumed
Examples	*E. coli* Nissle 1917 VSL#3 *Lactobacillus* species *Bifidobacterium* species Saccharomyces boulardii Prostora Max® Forti Flora® Proviable-DC®	Fructo-oligosaccharide (FOS) Galacto-oligosaccharide (GOS) Inulin Lactulose Psyllium Bran Beet pulp, pumpkin Resistant starch
Protective Mechanisms	Alters microbiota to suppress pathogens Improved intestinal barrier function Increased production of antimicrobial peptides Decreased expression of proinflammatory cytokines	Stimulates replication of beneficial bacteria (*Bifidobacterium*) Enhances production of SCFA (butyrate) Improved intestinal barrier function Decreases proinflammatory cytokines

Table 2. Basic Features of Probiotics and Prebiotics

Recent studies have also shown that dogs with IBD have distinctly different duodenal microbial communities compared to healthy dogs. Current treatments for IBD include the administration of nonspecific anti-inflammatory drugs which may confer serious side effects and do not address the underlying basis for disease, namely, altered microbial composition. The use of probiotics offers an attractive, physiologic, and non-toxic alternative to shift the balance to protective species and treat canine IBD. The authors (AEJ) have initiated a clinical trial to investigate the clinical, microbiologic, and anti-inflammatory effects of probiotic VSL#3 in the treatment of canine IBD. We hypothesize that VSL#3 used as an adjunct to standard therapy (i.e., elimination diet and prednisone) will induce a beneficial alteration of enteric bacteria leading to induction and maintenance of remission in dogs with IBD. A randomized, controlled clinical trial of eight weeks duration will assess the efficacy of standard therapy in conjunction with VSL#3 versus standard therapy alone in the management of canine IBD. There is a need for additional data to be generated to provide proof of efficacy in probiotic therapy before these agents can be applied to widespread clinical use. These studies will also provide highly relevant insight into the anti-inflammatory effects of probiotics for treatment of human and canine IBD.

Another popular probiotic is *E. coli* Nissle 1917 also known as Mutaflor®. This probiotic has been shown to be just as effective as mesalazine in achieving and maintaining remission of inflammation in UC patients [302-304]. It has recently been shown that when *E. coli* Nissle 1917 is genetically modified to produce the quorum-sensing molecule AI-2, it affected the beneficial probiotic properties of this organism [305]. Colonization of healthy newborn infants with *E. coli* Nissle 1917 has shown that the presence of pathogenic bacteria in the gut was significantly reduced compared to non-colonized infants [306]. *In vitro* studies have shown *E. coli* Nissle 1917 is able to reduce the invasive ability of multiple pathogenic organisms [307], and also to reduce the adherent and invasive ability of AIEC [308]. *E. coli* Nissle 1917 was also shown to either inhibit the growth (49 %) or overgrowth (30 %) of 79 % of uropathogenic organisms recovered from children with urinary tract infections [309]. Unlike VSL#3, Mutaflor® cannot be purchased in the U.S. due to its reclassification by the F.D.A. from a "medical food" (which is what VSL#3 is classified as) to a "biologic" [301, 310].

There are few reports on the use of probiotic bacteria in dogs and cats. Recent *in vitro* studies have confirmed the capacity of a lyophilized probiotic cocktail (e.g., three different *Lactobacillus* spp strains) to modulate the expression of regulatory versus pro-inflammatory cytokines in dogs with chronic enteropathies [311]. However, a clinical trial using this same probiotic cocktail fed to dogs with food-responsive diarrhea failed to induce consistent patterns of regulatory (e.g., beneficial) cytokine expression in spite of obvious clinical improvement [312]. One commercially-manufactured probiotic (FortiFlora™–*Enterococcus faecium* SF68, Nestle Purina) is reported to potentially control diarrhea and enhance immune responses in dogs and cats. Several recent trials attest to the short-term efficacy of probiotics in treating acute diarrhea in dogs and cats [313]. The link between the intestinal microbiota and gastrointestinal health in companion animals is now obvious. Future developments in the pharmabiotic field must include performance of randomized clinical trials to determine the role of probiotics and prebiotics in the management of canine chronic enteropathy. One large multicenter trial investigating the efficacy of VSL#3 in reducing inflammatory activity of canine IBD is presently underway

2.6.8. Prebiotics

Prebiotics are substances that can be used to promote specific changes in the microbiota. Administration has been shown to shift the microbiota in healthy adults; for example, individuals who consume either soluble corn fiber or polydextrose had increases in *F. prausnitzii* and those who consumed the soluble corn fiber had increases in *Roseburia* spp. [314]. As mentioned previously, both of these organisms metabolically produce butyrate and *F. prausnitzii* also has other anti-inflammatory properties. In animal models, prebiotics have been shown to be effective as well. The severity of DSS-induced colitis in rats was attenuated by administering inulin orally as evidenced by a reduction in histopathological scores and myeloperioxidase accumulation in the colons [315]. In addition, the acidity of the colonic contents increased in rats fed inulin as well as an increase in *Lactobacillus* spp. in the feces. In a multicenter trial feeding UC patients germinated barley foodstuff (GBF), patients consuming GBF had improved clinical activity index scores [316]. GBF has also been shown to be effective in maintaining remission [317] and reducing pro-inflammatory cytokine levels in UC patients [318]. In CD patients, dietary supplementation with fructo-oligosaccharide (FOS) reduced their disease activity index, increased fecal *Bifidobacterium* spp. levels as well as increased production of IL-10 and expression of TLR-2 and TLR-4 from lamina propria dendritic cells [319].

Scientific studies have also investigated the effects of dietary supplementation with prebiotics on the intestinal microbiota of healthy dogs and cats. In one study, FOS supplemented at 0.75 % dry matter produced qualitative and quantitative changes in the fecal flora of healthy cats [320]. Compared with samples from cats fed a basal diet, increased numbers of lactobacilli and *Bacteroides* spp. and decreased numbers of *E. coli* were associated with cats fed the FOS supplemented diet. However, bacteriologic examination of the duodenal juice in these same cats showed wide variation in the composition of the duodenal microbiota, across sampling periods, which was not affected by FOS supplementation [321]. Moreover, healthy Beagle dogs fed a 1 % FOS diet over a three-month trial showed inconsistent fecal excretion of *Lactobacillus* spp. and *Bifidobacterium* spp. [322]. While FOS supplementation has been shown to have health benefits, these studies demonstrate that FOS does not have an adverse affect on the microbiota and suggest that it may have positive physiological benefits as seen in humans. This observation and the lack of significant side effects associated with FOS supplementation provide evidence that FOS should be considered as an attractive alternative or adjunct therapy for IBD in dogs and cats.

3. Mouse models of IBD

Many different mouse models have been utilized in IBD research to elucidate the roles that bacteria, genetics, the immune response, and environment play in the induction and maintenance of IBD [323]. They fall into two main categories: chemically-induced and genetically-engineered models. The composition of the microbiota in the various mouse models is also discussed. Regardless of the strain of mouse employed in chemically-induced or genetically-engineered models, there are only five options for its microbiota—conventional, specific pathogen free, restricted, gnotobiotic, or germ-free. Note that the word gnotobiotic (gnostos–"known" bios –"life") indicates that all the organisms present, regardless of the numbers of species, are known and does not apply only to mice that are completely devoid of microbes (i.e., germfree).

3.1. Chemically-induced models

3.1.1. DSS

Dextran sulfate sodium (DSS) is formed by the esterification of dextran with chlorosulphonic acid [324]. Administered *ad libtum* in the drinking water, this compound causes enterocolitis in mice with disease severity being dependent on mouse strain, DSS molecular mass, and sulfur content [325-328]. Within three to seven days after the addition of DSS (1 to 10 % w/v) to the drinking water, mice exhibit loose stools, weight loss, and occult blood. Upon necropsy of mice treated with DSS, cecal atrophy and colonic shortening are noted, and histopathological examination reveals mucosal ulceration, inflammatory infiltrate, and hyperplastic epithelium in the colonic mucosa. It has also been reported that glandular dropout occurs prior to signs of inflammation. Although the exact mechanism of action for DSS-induced colitis is currently not known, it is thought to manifest epithelial toxicity [329, 330]. Other reports indicate that DSS increases mucosal permeability within three days of administration (before the appearance of inflammatory infiltrate) [331]. Studies have also shown that DSS is taken up by macrophages in the colon and mesenteric lymph node and by Kupffer cells in the liver [326, 330]. When macrophages become laden with DSS, they have a reduced ability to perform normal homeostatic functions such as tissue repair and phagocytosis of bacteria [332]. DSS was demonstrated to be cytotoxic to Caco-2 cells, binding to their nucleus, causing cell cycle arrest and reduced production of reactive oxygen species [333].

Microbial populations of the GIT are altered after DSS administration, with the microbiota of the treated mice having increased numbers of *Bacteroidaceae* and *Clostridium* spp. [326]. This result indicates that the changes to the microbiota may play a contributory role (e.g., reduction of butyrate production) in the induction of DSS-induced disease. However, DSS induces more severe colitis and increased mortality in GF mice as compared to their conventional counterparts [334, 335]. GF mice given either 5% or 1% DSS died at days three or 14, respectively, after the start of DSS administration [335]. Collectively, these studies indicate that the composition of the microbiota may influence the sensitivity of mice to DSS-induced colitis as well as support the idea that the resident microbiota affords cytoprotective benefits for the host.

3.1.2. TNBS (2,4,6,-trinitrobenzne sulfonic acid)

TNBS is a haptenating agent that causes a disease similar to CD when mixed with ethanol and administered rectally as an enema. Mice treated with TNBS develop a pan-colitis with the peak of clinical signs, such as diarrhea and rectal prolapse, occurring two to four weeks post-administration [112]. Microscopically, transmural inflammation is noted along with neutrophil infiltration, loss of goblet cells, edema, and granulomas. T cells isolated from the lamina propria secrete elevated levels of IFN-γ and IL-2 following stimulation with anti-CD3 and anti-CD28. However, administration of anti-IL-12 antibodies after induction of TNBS-induced colitis reduced the disease severity, and treated mice also showed reduced production of IFN-γ [112]. Further studies have shown that $CD4^+$ T cells recovered from mice with TNBS-induced colitis could induce mild colitis when adoptively transferred into naive control mice; the colitic lesions were characterized by inflammatory cell infiltrate that produced IFN-γ [336]. In that same study, researchers found that feeding mice TNBS-haptenized colonic protein caused the mice to develop oral tolerance. These mice subsequently failed to develop colitis after TNBS administration or the transfer of $CD4^+$ T cells from mice with TNBS-induced colitis. T cells from these tolerant mice secreted elevated amounts of TGF-β, IL-4, and IL-10 [336].

3.1.3. Oxazolone

Oxazolone is a haptenating agent that causes a disease in mice similar to UC when mixed with ethanol and administered rectally [337, 338]. SJL/J mice rapidly develop diarrhea and weight loss that peaks at day two post-administration with a 50 % mortality rate by day four. At day two, the distal half of the colon becomes hemorrhagic and edematous and histologically shows signs of superficial inflammation. There is epithelial cell erosion, goblet cell depletion, edema, and inflammatory cell infiltrate composed of neutrophils and eosinophils. This is similar to what is observed microscopically in the colonic tissues of human UC patients. These mice also develop elevated levels of IL-4 and IL-5, but no IFN-γ, indicating that oxazolone induces a Th2 response. Elevated levels of TGF-β are also noted and may play in a role in the induction of disease in only part of the colon. The model has also been examined for its role in determining efficacy of IBD treatments. BALB/c mice given either 5-aminosalicylic acid (5-ASA) or sodium prednisolone phosphate intra-rectally prior to and during induction of oxazolone colitis had decreased severity of disease [337]. The disease is self-limiting, and the mice that survive beyond day four show increased weight gain and are healthy by days 10-12 post-administration.

3.2. Genetically engineered models

3.2.1. IL-$10^{-/-}$

In 1993, Kuhn et al. discovered that mice deficient in the anti-inflammatory cytokine IL-10 spontaneously develop enterocolitis [213]. This model has been popular in IBD research and this genetic deficiency has been crossed onto many different genetic backgrounds of mouse [339-345]. The availability of different strains has highlighted the role that genetics plays in enterocolitis, as the severity of disease is strain dependent. The order of severity from most severe to least severe is as follows: C3Bir > 129 > BALB/c or NOD/Lt > C57BL/6 or C57BL/10. In addition to strain differences, development of entercolitis is also dependent on the microbiota, as GF IL-$10^{-/-}$ do not develop enterocolitis and disease is attenuated after administration of antibiotics to IL-$10^{-/-}$ mice harboring a conventional microbiota [346, 347]. The lack of IL-10 does not affect the development of B or T cells, but its absence does result in a lack of regulatory T cells [213, 348]. Studies to understand the development of disease in these mice have shown that B cells (while present in high numbers in the lamina propria) are not needed for the initiation of disease, but that disease is mediated by $CD4^+$ T cells [342, 349]. Transfer studies using RAG$2^{-/-}$ mice as recipients have specifically shown that naive $CD4^+$ T cells are capable of inducing colitis, and $CD45RB^{low}$ $CD4^+$ T cells from IL-$10^{-/-}$ mice can induce disease in these RAG$2^{-/-}$ mice

[348, 349]. This latter observation implicates IL-10 as a central mediator of regulatory T cells ($CD25^+$ $Foxp3^+$ $CD4^+$ T cells). It has also been shown that IL-12 and IFN-γ are needed for initiation but not the continuation of colitis [342, 350]. The increase in the production of IL-12 and IFN-γ along with undetectable levels of IL-4 indicates that the enterocolitis in these mice is mediated by a Th1 immune response, similar to that observed in humans with IBD [342, 346].

3.2.2. *Mdr1a*$^{-/-}$

In 1994, mice lacking the gene *mdr1a* were generated. This gene encodes a P-glycoprotein, which is a drug efflux pump, thus protecting host cells from the build-up of toxic compounds. It was noted later that these mice spontaneously develop a colitis similar to human IBD and that disease can be exacerbated by colonization with *Helicobacter bilis* [351, 352]. These *mdr1a*$^{-/-}$ mice have reduced growth rates compared to their WT counterparts and their histological lesions begin in the proximal colon and proceed distally as disease severity progresses. *Mdr1a*$^{-/-}$ males are more susceptible to the onset of severe disease than females [353, 354]. *Mdr1a*$^{-/-}$ mice also have increased epithelial permeability and reduced phosphorylation of both occludin and ZO-1, tight junction proteins, compared to WT counterparts [354]. They exhibit increased bacterial translocation with bacteria detected in both the spleen and lymph nodes that correlates with disease severity. Therefore, the induction of disease is associated with a defect in the epithelial barrier function of the GI tract. In addition to the similar disease progression found in IBD patients, studying these mice are of interest because the human MDR1 gene has been mapped on a loci that that is associated with susceptibility of IBD, although this relationship is under debate [355-358].

3.2.3. TRUC

TRUC mice are both T-bet$^{-/-}$ and RAG$^{-/-}$ and spontaneously develop colitis by four weeks of age [359, 360]. T-bet (T-box expressed in T cells) is a transcription factor that aids in the development of a Th1 response [359]. These mice have increased permeability of their colonic epithelium that increases with age and increased rate of epithelial cell death. Microscopically, there is inflammatory cell infiltrate, goblet cell dropout, crypt loss, and the presences of ulcers. The only cytokine elevated in these mice is TNF-α and disease can be ameliorated using an anti-TNF-α antibody. The microbiota also contributes to disease in this model, as treatment with antibiotics was able to "cure" the mice of their colitis. Additionally, the TRUC colitic microbiota can be horizontally transferred to both WT and RAG$^{-/-}$ mice, and 16S rRNA analysis of feces from TRUC mice revealed that the presence of *Klebsiella pneumoniae* and *Proteus mirabilis* correlate with colitis. Interestingly, GF TRUC mice colonized with these two organisms alone do not develop colitis unless a more complete microbiota is present [361].

3.3. $CD45RB^{hi}$ $CD4^+$ T-cell transfer model

C.B.-17 *scid* mice administered $CD45RB^{hi}$ $CD4^+$ T cells develop a wasting disease which is not seen if $CD45RB^{lo}$ $CD4^+$ T cells or $CD45RB^{hi}$ $CD8^+$ T cells are adoptively transferred [362-364]. Disease occurs three to five weeks post-administration and is limited to the large intestine. The mucosa, submucosa, and muscularis all presented with inflammatory cell infiltrates (macrophages and $CD4^+$ T cells predominately), and there was also a loss of goblet cells, epithelial cell hyperplasia, and deep fissure ulcers. Elevated levels of IFN-γ were present in these mice, and treatment with anti-IFN-γ or anti-TNF (α and β) antibodies ameliorated disease in these mice. However, the protection garnered by using the antibodies was not as great as when $CD45RB^{lo}$ $CD4^+$ T cells were transferred along with $CD45RB^{hi}$ $CD4^+$ T cells [362]. This disease type mimics CD with respect to the type of inflammatory response generated (Th1) and the type of intestinal inflammation present (transmural infiltrate of $CD4^+$ T cells) [365]. There is also a definite microbial component in this model of disease, as restricted microbiota mice have less severe disease as compared to their SPF counterparts [364].

3.4. Bacterial-induced models

3.4.1. Helicobacter spp.

Although not considered a microbial cause of IBD, the presence of *Helicobacter* spp. does adjuvant or predispose mice to the onset of colitis in some models. In our lab, we utilize a dual hit model of colitis consisting of both *Helicobacter bilis* colonization and low-dose (1.5%) DSS to elicit colitis, as shown in Figure 8 [366].

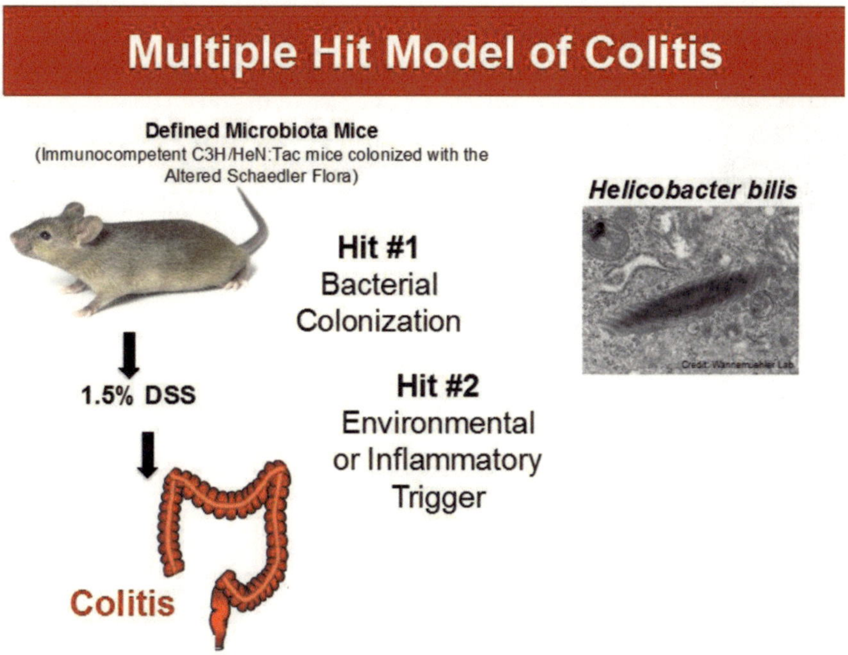

Figure 8. To increase sensitivity to a colitic insult, ASF-bearing C3H/HeN:Tac mice were colonized with a bacterial provocateur, *Helicobater bilis*. An otherwise non-colitic low dose of DSS is then administered resulting in colitis.

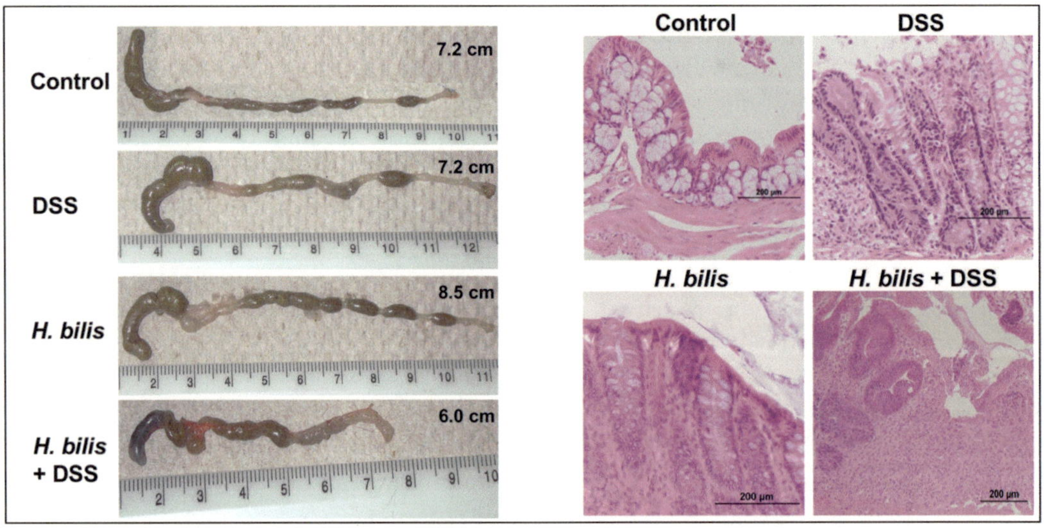

Figure 9. Mice colonized with *Helicobacter bilis* and subsequently administered a low dose of DSS exhibit colitis that is not seen with *H. bilis* or DSS alone. Disease is characterized grossly by colonic shortening, edema, cecal atrophy, enlarged lymphoid aggregates, and blood present in the contents. Microscopically, the disease presents with inflammatory cell infiltrate, crypt hyperplasia, glandular dropout, and cellular erosion

It has been noted that colonization of mice with *H. bilis* alone can change mucosal gene expression and alter the immune response in C3H/HeN mice bearing the altered Schaedler's flora (ASF) [366, 369]. Genes involved in T cell receptor signaling, the survival and activation of peripheral B cells, and chemotaxis are a few examples of the host genes that were upregulated by *H. bilis* colonization. Genes that were down regulated were involved in fatty acid metabolism and detoxification. After *H. bilis* colonization, serum antibodies directed at antigens derived from members of the ASF are induced [366, 369]. *H. hepaticus* colonization of A/JCr mice also induced changes in gene expression in the cecum, with female mice being more susceptible to the onset of disease [370, 371].

It appears that an over zealous host response to the introduction of the novel organism (i.e., provocateur) predisposes certain strains of mice for the onset of typholocoltiis following a secondary colitic insult. In a study comparing A/JCr mice (that develop mild inflammation) to C57BL/6 (who do not develop inflammation) mice, cecal gene expression profiles revealed that A/JCr mice had more genes differentially regulated (176) compared to C57BL/6 (80). Differentially expressed genes were predominantly those associated with immune response, chemotaxis, signal transduction, and antigen processing in the A/JCr mice while the genes upregulated in the C57BL/6 mice were predominately associated with immunoglobulin production.

In the *mdr1a*$^{-/-}$ mouse, it is not simply the presence of *Helicobacter* that results in the induction of colitis but the specific species of *Helicobacter* influences the induction of a differential immune response. In *mdr1a*$^{-/-}$ mice, *H. bilis* colonization causes colitis as early as three weeks post-infection, whereas *H. hepaticus* colonization ameliorated the severity of colitis in these mice compared to the uninfected control *mdr1a*$^{-/-}$ mice [352]. The disease phenotypes between spontaneous versus *Helicobacter*-induced colitis in *mdr1a*$^{-/-}$ mice were different, with epithelial ulceration not present in the *Helicobacter*-induced colitis. When *mdr1a*$^{-/-}$ mice were co-colonized with both *Helicobacter* species, the morbidity and mortality rate was between that of mice colonized by either *H. bilis* or *H. hepaticus* and the colitis that developed was characterized by dysplasia [372]. *H. bilis* was also able to out compete *H. hepaticus in vivo* as evidenced by recovery of higher numbers of *H. bilis,* suggesting that these two species may compete for similar niches in the GIT.

Additionally, colonization of IL-10$^{-/-}$ C57BL/6 mice with *Helicobacter* species results in the induction of colitis in otherwise disease-free mice [373]. It was also shown that the onset and severity of colitis was species specific in relation to colonization by *H. bilis* or *H. hepaticus* [374]. With respect to C3Bir.129 IL-10$^{-/-}$ mice, the presence of *Helicobacter* spp. is required for the spontaneous onset of disease [339]. Further studies show that colonization of RAG1$^{-/-}$ mice with *Helicobacter* species fails to elicit clinical signs of disease after nine months of colonization and only very mild colonic inflammation was detected at necropsy [374]. Taken together, these observations indicate that disease induction can be mediated by an aberrant adaptive immune response initiated by bacterial provocateurs entering an otherwise stable host-microbe environment.

3.4.2. *Brachyspira hyodysenteriae*

Similar to the need for the a resident microbiota in the TRUC model of colitis, mice colonized with *Brachyspira hyodysenteriae* also require the presence of a microbiota for the induction of typhlocolitis. *B. hyodysenteriae* is an anaerobic spirochete that is the causative agent of swine dysentery [375]. While the pathogenesis of *B. hyodysenteriae* is associated with the production of a ß-hemolysin [376], disease does not develop in the absence of a resident microbiota as was demonstrated by the inoculation of germfree pigs [377-379]. The importance of the microbiota was further demonstrated when the microbiota of C3H/HeSnJ or BALB/c mice was depleted by adding a cocktail of antibiotics (rifampicin, colistin, spectinomycin, spiramycin, and vancomycin) to their drinking water. As can be seen in Figure 10, the antibiotic cocktail depleted the numbers of Gram-positive, Gram-negative, and strict anaerobes by as much as 5 to 7 $\log_{10}$ (Nibbelink and Wannemuehler, unpublished observations). On day seven, antibiotic treated and sham treated mice were inoculated with 1 x 10^8 *B. hyodysenteirae* strain B204 and severity of disease was evaluated at 5, 10, and 15 days post-infection (DPI). As can be seen in Figure 11, the sham-treated mice developed severe typhlocolitis while the antibiotic treated mice had no lesions. At 15 DPI, the antibiotics were withdrawn from the drinking water of the remaining *B. hyodysenteriae*-infected mice to allow the microbiota to recover. On day 30 PI, the mice that had been treated with antibiotics through 15 DPI now presented with severe typhlocolitis. The presence and severity of typhlocolitis in these mice correlated with the presence of TNF-specific mRNA in the cecal tissue of the *B. hyodysenteriae*-infected mice (data not shown). Lastly, *B. hyodysenteriae*-induced typhlocolitis could also be prevented when the host's inflammatory response was inhibited [380, 381]. Collectively, these observations indicate that certain bacterial provocateurs (*K. pneumoniae, P. mirabilis,* and *B. hyodysenteriae*) may fail to induce disease in the absence of an appropriate resident microbiota. As depicted in Figure 12, the etiology of colitis is complex and may require the presence of a microbial provocateur, the resident microbiota, and a host inflammatory response.

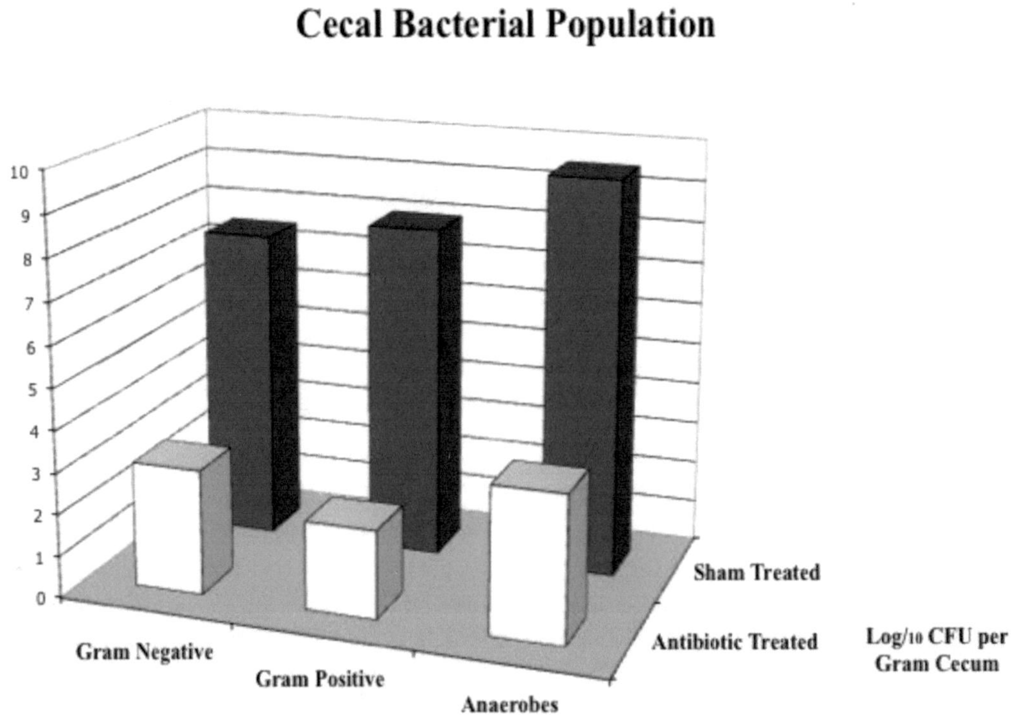

Figure 10. To assess the role of the microbiota in *Brachyspira hyodysenteriae*-induced typhlocolitis, C3H/HeSnJ mice were treated with an antibiotic cocktail to deplete the resident microbiota. Six days later, mice were infected with *B. hyodysenteriae*. The data indicate that there was a five to seven $\log_{10}$ reduction in the resident microbiota.

3.5. Conventional mice

The majority of commercially available mice harbor a "conventional" microbiota. This simply means that the composition of the community is unknown. There are different types of conventionally-reared mice. For example, Taconic Farms maintain two types of conventional microbiota mice, restricted flora™ (RF) and murine pathogen free™ (PF). RF mice are not colonized by β-hemolytic *Streptococcus* species, *K. pneumoniae, K. oxytoca, Pseudomonas aeruginosa,* or *Staphylococcus aureus.* Mice that are PF are *Helicobacter* free but can contain organisms not found in RF mice [382]. Additionally, mice on the same background purchased from different vendors can harbor different microbiota, as highlighted in work by Ivanov and colleagues demonstrating the presence of SFB in C57BL/6 mice from Taconic but not Jackson

http://dx.doi.org/10.5772/53920

Laboratories [54]. This lack of consistency in microbiota from mice of the same strain has even been identified at different facilities from the same vendor (Overstreet and Wannemuehler unpublished observation). Therefore, comparison of studies evaluating the microbiota of mice are difficult because there are hundreds of unknown bacterial species present in the murine microbiota and there is no standardized microbiota used by investigators. The advent of next-gen sequencing has helped to alleviate some of this challenge as all of the organisms in the gut can be identified based on 16S rRNA sequences. However, it still does not resolve the issue related to the use of disparate strains of mice with varying microbiota from different suppliers.

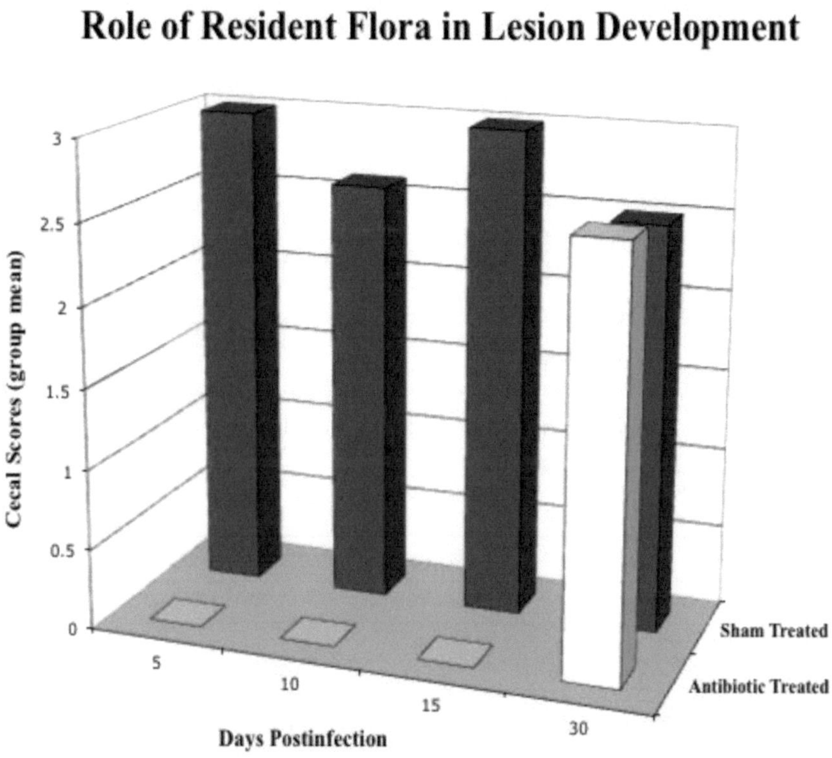

Figure 11. Assessment of *Brachyspira hyodysenteriae*-induced typhlocolitis in C3H/HeSnJ mice treated with an antibiotic cocktail. While *B. hyodysenteriae* colonized the antibiotic-treated mice to the same extent as it did the sham-treated mice, there was no evidence of typhlocolitis in the antibiotic treated mice through 15 days post-infection (DPI). However, 15 days after the antibiotics were withdrawn (30 DPI), the mice that had been treated with the antibiotics had developed severe disease once the microbiota recovered.

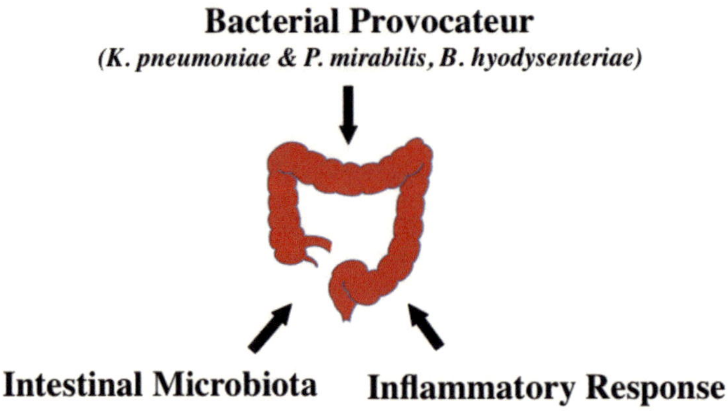

Figure 12. The pathogenesis of inflammatory bowel disease is complex. Studies from animal models indicate that the etiology of disease involves the presence of a bacterial provocateur, the resident microbiota, and the host response.

3.6. Germfree mice

GF mice are completely devoid of microbial life. As mentioned previously, this does grossly affect the anatomy of these mice, which is most evident by the enlarged cecum being the most prominent feature [34]. The discovery that many GF mouse strains that carry genetic deficiencies associated with IBD (notably the IL-$10^{-/-}$) do not develop colitis has led to the popularity of GF models to study the role of bacteria in the pathogenesis of IBD [346]. To determine if an organism is capable of initiating colitis, GF mice are monoassociated with a single bacterial species and then monitored for clinical signs of disease. Some of the bacterial strains used to date to evaluate their ability to induce disease in IL-$10^{-/-}$ mice are shown in Table 3.

Organism	Colitis Severity	Time of Disease Onset	Reference
Enterococcus faecalis	Severe	10-12 weeks p.i.	[383, 384]
Escherichia coli (from WT SPF mouse)	Moderate	3 weeks p.i.	[383]
Pseudomonas flourescens	No disease	-	[383]
Helicobacter hepaticus	No disease	-	[385]
Lactococcus lactis	No disease	-	[384]
Viridans group *Streptococcus*	No disease	-	[386]
Clostridium sordellii	No disease	-	[386]
Bacteroides vulgatus	No disease	-	[386]
Bifidobacterium animalis	Mild	23 weeks p.i.	[387]
Bifidobacterium infantis	No disease	-	[387]

Table 3. Bacterial strains used to monoassociate GF mice to examine the ability of the strain to induce colitis

Although the information gathered from these studies has been useful in analyzing the immune response to specific organisms, trying to relate the resultant disease to that characteristic of IBD is marginal at best because of the differences in the complexities of the microbiota. IBD itself is a multi-factorial disease and it has been fairly well-established that the role of bacteria in IBD is associated with a shift in community dynamics (i.e., dysbiosis) and not the presence/absence of one particular species. A perfect example of this complexity is the fact that *K. pneumonia* and *P. mirabilis* fail to induce colitis in GF TRUC mice (Figure 12) [361].

3.7. Defined microbiota mice

Also referred to as gnotobiotic, defined microbiota (DM) mice have a microbiota in which all members are known and are housed in flexible film isolators to maintain this status [388]. One of the most established DM mouse models harbors the "Altered Schaedler Flora" (ASF). Developed by Dr. Rodger Orcutt and colleagues as a request from the National Cancer Institute, these eight microbial species were originally used to standardized the microbiota of the rodents used as founders in their breeding colonies [389]. He chose to modify his mentor's (Dr. Russ Schaedler) cocktail of organisms by eliminating facultative anaerobes (*Escherichia coli* var. mutabilis and *Streptococcus fecalis*) and the anaerobic *Streptococcus* and *Clostridia* spp. that formed the original "Schaedler Flora". Dr. Orcutt added four additional species (see Table 4 below). This resulted in an anaerobic community devoid of any cocci or spore-forming blunt ended rods, which comprise the main isolator contaminants, making it easier to monitor for contamination of the gnotobiotic isolator. This new community was dubbed the "Altered Schaedler Flora" and was utilized in the breeding stock by major commercial mouse vendors in the US in that era. The ASF consists of members with different morphologies so that identification using fecal smears for microscopic evaluation was possible. The members, whose full genomes have yet to be sequenced, have had 16S rRNA sequencing performed to assist with the identification of the organisms [390].

Multiple studies have demonstrated the stability of this community both when maintained under gnotobiotic housing conditions or when part of a conventionalized microbiota [391-394]. In our own lab, all eight ASF members have been stably maintained in our breeding colony for over 12 years, indicating the remarkable stability of this model microbial community over time. PCR primers have been developed for each of the eight ASF members as well as group-specific FISH probes [391, 394]. Therefore, the effects of any perturbation of the ASF, such as with antibiotics, inflammation, or CAM treatments can be monitored by bacterial abundance as well as spatial redistribution using qPCR and FISH, respectively. All of the organisms can be cultured and whole cell sonicates produced to measure the immune response to each organism individually (something that is impossible to do with a conventional microbiota). Additionally, this community, although limited in scope, is able to synthesize all the metabolites needed by the mouse and maintains near normal cecal shape and size, something not possible in GF mice. It is important to note, however, that some of the characteristics of ASF mice are more similar to GF than conventional mice. Both ASF and GF mice have high fecal tryptic activity and possess the ability to degrade mucin and β-aspartylglycine. They also cannot convert bilirubin to urobilinogens or cholesterol to coprostanol [395]. Interestingly, this same research team compared these parameters in CD patients versus healthy subjects and the characteristics of the microbial metabolism associated with the microbiota of CD patients were very similar to those of the ASF [396]. This study suggests that there is benefit to the use of the ASF in mouse models of IBD.

Other defined microbiota mouse studies have been published [397-400]. A study using ten bacterial species specifically chosen for their metabolic function were used to colonize GF mice [397]. Using microbial RNA-seq, the authors were able to build a model relating perturbation of the microbial community to changes in diet. By modeling the functional capacity of a gnotobiotic community under different conditions, this model and similar approaches can be used to unravel the operational dynamics of the gut microbiome with respect to nutrient utilization such that the microbiota might be manipulated to improve human and animal health [397]. Another study colonized mice with *E. rectale* and *B. thetaiotamicron*, and the authors then assessed changes in bacterial gene expression using Affymetrix GeneChips to show that the cross-talk between these two organisms affected up- and down-regulated genes in response to one another.

Strain	Identity
ASF356	Most closely related to *Clostridium propionicum* (92% max identity) [390] Member of *Clostridium* cluster XIV
ASF360	*Lactobacillus intestinalis* (99% max identity) [401]
ASF361	*Lactobacillus murinus [390]*
ASF457	*Mucispirillum schaedleri [402]*
ASF492	*Eubacterium plexicaudatum* [403] Member of *Clostridium* cluster XIV
ASF500	*Clostridium* sp. with no known related organism in GenBank Database [390]
ASF502	Most closely related to *Ruminococcus gnavus* (92% max identity) [390] Member of *Clostridium* cluster XIV
ASF519	*Parabacteroides goldsteinii* (99% max identity) [404, 405]

Table 4. Members of the altered Schaedler flora

Three human commensals, *E. coli, B. longum,* and *L. johnsonii,* have also been used to colonize GF mice to create a gnotobiotic community [398]. This community was used to identify the effects that the introduction of novel organisms has on the community dynamic. When colonized with a second *Lactobacillus, L. paracasei,* it was noted that both *Lactobacillus* spp. were able to co-habitate reaching similar fecal titers. However, that was not the same when a fifth organism was added, a second *B. longum* strain. This new strain was only maintained in the mouse at detectable levels for three days. Lastly, a second *E. coli* strain was added to the original community of three. This new *E. coli* reached the highest titer of any organism in the community. This addition caused the reduction of the original *E. coli* to drop to undetectable levels at day two post-addition. Later *L. johnsonii* also reached undetectable levels. *B. longum* decreased initially but them returned to normal titer levels. Lastly, when the original tri-associated mice were exposed to conventional mouse feces, the numbers of the original three organisms decreased.

In this chapter, we have discussed the three most common types of microbiota available for use in IBD research. Because it is clear that IBD is associated with an imbalance in the microbial community, the use of GF mice (which cannot mimic a "community" dynamic) may be less useful in unraveling the complexities of a multifactorial disease in place of defined microbiota and conventional microbiota mice. Ideally, one would want to use a simplified community (such as the ASF) where the actions of all organisms can be assessed. To understand the dynamic interactions that occur between microbes and between the microbes and the host, it will be important to start with what is known in order to begin the unraveling the enigmatic nature of gut health and disease.

Author details

Anne-Marie C. Overstreet[1], Amanda E. Ramer-Tait[3], Albert E. Jergens[2] and Michael J. Wannemuehler[1]

1 Department of Veterinary Microbiology and Preventive Medicine, Iowa State University, Ames, IA, USA

2 Department of Veterinary Clinical Sciences, Iowa State University, Ames, IA, USA

3 Department of Food Science and Technology, University of Nebraska-Lincoln, Lincoln, NE, USA

References

[1] Whitman, W.B., Coleman, D.C., and Wiebe, W.J., Prokaryotes: the unseen majority. Proceedings of the National Academy of Sciences of the United States of America, 1998. 95(12): p. 6578-83.

[2] Savage, D.C., Microbial ecology of the gastrointestinal tract. Annual Review of Microbiology, 1977. 31: p. 107-33.

[3] Zhu, B., Wang, X., and Li, L., Human gut microbiome: the second genome of human body. Protein & Cell, 2010. 1(8): p. 718-25.

[4] Structure, function and diversity of the healthy human microbiome. Nature, 2012. 486(7402): p. 207-14.

[5] Turnbaugh, P.J., Ley, R.E., Hamady, M., Fraser-Liggett, C.M., Knight, R., et al., The human microbiome project. Nature, 2007. 449(7164): p. 804-10.

[6] Peterson, J., Garges, S., Giovanni, M., McInnes, P., Wang, L., et al., The NIH Human Microbiome Project. Genome research, 2009. 19(12): p. 2317-23.

[7] Moore, S.J. and Warren, M.J., The anaerobic biosynthesis of vitamin B12. Biochemical Society Transactions, 2012. 40(3): p. 581-6.

[8] Rossi, M., Amaretti, A., and Raimondi, S., Folate production by probiotic bacteria. Nutrients, 2011. 3(1): p. 118-34.

[9] LeBlanc, J.G., Laino, J.E., del Valle, M.J., Vannini, V., van Sinderen, D., et al., B-group vitamin production by lactic acid bacteria--current knowledge and potential applications. Journal of Applied Microbiology, 2011. 111(6): p. 1297-309.

[10] Morishita, T., Tamura, N., Makino, T., and Kudo, S., Production of menaquinones by lactic acid bacteria. Journal of Dairy Science, 1999. 82(9): p. 1897-903.

[11] Turnbaugh, P.J., Ley, R.E., Mahowald, M.A., Magrini, V., Mardis, E.R., et al., An obesity-associated gut microbiome with increased capacity for energy harvest. Nature, 2006. 444(7122): p. 1027-31.

[12] Nicholson, J.K., Holmes, E., Kinross, J., Burcelin, R., Gibson, G., et al., Host-gut microbiota metabolic interactions. Science, 2012. 336(6086): p. 1262-7.

[13] Bene, L., Falus, A., Baffy, N., and Fulop, A.K., Cellular and molecular mechanisms in the two major forms of inflammatory bowel disease. Pathology Oncology Research, 2011. 17(3): p. 463-72.

[14] Eckburg, P.B., Bik, E.M., Bernstein, C.N., Purdom, E., Dethlefsen, L., et al., Diversity of the human intestinal microbial flora. Science, 2005. 308(5728): p. 1635-8.

[15] Hold, G.L., Pryde, S.E., Russell, V.J., Furrie, E., and Flint, H.J., Assessment of microbial diversity in human colonic samples by 16S rDNA sequence analysis. FEMS Microbiology Ecology, 2002. 39(1): p. 33-9.

[16] O'Hara, A.M. and Shanahan, F., The gut flora as a forgotten organ. EMBO Reports, 2006. 7(7): p. 688-93.

[17] Suau, A., Bonnet, R., Sutren, M., Godon, J.J., Gibson, G.R., et al., Direct analysis of genes encoding 16S rRNA from complex communities reveals many novel molecular species within the human gut. Applied and Environmental Microbiology, 1999. 65(11): p. 4799-807.

[18] Frank, D.N., St Amand, A.L., Feldman, R.A., Boedeker, E.C., Harpaz, N., et al., Molecular-phylogenetic characterization of microbial community imbalances in human inflammatory bowel diseases. Proceedings of the National Academy of Sciences of the United States of America, 2007. 104(34): p. 13780-5.

[19] Miller, T.L. and Wolin, M.J., Enumeration of *Methanobrevibacter smithii* in human feces. Archives of Microbiology, 1982. 131(1): p. 14-8.

[20] Schaedler, R.W., Dubos, R., and Costello, R., The Development of the Bacterial Flora in the Gastrointestinal Tract of Mice. The Journal of Experimental Medicine, 1965. 122: p. 59-66.

[21] Savage, D.C., Factors involved in colonization of the gut epithelial surface. The American Journal of Clinical Nutrition, 1978. 31(10 Suppl): p. S131-S135.

[22] Dominguez-Bello, M.G., Costello, E.K., Contreras, M., Magris, M., Hidalgo, G., et al., Delivery mode shapes the acquisition and structure of the initial microbiota across multiple body habitats in newborns. Proceedings of the National Academy of Sciences of the United States of America, 2010. 107(26): p. 11971-5.

[23] Gronlund, M.-M., Lehtonen, O.-P., Eerola, E., and Kero, P., Fecal Microflora in Healthy Infants Born by Different Methods of Delivery: Permanent Changes in Intestinal Flora After Cesarean Delivery. Journal of Pediatric Gastroenterology and Nutrition, 1999. 28(1): p. 19-25.

[24] Dominguez-Bello, M.G., Blaser, M.J., Ley, R.E., and Knight, R., Development of the human gastrointestinal microbiota and insights from high-throughput sequencing. Gastroenterology, 2011. 140(6): p. 1713-9.

[25] Lindsay, J.A., *Clostridium perfringens* type A enterotoxin (CPE): more than just explosive diarrhea. Critical Reviews in Microbiology, 1996. 22(4): p. 257-77.

[26] Watson, J., Jones, R., and Cortes, C., Community-Associated Methicillin-Resistant *Staphylococcus aureus* Infection among Healthy newborns-Chicago and Los Angeles County, 2004. Journal of the American Medical Association, 2006. 296(1): p. 36-38.

[27] van Nimwegen, F.A., Penders, J., Stobberingh, E.E., Postma, D.S., Koppelman, G.H., et al., Mode and place of delivery, gastrointestinal microbiota, and their influence on asthma and atopy. The Journal of Allergy and Clinical Immunology, 2011. 128(5): p. 948-55 e1-3.

[28] Magnus, M.C., Haberg, S.E., Stigum, H., Nafstad, P., London, S.J., et al., Delivery by Cesarean section and early childhood respiratory symptoms and disorders: the Norwegian mother and child cohort study. American Journal of Epidemiology, 2011. 174(11): p. 1275-85.

[29] Bezirtzoglou, E., Tsiotsias, A., and Welling, G.W., Microbiota profile in feces of breast- and formula-fed newborns by using fluorescence in situ hybridization (FISH). Anaerobe, 2011. 17(6): p. 478-82.

[30] Fallani, M., Amarri, S., Uusijarvi, A., Adam, R., Khanna, S., et al., Determinants of the human infant intestinal microbiota after the introduction of first complementary foods in infant samples from five European centres. Microbiology, 2011. 157(Pt 5): p. 1385-92.

[31] Thompson, G.R. and Trexler, P.C., Gastrointestinal structure and function in germ-free or gnotobiotic animals. Gut, 1971. 12(3): p. 230-5.

[32] Lesher, S., Walburg, H.E., Jr., and Sacher, G.A., Jr., Generation Cycle in the Duodenal Crypt Cells of Germ-Free and Conventional Mice. Nature, 1964. 202: p. 884-6.

[33] Savage, D.C., Siegel, J.E., Snellen, J.E., and Whitt, D.D., Transit time of epithelial cells in the small intestines of germfree mice and ex-germfree mice associated with indigenous microorganisms. Applied and Environmental Microbiology, 1981. 42(6): p. 996-1001.

[34] Schaedler, R.W., Dubs, R., and Costello, R., Association of Germfree Mice with Bacteria Isolated from Normal Mice. The Journal of Experimental Medicine, 1965. 122: p. 77-82.

[35] Wostmann, B.S. and Bruckner-Kardoss, E., Oxidation-reduction potentials in cecal contents of germfree and conventional rats. Proceedings of the Society for Experimental Biology and Medicine, 1966. 121(4): p. 1111-4.

[36] Gustafsson, B.E., Daft, F.S., Mc, D.E., Smith, J.C., and Fitzgerald, R.J., Effects of vitamin K-active compounds and intestinal microorganisms in vitamin K-deficient germfree rats. The Journal of Nutrition, 1962. 78: p. 461-8.

[37] Abrams, G.D. and Bishop, J.E., Effect of the normal microbial flora on the resistance of the small intestine to infection. Journal of Bacteriology, 1966. 92(6): p. 1604-8.

[38] Coates, M.E., Gnotobiotic animals in nutrition research. The Proceedings of the Nutrition Society, 1973. 32(2): p. 53-8.

[39] Bauer, H., Horowitz, R.E., Levenson, S.M., and Popper, H., The response of the lymphatic tissue to the microbial flora. Studies on germfree mice. The American Journal of Pathology, 1963. 42: p. 471-83.

[40] Horowitz, R.E., Bauer, H., Paronetto, F., Abrams, G.D., Watkins, K.C., et al., The Response of the Lymphatic Tissue to Bacterial Antigen. Studies in Germfree Mice. The American Journal of Pathology, 1964. 44: p. 747-61.

[41] Bauer, H., Paronetto, F., Burns, W.A., and Einheber, A., The enhancing effect of the microbial flora on macrophage function and the immune response. A study in germfree mice. The Journal of Experimental Medicine, 1966. 123(6): p. 1013-24.

[42] Johansson, M.E., Larsson, J.M., and Hansson, G.C., The two mucus layers of colon are organized by the MUC2 mucin, whereas the outer layer is a legislator of host-microbial interactions. Proceedings of the National Academy of Sciences of the United States of America, 2011. 108 Suppl 1: p. 4659-65.

[43] Atuma, C., Strugala, V., Allen, A., and Holm, L., The adherent gastrointestinal mucus gel layer: thickness and physical state *in vivo*. American Journal of Physiology, 2001. 280(5): p. G922-9.

[44] Hansson, G.C. and Johansson, M.E., The inner of the two Muc2 mucin-dependent mucus layers in colon is devoid of bacteria. Gut Microbes, 2010. 1(1): p. 51-54.

[45] Van der Sluis, M., De Koning, B.A., De Bruijn, A.C., Velcich, A., Meijerink, J.P., et al., Muc2-deficient mice spontaneously develop colitis, indicating that MUC2 is critical for colonic protection. Gastroenterology, 2006. 131(1): p. 117-29.

[46] Edelblum, K.L. and Turner, J.R., The tight junction in inflammatory disease: communication breakdown. Current Opinion in Pharmacology, 2009. 9(6): p. 715-20.

[47] Garcia-Lafuente, A., Antolin, M., Guarner, F., Crespo, E., Salas, A., et al., Incrimination of anaerobic bacteria in the induction of experimental colitis. The American Journal of Physiology, 1997. 272(1 Pt 1): p. G10-5.

[48] Wlodarska, M., Willing, B., Keeney, K.M., Menendez, A., Bergstrom, K.S., et al., Antibiotic treatment alters the colonic mucus layer and predisposes the host to exacerbated *Citrobacter rodentium*-induced colitis. Infection and Immunity, 2011. 79(4): p. 1536-45.

[49] Sturm, A. and Dignass, A.U., Epithelial restitution and wound healing in inflammatory bowel disease. World Journal of Gastroenterology 2008. 14(3): p. 348-53.

[50] Kim, Y.S. and Ho, S.B., Intestinal goblet cells and mucins in health and disease: recent insights and progress. Current Gastroenterology Reports, 2010. 12(5): p. 319-30.

[51] Round, J.L., Lee, S.M., Li, J., Tran, G., Jabri, B., et al., The Toll-like receptor 2 pathway establishes colonization by a commensal of the human microbiota. Science, 2011. 332(6032): p. 974-7.

[52] Round, J.L. and Mazmanian, S.K., Inducible Foxp3+ regulatory T-cell development by a commensal bacterium of the intestinal microbiota. Proceedings of the National Academy of Sciences of the United States of America, 2010. 107(27): p. 12204-9.

[53] Atarashi, K., Tanoue, T., Shima, T., Imaoka, A., Kuwahara, T., et al., Induction of colonic regulatory T cells by indigenous *Clostridium* species. Science, 2011. 331(6015): p. 337-41.

[54] Ivanov, II, Atarashi, K., Manel, N., Brodie, E.L., Shima, T., et al., Induction of intestinal Th17 cells by segmented filamentous bacteria. Cell, 2009. 139(3): p. 485-98.

[55] Backhed, F., Ding, H., Wang, T., Hooper, L.V., Koh, G.Y., et al., The gut microbiota as an environmental factor that regulates fat storage. Proceedings of the National Academy of Sciences of the United States of America, 2004. 101(44): p. 15718-23.

[56] Oresic, M., Seppanen-Laakso, T., Yetukuri, L., Backhed, F., and Hanninen, V., Gut microbiota affects lens and retinal lipid composition. Experimental Eye Research, 2009. 89(5): p. 604-7.

[57] Rubinstein, R., Howard, A.V., and Wrong, O.M., *In vivo* dialysis of faeces as a method of stool analysis. IV. The organic anion component. Clinical Science, 1969. 37(2): p. 549-64.

[58] Barcenilla, A., Pryde, S.E., Martin, J.C., Duncan, S.H., Stewart, C.S., et al., Phylogenetic relationships of butyrate-producing bacteria from the human gut. Applied and Environmental Microbiology, 2000. 66(4): p. 1654-61.

[59] Hold, G.L., Schwiertz, A., Aminov, R.I., Blaut, M., and Flint, H.J., Oligonucleotide probes that detect quantitatively significant groups of butyrate-producing bacteria in human feces. Applied and Environmental Microbiology, 2003. 69(7): p. 4320-4.

[60] Suau, A., Rochet, V., Sghir, A., Gramet, G., Brewaeys, S., et al., *Fusobacterium prausnitzii* and related species represent a dominant group within the human fecal flora. Systematic and Applied Microbiology, 2001. 24(1): p. 139-45.

[61] Louis, P. and Flint, H.J., Diversity, metabolism and microbial ecology of butyrate-producing bacteria from the human large intestine. FEMS Microbiology Letters, 2009. 294(1): p. 1-8.

[62] Twarog, R. and Wolfe, R.S., Role of butyryl phosphate in the energy metabolism of *Clostridium Tetanomorphum*. Journal of Bacteriology, 1963. 86: p. 112-7.

[63] Twarog, R. and Wolfe, R.S., Enzymatic phosphorylation of butyrate. The Journal of Biological Chemistry, 1962. 237: p. 2474-7.

[64] Louis, P., Duncan, S.H., McCrae, S.I., Millar, J., Jackson, M.S., et al., Restricted distribution of the butyrate kinase pathway among butyrate-producing bacteria from the human colon. Journal of Bacteriology, 2004. 186(7): p. 2099-106.

[65] Duncan, S.H., Barcenilla, A., Stewart, C.S., Pryde, S.E., and Flint, H.J., Acetate utilization and butyryl coenzyme A (CoA):acetate-CoA transferase in butyrate-producing bacteria from the human large intestine. Applied and Environmental Microbiology, 2002. 68(10): p. 5186-90.

[66] Roediger, W.E., Role of anaerobic bacteria in the metabolic welfare of the colonic mucosa in man. Gut, 1980. 21(9): p. 793-8.

[67] Roediger, W.E., Utilization of nutrients by isolated epithelial cells of the rat colon. Gastroenterology, 1982. 83(2): p. 424-9.

[68] Fitch, M.D. and Fleming, S.E., Metabolism of short-chain fatty acids by rat colonic mucosa *in vivo*. The American Journal of Physiology, 1999. 277(1 Pt 1): p. G31-40.

[69] Clausen, M.R. and Mortensen, P.B., Kinetic studies on colonocyte metabolism of short chain fatty acids and glucose in ulcerative colitis. Gut, 1995. 37(5): p. 684-9.

[70] Donohoe, D.R., Garge, N., Zhang, X., Sun, W., O'Connell, T.M., et al., The microbiome and butyrate regulate energy metabolism and autophagy in the mammalian colon. Cell Metabolism, 2011. 13(5): p. 517-26.

[71] Mihaylova, M.M. and Shaw, R.J., The AMPK signalling pathway coordinates cell growth, autophagy and metabolism. Nature Cell biology, 2011. 13(9): p. 1016-23.

[72] Sealy, L. and Chalkley, R., The effect of sodium butyrate on histone modification. Cell, 1978. 14(1): p. 115-21.

[73] Riggs, M.G., Whittaker, R.G., Neumann, J.R., and Ingram, V.M., n-Butyrate causes histone modification in HeLa and Friend erythroleukaemia cells. Nature, 1977. 268(5619): p. 462-4.

[74] Kouraklis, G. and Theocharis, S., Histone deacetylase inhibitors: a novel target of anticancer therapy (review). Oncology Reports, 2006. 15(2): p. 489-94.

[75] Della Ragione, F., Criniti, V., Della Pietra, V., Borriello, A., Oliva, A., et al., Genes modulated by histone acetylation as new effectors of butyrate activity. FEBS Letters, 2001. 499(3): p. 199-204.

[76] Siavoshian, S., Segain, J.P., Kornprobst, M., Bonnet, C., Cherbut, C., et al., Butyrate and trichostatin A effects on the proliferation/differentiation of human intestinal epithelial cells: induction of cyclin D3 and p21 expression. Gut, 2000. 46(4): p. 507-14.

[77] Segain, J.P., Raingeard de la Bletiere, D., Bourreille, A., Leray, V., Gervois, N., et al., Butyrate inhibits inflammatory responses through NFkappaB inhibition: implications for Crohn's disease. Gut, 2000. 47(3): p. 397-403.

[78] Venkatraman, A., Ramakrishna, B.S., Shaji, R.V., Kumar, N.S., Pulimood, A., et al., Amelioration of dextran sulfate colitis by butyrate: role of heat shock protein 70 and NF-kappaB. American Journal of Physiology. Gastrointestinal and Liver Physiology, 2003. 285(1): p. G177-84.

[79] Luhrs, H., Gerke, T., Muller, J.G., Melcher, R., Schauber, J., et al., Butyrate inhibits NF-kappaB activation in lamina propria macrophages of patients with ulcerative colitis. Scandinavian Journal of Gastroenterology, 2002. 37(4): p. 458-66.

[80] Tong, X., Yin, L., and Giardina, C., Butyrate suppresses Cox-2 activation in colon cancer cells through HDAC inhibition. Biochemical and Biophysical Research Communications, 2004. 317(2): p. 463-71.

[81] Tehrani, A.B., Nezami, B.G., Gewirtz, A., and Srinivasan, S., Obesity and its associated disease: a role for microbiota? Neurogastroenterology and Motility 2012. 24(4): p. 305-11.

[82] Bradley, W.D., Zwingelstein, C., and Rondinone, C.M., The emerging role of the intestine in metabolic diseases. Archives of Physiology and Biochemistry, 2011. 117(3): p. 165-76.

[83] Dorer, M.S., Talarico, S., and Salama, N.R., *Helicobacter pylori's* unconventional role in health and disease. PLoS Pathogens, 2009. 5(10): p. e1000544.

[84] Hammer, H.F., Gut microbiota and inflammatory bowel disease. Digestive Diseases, 2011. 29(6): p. 550-3.

[85] Kaur, N., Chen, C.C., Luther, J., and Kao, J.Y., Intestinal dysbiosis in inflammatory bowel disease. Gut Microbes, 2011. 2(4): p. 211-6.

[86] Vanderploeg, R., Panaccione, R., Ghosh, S., and Rioux, K., Influences of intestinal bacteria in human inflammatory bowel disease. Infectious Disease Clinics of North America, 2010. 24(4): p. 977-93, ix.

[87] Nell, S., Suerbaum, S., and Josenhans, C., The impact of the microbiota on the pathogenesis of IBD: lessons from mouse infection models. Nature Reviews: Microbiology, 2010. 8(8): p. 564-77.

[88] Meadows, R., Gut bacteria may override genetic protections against diabetes. PLoS Biology, 2011. 9(12): p. e1001215.

[89] Harris, K., Kassis, A., Major, G., and Chou, C.J., Is the gut microbiota a new factor contributing to obesity and its metabolic disorders? Journal of Obesity, 2012. 2012: p. 879151.

[90] Crohn, B.B., Ginzburg, L., and Oppenheimer, G.D., Landmark article Oct 15, 1932. Regional ileitis. A pathological and clinical entity. By Burril B. Crohn, Leon Ginzburg, and Gordon D. Oppenheimer. The Journal of the American Medical Association, 1984. 251(1): p. 73-9.

[91] Molodecky, N.A., Soon, I.S., Rabi, D.M., Ghali, W.A., Ferris, M., et al., Increasing incidence and prevalence of the inflammatory bowel diseases with time, based on systematic review. Gastroenterology, 2012. 142(1): p. 46-54 e42; quiz e30.

[92] Lees, C.W., Barrett, J.C., Parkes, M., and Satsangi, J., New IBD genetics: common pathways with other diseases. Gut, 2011. 60(12): p. 1739-53.

[93] Franke, A., McGovern, D.P., Barrett, J.C., Wang, K., Radford-Smith, G.L., et al., Genome-wide meta-analysis increases to 71 the number of confirmed Crohn's disease susceptibility loci. Nature Genetics, 2010. 42(12): p. 1118-25.

[94] Anderson, C.A., Boucher, G., Lees, C.W., Franke, A., D'Amato, M., et al., Meta-analysis identifies 29 additional ulcerative colitis risk loci, increasing the number of confirmed associations to 47. Nature Genetics, 2011. 43(3): p. 246-52.

[95] Cadwell, K., Liu, J.Y., Brown, S.L., Miyoshi, H., Loh, J., et al., A key role for autophagy and the autophagy gene *Atg16l1* in mouse and human intestinal Paneth cells. Nature, 2008. 456(7219): p. 259-63.

[96] Biswas, A., Petnicki-Ocwieja, T., and Kobayashi, K.S., Nod2: a key regulator linking microbiota to intestinal mucosal immunity. Journal of Molecular Medicine, 2012. 90(1): p. 15-24.

[97] Ogura, Y., Inohara, N., Benito, A., Chen, F.F., Yamaoka, S., et al., Nod2, a Nod1/Apaf-1 family member that is restricted to monocytes and activates NF-kappaB. The Journal of Biological Chemistry, 2001. 276(7): p. 4812-8.

[98] Tada, H., Aiba, S., Shibata, K., Ohteki, T., and Takada, H., Synergistic effect of Nod1 and Nod2 agonists with toll-like receptor agonists on human dendritic cells to generate interleukin-12 and T helper type 1 cells. Infection and Immunity, 2005. 73(12): p. 7967-76.

[99] Hisamatsu, T., Suzuki, M., Reinecker, H.C., Nadeau, W.J., McCormick, B.A., et al., CARD15/NOD2 functions as an antibacterial factor in human intestinal epithelial cells. Gastroenterology, 2003. 124(4): p. 993-1000.

[100] Uehara, A., Fujimoto, Y., Fukase, K., and Takada, H., Various human epithelial cells express functional Toll-like receptors, NOD1 and NOD2 to produce anti-microbial peptides, but not proinflammatory cytokines. Molecular Immunology, 2007. 44(12): p. 3100-11.

[101] Inohara, N., Koseki, T., Lin, J., del Peso, L., Lucas, P.C., et al., An induced proximity model for NF-kappa B activation in the Nod1/RICK and RIP signaling pathways. The Journal of Biological Chemistry, 2000. 275(36): p. 27823-31.

[102] Petnicki-Ocwieja, T., Hrncir, T., Liu, Y.J., Biswas, A., Hudcovic, T., et al., Nod2 is required for the regulation of commensal microbiota in the intestine. Proceedings of the National Academy of Sciences of the United States of America, 2009. 106(37): p. 15813-8.

[103] Hampe, J., Franke, A., Rosenstiel, P., Till, A., Teuber, M., et al., A genome-wide association scan of nonsynonymous SNPs identifies a susceptibility variant for Crohn disease in ATG16L1. Nature Genetics, 2007. 39(2): p. 207-11.

[104] Deretic, V., Autophagy in innate and adaptive immunity. Trends in Immunology, 2005. 26(10): p. 523-8.

[105] Rioux, J.D., Xavier, R.J., Taylor, K.D., Silverberg, M.S., Goyette, P., et al., Genome-wide association study identifies new susceptibility loci for Crohn disease and implicates autophagy in disease pathogenesis. Nature Genetics, 2007. 39(5): p. 596-604.

[106] Lapaquette, P., Bringer, M.A., and Darfeuille-Michaud, A., Defects in autophagy favour adherent-invasive *Escherichia coli* persistence within macrophages leading to increased pro-inflammatory response. Cellular Microbiology, 2012. 14(6): p. 791-807.

[107] Kuballa, P., Huett, A., Rioux, J.D., Daly, M.J., and Xavier, R.J., Impaired autophagy of an intracellular pathogen induced by a Crohn's disease associated ATG16L1 variant. PloS One, 2008. 3(10): p. e3391.

[108] Sartor, R.B., Mechanisms of disease: pathogenesis of Crohn's disease and ulcerative colitis. Nature Clinical Practice. Gastroenterology & Hepatology, 2006. 3(7): p. 390-407.

[109] Fuss, I.J., Neurath, M., Boirivant, M., Klein, J.S., de la Motte, C., et al., Disparate CD4+ lamina propria (LP) lymphokine secretion profiles in inflammatory bowel disease. Crohn's disease LP cells manifest increased secretion of IFN-gamma, whereas ulcerative colitis LP cells manifest increased secretion of IL-5. Journal of Immunology, 1996. 157(3): p. 1261-70.

[110] Monteleone, G., Biancone, L., Marasco, R., Morrone, G., Marasco, O., et al., Interleukin 12 is expressed and actively released by Crohn's disease intestinal lamina propria mononuclear cells. Gastroenterology, 1997. 112(4): p. 1169-78.

[111] Okazawa, A., Kanai, T., Watanabe, M., Yamazaki, M., Inoue, N., et al., Th1-mediated intestinal inflammation in Crohn's disease may be induced by activation of lamina propria lymphocytes through synergistic stimulation of interleukin-12 and interleukin-18 without T cell receptor engagement. The American Journal of Gastroenterology, 2002. 97(12): p. 3108-17.

[112] Neurath, M.F., Fuss, I., Kelsall, B.L., Stuber, E., and Strober, W., Antibodies to interleukin 12 abrogate established experimental colitis in mice. The Journal of Experimental Medicine, 1995. 182(5): p. 1281-90.

[113] Fuss, I.J., Heller, F., Boirivant, M., Leon, F., Yoshida, M., et al., Nonclassical CD1d-restricted NK T cells that produce IL-13 characterize an atypical Th2 response in ulcerative colitis. The Journal of Clinical Investigation, 2004. 113(10): p. 1490-7.

[114] Fujino, S., Andoh, A., Bamba, S., Ogawa, A., Hata, K., et al., Increased expression of interleukin 17 in inflammatory bowel disease. Gut, 2003. 52(1): p. 65-70.

[115] Kobayashi, T., Okamoto, S., Hisamatsu, T., Kamada, N., Chinen, H., et al., IL23 differentially regulates the Th1/Th17 balance in ulcerative colitis and Crohn's disease. Gut, 2008. 57(12): p. 1682-9.

[116] Olsen, T., Rismo, R., Cui, G., Goll, R., Christiansen, I., et al., TH1 and TH17 interactions in untreated inflamed mucosa of inflammatory bowel disease, and their potential to mediate the inflammation. Cytokine, 2011. 56(3): p. 633-40.

[117] Nielsen, O.H., Kirman, I., Rudiger, N., Hendel, J., and Vainer, B., Upregulation of interleukin-12 and -17 in active inflammatory bowel disease. Scandinavian Journal of Gastroenterology, 2003. 38(2): p. 180-5.

[118] Cho, J.H. and Brant, S.R., Recent insights into the genetics of inflammatory bowel disease. Gastroenterology, 2011. 140(6): p. 1704-12.

[119] Newman, W.G., Zhang, Q., Liu, X., Amos, C.I., and Siminovitch, K.A., Genetic variants in *IL-23R* and *ATG16L1* independently predispose to increased susceptibility to Crohn's disease in a Canadian population. Journal of Clinical Gastroenterology, 2009. 43(5): p. 444-7.

[120] McGeachy, M.J. and Cua, D.J., Th17 cell differentiation: the long and winding road. Immunity, 2008. 28(4): p. 445-53.

[121] Oppmann, B., Lesley, R., Blom, B., Timans, J.C., Xu, Y., et al., Novel p19 protein engages IL-12p40 to form a cytokine, IL-23, with biological activities similar as well as distinct from IL-12. Immunity, 2000. 13(5): p. 715-25.

[122] Parham, C., Chirica, M., Timans, J., Vaisberg, E., Travis, M., et al., A receptor for the heterodimeric cytokine IL-23 is composed of IL-12Rbeta1 and a novel cytokine receptor subunit, IL-23R. Journal of Immunology, 2002. 168(11): p. 5699-708.

[123] Elson, C.O., Cong, Y., Weaver, C.T., Schoeb, T.R., McClanahan, T.K., et al., Monoclonal anti-interleukin 23 reverses active colitis in a T cell-mediated model in mice. Gastroenterology, 2007. 132(7): p. 2359-70.

[124] Ahern, P.P., Schiering, C., Buonocore, S., McGeachy, M.J., Cua, D.J., et al., Interleukin-23 drives intestinal inflammation through direct activity on T cells. Immunity, 2010. 33(2): p. 279-88.

[125] Liu, Z., Feng, B.S., Yang, S.B., Chen, X., Su, J., et al., Interleukin (IL)-23 suppresses IL-10 in inflammatory bowel disease. The Journal of Biological Chemistry, 2012. 287(5): p. 3591-7.

[126] Macpherson, A., Khoo, U.Y., Forgacs, I., Philpott-Howard, J., and Bjarnason, I., Mucosal antibodies in inflammatory bowel disease are directed against intestinal bacteria. Gut, 1996. 38(3): p. 365-75.

[127] Scott, M.G., Nahm, M.H., Macke, K., Nash, G.S., Bertovich, M.J., et al., Spontaneous secretion of IgG subclasses by intestinal mononuclear cells: differences between ulcerative colitis, Crohn's disease, and controls. Clinical and Experimental Immunology, 1986. 66(1): p. 209-15.

[128] MacDermott, R.P., Nash, G.S., and Nahm, M.H., Antibody secretion by human intestinal mononuclear cells from normal controls and inflammatory bowel disease patients. Immunological Investigations, 1989. 18(1-4): p. 449-57.

[129] MacDermott, R.P., Nash, G.S., Auer, I.O., Shlien, R., Lewis, B.S., et al., Alterations in serum immunoglobulin G subclasses in patients with ulcerative colitis and Crohn's disease. Gastroenterology, 1989. 96(3): p. 764-8.

[130] Philipsen, E.K., Bondesen, S., Andersen, J., and Larsen, S., Serum immunoglobulin G subclasses in patients with ulcerative colitis and Crohn's disease of different disease activities. Scandinavian Journal of Gastroenterology, 1995. 30(1): p. 50-3.

[131] Vecchi, M., Spina, L., Cavallaro, F., and Pastorelli, L., Do Antibodies Have a Role in IBD Pathogenesis? Inflammatory Bowel Diseases, 2008. 14(S2): p. S95-S96.

[132] Orholm, M., Binder, V., Sorensen, T.I., Rasmussen, L.P., and Kyvik, K.O., Concordance of inflammatory bowel disease among Danish twins. Results of a nationwide study. Scandinavian Journal of Gastroenterology, 2000. 35(10): p. 1075-81.

[133] Halfvarson, J., Bodin, L., Tysk, C., Lindberg, E., and Jarnerot, G., Inflammatory bowel disease in a Swedish twin cohort: a long-term follow-up of concordance and clinical characteristics. Gastroenterology, 2003. 124(7): p. 1767-73.

[134] Ng, S.C., Woodrow, S., Patel, N., Subhani, J., and Harbord, M., Role of genetic and environmental factors in British twins with inflammatory bowel disease. Inflammatory Bowel Diseases, 2012. 18(4): p. 725-36.

[135] Lindberg, E., Tysk, C., Andersson, K., and Jarnerot, G., Smoking and inflammatory bowel disease. A case control study. Gut, 1988. 29(3): p. 352-7.

[136] Halfvarson, J., Jess, T., Magnuson, A., Montgomery, S.M., Orholm, M., et al., Environmental factors in inflammatory bowel disease: a co-twin control study of a Swedish-Danish twin population. Inflammatory Bowel Diseases, 2006. 12(10): p. 925-33.

[137] Mahid, S.S., Minor, K.S., Soto, R.E., Hornung, C.A., and Galandiuk, S., Smoking and inflammatory bowel disease: a meta-analysis. Mayo Clinic Proceedings, 2006. 81(11): p. 1462-71.

[138] Radford-Smith, G.L., Edwards, J.E., Purdie, D.M., Pandeya, N., Watson, M., et al., Protective role of appendicectomy on onset and severity of ulcerative colitis and Crohn's disease. Gut, 2002. 51(6): p. 808-13.

[139] Cosnes, J., Carbonnel, F., Beaugerie, L., Blain, A., Reijasse, D., et al., Effects of appendicectomy on the course of ulcerative colitis. Gut, 2002. 51(6): p. 803-7.

[140] Castiglione, F., Diaferia, M., Morace, F., Labianca, O., Meucci, C., et al., Risk factors for inflammatory bowel diseases according to the "hygiene hypothesis": a case-control, multi-centre, prospective study in Southern Italy. Journal of Crohn's & Colitis, 2012. 6(3): p. 324-9.

[141] Krieglstein, C.F., Cerwinka, W.H., Laroux, F.S., Grisham, M.B., Schurmann, G., et al., Role of appendix and spleen in experimental colitis. The Journal of Surgical Research, 2001. 101(2): p. 166-75.

[142] Mizoguchi, A., Mizoguchi, E., Chiba, C., and Bhan, A.K., Role of appendix in the development of inflammatory bowel disease in TCR-alpha mutant mice. The Journal of Experimental Medicine, 1996. 184(2): p. 707-15.

[143] Godet, P.G., May, G.R., and Sutherland, L.R., Meta-analysis of the role of oral contraceptive agents in inflammatory bowel disease. Gut, 1995. 37(5): p. 668-73.

[144] Klement, E., Cohen, R.V., Boxman, J., Joseph, A., and Reif, S., Breastfeeding and risk of inflammatory bowel disease: a systematic review with meta-analysis. The American Journal of Clinical Nutrition, 2004. 80(5): p. 1342-52.

[145] Han, D.Y., Fraser, A.G., Dryland, P., and Ferguson, L.R., Environmental factors in the development of chronic inflammation: a case-control study on risk factors for Crohn's disease within New Zealand. Mutation Research, 2010. 690(1-2): p. 116-22.

[146] Gilat, T., Hacohen, D., Lilos, P., and Langman, M.J., Childhood factors in ulcerative colitis and Crohn's disease. An international cooperative study. Scandinavian Journal of Gastroenterology, 1987. 22(8): p. 1009-24.

[147] Hviid, A., Svanstrom, H., and Frisch, M., Antibiotic use and inflammatory bowel diseases in childhood. Gut, 2011. 60(1): p. 49-54.

[148] Hildebrand, H., Malmborg, P., Askling, J., Ekbom, A., and Montgomery, S.M., Early-life exposures associated with antibiotic use and risk of subsequent Crohn's disease. Scandinavian Journal of Gastroenterology, 2008. 43(8): p. 961-6.

[149] Card, T., Logan, R.F., Rodrigues, L.C., and Wheeler, J.G., Antibiotic use and the development of Crohn's disease. Gut, 2004. 53(2): p. 246-50.

[150] Shaw, S.Y., Blanchard, J.F., and Bernstein, C.N., Association between the use of antibiotics and new diagnoses of Crohn's disease and ulcerative colitis. The American Journal of Gastroenterology, 2011. 106(12): p. 2133-42.

[151] Jernberg, C., Lofmark, S., Edlund, C., and Jansson, J.K., Long-term ecological impacts of antibiotic administration on the human intestinal microbiota. The ISME journal, 2007. 1(1): p. 56-66.

[152] Sartor, R.B., Does *Mycobacterium avium* subspecies *paratuberculosis* cause Crohn's disease? Gut, 2005. 54(7): p. 896-8.

[153] Singh, A.V., Singh, S.V., Singh, P.K., and Sohal, J.S., Is *Mycobacterium avium* subsp. *paratuberculosis*, the cause of Johne's disease in animals, a good candidate for Crohn's disease in man? Indian Journal of Gastroenterology 2010. 29(2): p. 53-8.

[154] Chiodini, R.J., Van Kruiningen, H.J., Merkal, R.S., Thayer, W.R., Jr., and Coutu, J.A., Characteristics of an unclassified *Mycobacterium* species isolated from patients with Crohn's disease. Journal of Clinical Microbiology, 1984. 20(5): p. 966-71.

[155] Thorel, M.F., Krichevsky, M., and Levy-Frebault, V.V., Numerical taxonomy of mycobactin-dependent mycobacteria, emended description of *Mycobacterium avium*, and description of *Mycobacterium avium* subsp. *avium* subsp. nov., *Mycobacterium avium* subsp. *paratuberculosis* subsp. nov., and *Mycobacterium avium* subsp. *silvaticum* subsp. nov. International Journal of Systematic Bacteriology, 1990. 40(3): p. 254-60.

[156] Sanderson, J.D., Moss, M.T., Tizard, M.L., and Hermon-Taylor, J., *Mycobacterium paratuberculosis* DNA in Crohn's disease tissue. Gut, 1992. 33(7): p. 890-6.

[157] Dell'Isola, B., Poyart, C., Goulet, O., Mougenot, J.F., Sadoun-Journo, E., et al., Detection of *Mycobacterium paratuberculosis* by polymerase chain reaction in children with Crohn's disease. The Journal of Infectious Diseases, 1994. 169(2): p. 449-51.

[158] Fidler, H.M., Thurrell, W., Johnson, N.M., Rook, G.A., and McFadden, J.J., Specific detection of *Mycobacterium paratuberculosis* DNA associated with granulomatous tissue in Crohn's disease. Gut, 1994. 35(4): p. 506-10.

[159] Lisby, G., Andersen, J., Engbaek, K., and Binder, V., *Mycobacterium paratuberculosis* in intestinal tissue from patients with Crohn's disease demonstrated by a nested primer polymerase chain reaction. Scandinavian Journal of Gastroenterology, 1994. 29(10): p. 923-9.

[160] Suenaga, K., Yokoyama, Y., Okazaki, K., and Yamamoto, Y., Mycobacteria in the intestine of Japanese patients with inflammatory bowel disease. The American Journal of Gastroenterology, 1995. 90(1): p. 76-80.

[161] Murray, A., Oliaro, J., Schlup, M.M., and Chadwick, V.S., *Mycobacterium paratuberculosis* and inflammatory bowel disease: frequency distribution in serial colonoscopic biopsies using the polymerase chain reaction. Microbios, 1995. 83(337): p. 217-28.

[162] Roholl, P.J., Herrewegh, A., and van Soolingen, D., Positive IS900 *in situ* hybridization signals as evidence for role of *Mycobacterium avium* subsp. *paratuberculosis* in etiology of Crohn's disease. Journal of Clinical Microbiology, 2002. 40(8): p. 3112; author reply 3112-3.

[163] Rowbotham, D.S., Mapstone, N.P., Trejdosiewicz, L.K., Howdle, P.D., and Quirke, P., *Mycobacterium paratuberculosis* DNA not detected in Crohn's disease tissue by fluorescent polymerase chain reaction. Gut, 1995. 37(5): p. 660-7.

[164] Frank, T.S. and Cook, S.M., Analysis of paraffin sections of Crohn's disease for *Mycobacterium paratuberculosis* using polymerase chain reaction. Modern Pathology 1996. 9(1): p. 32-5.

[165] Dumonceau, J.M., Van Gossum, A., Adler, M., Fonteyne, P.A., Van Vooren, J.P., et al., No *Mycobacterium paratuberculosis* found in Crohn's disease using polymerase chain reaction. Digestive Diseases and Sciences, 1996. 41(2): p. 421-6.

[166] Al-Shamali, M., Khan, I., Al-Nakib, B., Al-Hassan, F., and Mustafa, A.S., A multiplex polymerase chain reaction assay for the detection of *Mycobacterium paratuberculosis* DNA in Crohn's disease tissue. Scandinavian Journal of Gastroenterology, 1997. 32(8): p. 819-23.

[167] Chiba, M., Fukushima, T., Horie, Y., Iizuka, M., and Masamune, O., No *Mycobacterium paratuberculosis* detected in intestinal tissue, including Peyer's patches and lymph follicles, of Crohn's disease. Journal of Gastroenterology, 1998. 33(4): p. 482-7.

[168] Cellier, C., De Beenhouwer, H., Berger, A., Penna, C., Carbonnel, F., et al., *Mycobacterium paratuberculosis* and *Mycobacterium avium* subsp. *silvaticum* DNA cannot be detected by PCR in Crohn's disease tissue. Gastroenterologie Clinique et Biologique, 1998. 22(8-9): p. 675-8.

[169] Kanazawa, K., Haga, Y., Funakoshi, O., Nakajima, H., Munakata, A., et al., Absence of *Mycobacterium paratuberculosis* DNA in intestinal tissues from Crohn's disease by nested polymerase chain reaction. Journal of Gastroenterology, 1999. 34(2): p. 200-6.

[170] Thayer, W.R., Jr., Coutu, J.A., Chiodini, R.J., Van Kruiningen, H.J., and Merkal, R.S., Possible role of mycobacteria in inflammatory bowel disease. II. Mycobacterial antibodies in Crohn's disease. Digestive Diseases and Sciences, 1984. 29(12): p. 1080-5.

[171] Elsaghier, A., Prantera, C., Moreno, C., and Ivanyi, J., Antibodies to *Mycobacterium paratuberculosis*-specific protein antigens in Crohn's disease. Clinical and Experimental Immunology, 1992. 90(3): p. 503-8.

[172] Vannuffel, P., Dieterich, C., Naerhuyzen, B., Gilot, P., Coene, M., et al., Occurrence, in Crohn's disease, of antibodies directed against a species-specific recombinant polypeptide of *Mycobacterium paratuberculosis*. Clinical and Diagnostic Laboratory Immunology, 1994. 1(2): p. 241-3.

[173] Kreuzpaintner, G., Das, P.K., Stronkhorst, A., Slob, A.W., and Strohmeyer, G., Effect of intestinal resection on serum antibodies to the mycobacterial 45/48 kilodalton doublet antigen in Crohn's disease. Gut, 1995. 37(3): p. 361-6.

[174] Naser, S., Shafran, I., and El-Zaatari, F., *Mycobacterium avium* subsp. *paratuberculosis* in Crohn's disease is serologically positive. Clinical and Diagnostic Laboratory Immunology, 1999. 6(2): p. 282.

[175] Suenaga, K., Yokoyama, Y., Nishimori, I., Sano, S., Morita, M., et al., Serum antibodies to *Mycobacterium paratuberculosis* in patients with Crohn's disease. Digestive Diseases and Sciences, 1999. 44(6): p. 1202-7.

[176] Naser, S.A., Hulten, K., Shafran, I., Graham, D.Y., and El-Zaatari, F.A., Specific seroreactivity of Crohn's disease patients against p35 and p36 antigens of *M. avium* subsp. *paratuberculosis*. Veterinary Microbiology, 2000. 77(3-4): p. 497-504.

[177] Cho, S.N., Brennan, P.J., Yoshimura, H.H., Korelitz, B.I., and Graham, D.Y., Mycobacterial aetiology of Crohn's disease: serologic study using common mycobacterial antigens and a species-specific glycolipid antigen from *Mycobacterium paratuberculosis*. Gut, 1986. 27(11): p. 1353-6.

[178] McFadden, J.J. and Houdayer, C., No evidence for antibodies to mycobacterial A60 antigen in Crohn's disease sera by enzyme-linked immunoabsorbent assay (ELISA). Journal of Medical Microbiology, 1988. 25(4): p. 295-8.

[179] Tanaka, K., Wilks, M., Coates, P.J., Farthing, M.J., Walker-Smith, J.A., et al., *Mycobacterium paratuberculosis* and Crohn's disease. Gut, 1991. 32(1): p. 43-5.

[180] Brunello, F., Pera, A., Martini, S., Marino, L., Astegiano, M., et al., Antibodies to *Mycobacterium paratuberculosis* in patients with Crohn's disease. Digestive Diseases and Sciences, 1991. 36(12): p. 1741-5.

[181] Stainsby, K.J., Lowes, J.R., Allan, R.N., and Ibbotson, J.P., Antibodies to *Mycobacterium paratuberculosis* and nine species of environmental mycobacteria in Crohn's disease and control subjects. Gut, 1993. 34(3): p. 371-4.

[182] Walmsley, R.S., Ibbotson, J.P., Chahal, H., and Allan, R.N., Antibodies against *Mycobacterium paratuberculosis* in Crohn's disease. QJM : Monthly Journal of the Association of Physicians, 1996. 89(3): p. 217-21.

[183] Sechi, L.A., Gazouli, M., Ikonomopoulos, J., Lukas, J.C., Scanu, A.M., et al., *Mycobacterium avium* subsp. *paratuberculosis*, genetic susceptibility to Crohn's disease, and Sardinians: the way ahead. Journal of Clinical Microbiology, 2005. 43(10): p. 5275-7.

[184] Singh, S. and Gopinath, K., *Mycobacterium avium* subspecies *Paratuberculosis* and Crohn's Regional Ileitis: How Strong is Association? Journal of Laboratory Physicians, 2011. 3(2): p. 69-74.

[185] Chiodini, R.J., Chamberlin, W.M., Sarosiek, J., and McCallum, R.W., Crohn's disease and the mycobacterioses: a quarter century later. Causation or simple association? Critical Reviews in Microbiology, 2012. 38(1): p. 52-93.

[186] Darfeuille-Michaud, A., Neut, C., Barnich, N., Lederman, E., Di Martino, P., et al., Presence of adherent *Escherichia coli* strains in ileal mucosa of patients with Crohn's disease. Gastroenterology, 1998. 115(6): p. 1405-13.

[187] Darfeuille-Michaud, A., Boudeau, J., Bulois, P., Neut, C., Glasser, A.L., et al., High prevalence of adherent-invasive *Escherichia coli* associated with ileal mucosa in Crohn's disease. Gastroenterology, 2004. 127(2): p. 412-21.

[188] Boudeau, J., Barnich, N., and Darfeuille-Michaud, A., Type 1 pili-mediated adherence of *Escherichia coli* strain LF82 isolated from Crohn's disease is involved in bacterial invasion of intestinal epithelial cells. Molecular Microbiology, 2001. 39(5): p. 1272-84.

[189] Barnich, N., Carvalho, F.A., Glasser, A.L., Darcha, C., Jantscheff, P., et al., CEACAM6 acts as a receptor for adherent-invasive *E. coli*, supporting ileal mucosa colonization in Crohn disease. The Journal of Clinical Investigation, 2007. 117(6): p. 1566-74.

[190] Boudeau, J., Glasser, A.L., Masseret, E., Joly, B., and Darfeuille-Michaud, A., Invasive ability of an *Escherichia coli* strain isolated from the ileal mucosa of a patient with Crohn's disease. Infection and Immunity, 1999. 67(9): p. 4499-509.

[191] Glasser, A.L., Boudeau, J., Barnich, N., Perruchot, M.H., Colombel, J.F., et al., Adherent invasive *Escherichia coli* strains from patients with Crohn's disease survive and replicate within macrophages without inducing host cell death. Infection and Immunity, 2001. 69(9): p. 5529-37.

[192] Meconi, S., Vercellone, A., Levillain, F., Payre, B., Al Saati, T., et al., Adherent-invasive *Escherichia coli* isolated from Crohn's disease patients induce granulomas *in vitro*. Cellular Microbiology, 2007. 9(5): p. 1252-61.

[193] Mansfield, C.S., James, F.E., Craven, M., Davies, D.R., O'Hara, A.J., et al., Remission of histiocytic ulcerative colitis in Boxer dogs correlates with eradication of invasive

intramucosal *Escherichia coli*. Journal of Veterinary Internal Medicine, 2009. 23(5): p. 964-9.

[194] Swidsinski, A., Ladhoff, A., Pernthaler, A., Swidsinski, S., Loening-Baucke, V., et al., Mucosal flora in inflammatory bowel disease. Gastroenterology, 2002. 122(1): p. 44-54.

[195] Kleessen, B., Kroesen, A.J., Buhr, H.J., and Blaut, M., Mucosal and invading bacteria in patients with inflammatory bowel disease compared with controls. Scandinavian Journal of Gastroenterology, 2002. 37(9): p. 1034-41.

[196] Schultsz, C., Van Den Berg, F.M., Ten Kate, F.W., Tytgat, G.N., and Dankert, J., The intestinal mucus layer from patients with inflammatory bowel disease harbors high numbers of bacteria compared with controls. Gastroenterology, 1999. 117(5): p. 1089-97.

[197] Takaishi, H., Matsuki, T., Nakazawa, A., Takada, T., Kado, S., et al., Imbalance in intestinal microflora constitution could be involved in the pathogenesis of inflammatory bowel disease. International Journal of Medical Microbiology 2008. 298(5-6): p. 463-72.

[198] Swidsinski, A., Weber, J., Loening-Baucke, V., Hale, L.P., and Lochs, H., Spatial organization and composition of the mucosal flora in patients with inflammatory bowel disease. Journal of Clinical Microbiology, 2005. 43(7): p. 3380-9.

[199] Marteau, P., Pochart, P., Dore, J., Bera-Maillet, C., Bernalier, A., et al., Comparative study of bacterial groups within the human cecal and fecal microbiota. Applied and Environmental Microbiology, 2001. 67(10): p. 4939-42.

[200] Zoetendal, E.G., von Wright, A., Vilpponen-Salmela, T., Ben-Amor, K., Akkermans, A.D., et al., Mucosa-associated bacteria in the human gastrointestinal tract are uniformly distributed along the colon and differ from the community recovered from feces. Applied and Environmental Microbiology, 2002. 68(7): p. 3401-7.

[201] Andoh, A., Kuzuoka, H., Tsujikawa, T., Nakamura, S., Hirai, F., et al., Multicenter analysis of fecal microbiota profiles in Japanese patients with Crohn's disease. Journal of Gastroenterology, 2012.

[202] Sokol, H., Seksik, P., Rigottier-Gois, L., Lay, C., Lepage, P., et al., Specificities of the fecal microbiota in inflammatory bowel disease. Inflammatory Bowel Diseases, 2006. 12(2): p. 106-11.

[203] Sokol, H., Seksik, P., Furet, J.P., Firmesse, O., Nion-Larmurier, I., et al., Low counts of *Faecalibacterium prausnitzii* in colitis microbiota. Inflammatory Bowel Diseases, 2009. 15(8): p. 1183-9.

[204] Willing, B.P., Dicksved, J., Halfvarson, J., Andersson, A.F., Lucio, M., et al., A pyrosequencing study in twins shows that gastrointestinal microbial profiles vary with in-

flammatory bowel disease phenotypes. Gastroenterology, 2010. 139(6): p. 1844-1854 e1.

[205] Willing, B., Halfvarson, J., Dicksved, J., Rosenquist, M., Jarnerot, G., et al., Twin studies reveal specific imbalances in the mucosa-associated microbiota of patients with ileal Crohn's disease. Inflammatory Bowel Diseases, 2009. 15(5): p. 653-60.

[206] Scanlan, P.D., Shanahan, F., O'Mahony, C., and Marchesi, J.R., Culture-independent analyses of temporal variation of the dominant fecal microbiota and targeted bacterial subgroups in Crohn's disease. Journal of Clinical Microbiology, 2006. 44(11): p. 3980-8.

[207] Sokol, H., Pigneur, B., Watterlot, L., Lakhdari, O., Bermudez-Humaran, L.G., et al., *Faecalibacterium prausnitzii* is an anti-inflammatory commensal bacterium identified by gut microbiota analysis of Crohn disease patients. Proceedings of the National Academy of Sciences of the United States of America, 2008. 105(43): p. 16731-6.

[208] Martinez-Medina, M., Aldeguer, X., Gonzalez-Huix, F., Acero, D., and Garcia-Gil, L.J., Abnormal microbiota composition in the ileocolonic mucosa of Crohn's disease patients as revealed by polymerase chain reaction-denaturing gradient gel electrophoresis. Inflammatory Bowel Dseases, 2006. 12(12): p. 1136-45.

[209] Swidsinski, A., Loening-Baucke, V., Vaneechoutte, M., and Doerffel, Y., Active Crohn's disease and ulcerative colitis can be specifically diagnosed and monitored based on the biostructure of the fecal flora. Inflammatory Bowel Diseases, 2008. 14(2): p. 147-61.

[210] Lupp, C., Robertson, M.L., Wickham, M.E., Sekirov, I., Champion, O.L., et al., Host-mediated inflammation disrupts the intestinal microbiota and promotes the overgrowth of *Enterobacteriaceae*. Cell Host & Microbe, 2007. 2(2): p. 119-29.

[211] Luperchio, S.A. and Schauer, D.B., Molecular pathogenesis of *Citrobacter rodentium* and transmissible murine colonic hyperplasia. Microbes and Infection 2001. 3(4): p. 333-40.

[212] Mansfield, L.S., Bell, J.A., Wilson, D.L., Murphy, A.J., Elsheikha, H.M., et al., C57BL/6 and congenic interleukin-10-deficient mice can serve as models of *Campylobacter jejuni* colonization and enteritis. Infection and Immunity, 2007. 75(3): p. 1099-115.

[213] Kuhn, R., Lohler, J., Rennick, D., Rajewsky, K., and Muller, W., Interleukin-10-deficient mice develop chronic enterocolitis. Cell, 1993. 75(2): p. 263-74.

[214] Jergens, A.E. and Simpson, K.W., Inflammatory bowel disease in veterinary medicine. Frontiers in Bioscience, 2012. 4: p. 1404-19.

[215] Jergens, A.E., Moore, F.M., Haynes, J.S., and Miles, K.G., Idiopathic inflammatory bowel disease in dogs and cats: 84 cases (1987-1990). Journal of the American Veterinary Medical Association, 1992. 201(10): p. 1603-8.

[216] Jergens, A.E., Inflammatory bowel disease. Current perspectives. The Veterinary Clinics of North America. Small Animal Practice, 1999. 29(2): p. 501-21, vii.

[217] German, A.J., Hall, E.J., and Day, M.J., Immune cell populations within the duodenal mucosa of dogs with enteropathies. Journal of Veterinary Internal Medicine, 2001. 15(1): p. 14-25.

[218] Kathrani, A., House, A., Catchpole, B., Murphy, A., German, A., et al., Polymorphisms in the TLR4 and TLR5 gene are significantly associated with inflammatory bowel disease in German shepherd dogs. PloS one, 2010. 5(12): p. e15740.

[219] Allenspach, K., House, A., Smith, K., McNeill, F.M., Hendricks, A., et al., Evaluation of mucosal bacteria and histopathology, clinical disease activity and expression of Toll-like receptors in German shepherd dogs with chronic enteropathies. Veterinary Microbiology, 2010. 146(3-4): p. 326-35.

[220] Simpson, K.W., Dogan, B., Rishniw, M., Goldstein, R.E., Klaessig, S., et al., Adherent and invasive *Escherichia coli* is associated with granulomatous colitis in boxer dogs. Infection and Immunity, 2006. 74(8): p. 4778-92.

[221] Baumgart, M., Dogan, B., Rishniw, M., Weitzman, G., Bosworth, B., et al., Culture independent analysis of ileal mucosa reveals a selective increase in invasive *Escherichia coli* of novel phylogeny relative to depletion of *Clostridiales* in Crohn's disease involving the ileum. The ISME journal, 2007. 1(5): p. 403-18.

[222] Craven, M., Mansfield, C.S., and Simpson, K.W., Granulomatous colitis of boxer dogs. The Veterinary Clinics of North America: Small Animal Practice, 2011. 41(2): p. 433-45.

[223] Kathrani, A., Schmitz, S., Priestnall, S.L., Smith, K.C., Werling, D., et al., CD11c+ cells are significantly decreased in the duodenum, ileum and colon of dogs with inflammatory bowel disease. Journal of Comparative Pathology, 2011. 145(4): p. 359-66.

[224] Xenoulis, P.G., Palculict, B., Allenspach, K., Steiner, J.M., Van House, A.M., et al., Molecular-phylogenetic characterization of microbial communities imbalances in the small intestine of dogs with inflammatory bowel disease. FEMS microbiology ecology, 2008. 66(3): p. 579-89.

[225] Suchodolski, J.S., Xenoulis, P.G., Paddock, C.G., Steiner, J.M., and Jergens, A.E., Molecular analysis of the bacterial microbiota in duodenal biopsies from dogs with idiopathic inflammatory bowel disease. Veterinary Microbiology, 2010. 142(3-4): p. 394-400.

[226] Sartor, R.B., Microbial influences in inflammatory bowel diseases. Gastroenterology, 2008. 134(2): p. 577-94.

[227] Suchodolski, J.S., Dowd, S.E., Wilke, V., Steiner, J.M., and Jergens, A.E., 16S rRNA gene pyrosequencing reveals bacterial dysbiosis in the duodenum of dogs with idiopathic inflammatory bowel disease. PloS one, 2012. 7(6): p. e39333.

[228] Craven, M., Simpson, J.W., Ridyard, A.E., and Chandler, M.L., Canine inflammatory bowel disease: retrospective analysis of diagnosis and outcome in 80 cases (1995-2002). The Journal of Small Animal Practice, 2004. 45(7): p. 336-42.

[229] Allenspach, K., Wieland, B., Grone, A., and Gaschen, F., Chronic enteropathies in dogs: evaluation of risk factors for negative outcome. Journal of Veterinary Internal Medicine 2007. 21(4): p. 700-8.

[230] Simpson, K.W. and Jergens, A.E., Pitfalls and progress in the diagnosis and management of canine inflammatory bowel disease. The Veterinary Clinics of North America. Small Animal Practice, 2011. 41(2): p. 381-98.

[231] Best, W.R., Becktel, J.M., Singleton, J.W., and Kern, F., Jr., Development of a Crohn's disease activity index. National Cooperative Crohn's Disease Study. Gastroenterology, 1976. 70(3): p. 439-44.

[232] Harvey, R.F. and Bradshaw, J.M., A simple index of Crohn's-disease activity. Lancet, 1980. 1(8167): p. 514.

[233] van Hees, P.A., van Elteren, P.H., van Lier, H.J., and van Tongeren, J.H., An index of inflammatory activity in patients with Crohn's disease. Gut, 1980. 21(4): p. 279-86.

[234] Jergens, A.E., Schreiner, C.A., Frank, D.E., Niyo, Y., Ahrens, F.E., et al., A scoring index for disease activity in canine inflammatory bowel disease. Journal of Veterinary Internal Medicine, 2003. 17(3): p. 291-7.

[235] Jergens, A.E., Crandell, J., Morrison, J.A., Deitz, K., Pressel, M., et al., Comparison of oral prednisone and prednisone combined with metronidazole for induction therapy of canine inflammatory bowel disease: a randomized-controlled trial. Journal of Veterinary Internal Medicine, 2010. 24(2): p. 269-77.

[236] Washabau, R.J., Day, M.J., Willard, M.D., Hall, E.J., Jergens, A.E., et al., Endoscopic, biopsy, and histopathologic guidelines for the evaluation of gastrointestinal inflammation in companion animals. Journal of Veterinary Internal Medicine, 2010. 24(1): p. 10-26.

[237] Trepanier, L., Idiopathic inflammatory bowel disease in cats. Rational treatment selection. Journal of Feline Medicine and Surgery, 2009. 11(1): p. 32-8.

[238] Kirkness, E.F., Bafna, V., Halpern, A.L., Levy, S., Remington, K., et al., The dog genome: survey sequencing and comparative analysis. Science, 2003. 301(5641): p. 1898-903.

[239] Allenspach, K., Tests to investigate gastrointestinal diseases in dogs--which markers are actually useful for the practitioner? The Journal of Small Animal Practice, 2007. 48(11): p. 607-8.

[240] Mowat, C., Cole, A., Windsor, A., Ahmad, T., Arnott, I., et al., Guidelines for the management of inflammatory bowel disease in adults. Gut, 2011. 60(5): p. 571-607.

[241] Khan, K.J., Ullman, T.A., Ford, A.C., Abreu, M.T., Abadir, A., et al., Antibiotic therapy in inflammatory bowel disease: a systematic review and meta-analysis. The American Journal of Gastroenterology, 2011. 106(4): p. 661-73.

[242] Guslandi, M., Rifaximin in the treatment of inflammatory bowel disease. World Journal of Gastroenterology 2011. 17(42): p. 4643-6.

[243] Scarpignato, C. and Pelosini, I., Rifaximin, a poorly absorbed antibiotic: pharmacology and clinical potential. Chemotherapy, 2005. 51 Suppl 1: p. 36-66.

[244] Maccaferri, S., Vitali, B., Klinder, A., Kolida, S., Ndagijimana, M., et al., Rifaximin modulates the colonic microbiota of patients with Crohn's disease: an *in vitro* approach using a continuous culture colonic model system. The Journal of Antimicrobial Chemotherapy, 2010. 65(12): p. 2556-65.

[245] Lahat, G., Halperin, D., Barazovsky, E., Shalit, I., Rabau, M., et al., Immunomodulatory effects of ciprofloxacin in TNBS-induced colitis in mice. Inflammatory Bowel Diseases, 2007. 13(5): p. 557-65.

[246] Dalhoff, A., Immunomodulatory activities of fluoroquinolones. Infection, 2005. 33 Suppl 2: p. 55-70.

[247] Barry, V.C., Belton, J.G., Conalty, M.L., Denneny, J.M., Edward, D.W., et al., A new series of phenazines (rimino-compounds) with high antituberculosis activity. Nature, 1957. 179(4568): p. 1013-5.

[248] Arbiser, J.L. and Moschella, S.L., Clofazimine: a review of its medical uses and mechanisms of action. Journal of the American Academy of Dermatology, 1995. 32(2 Pt 1): p. 241-7.

[249] Cholo, M.C., Steel, H.C., Fourie, P.B., Germishuizen, W.A., and Anderson, R., Clofazimine: current status and future prospects. The Journal of Antimicrobial Chemotherapy, 2012. 67(2): p. 290-8.

[250] Van Rensburg, C.E., Joone, G.K., O'Sullivan, J.F., and Anderson, R., Antimicrobial activities of clofazimine and B669 are mediated by lysophospholipids. Antimicrobial Agents and Chemotherapy, 1992. 36(12): p. 2729-35.

[251] Sarracent, J. and Finlay, C.M., The action of Clofazimine on the level of lysosomal enzymes of cultured macrophages. Clinical and Experimental Immunology, 1982. 48(1): p. 261-7.

[252] Sarracent, J. and Finlay, C.M., Phagocytosis and intracellular degradation of 125I-labelled immune complexes by Clofazimine treated macrophage cultures. Clinical and Experimental Immunology, 1982. 48(1): p. 268-72.

[253] Ren, Y.R., Pan, F., Parvez, S., Fleig, A., Chong, C.R., et al., Clofazimine inhibits human Kv1.3 potassium channel by perturbing calcium oscillation in T lymphocytes. PloS One, 2008. 3(12): p. e4009.

[254] Triantafillidis, J.K., Merikas, E., and Georgopoulos, F., Current and emerging drugs for the treatment of inflammatory bowel disease. Drug Design, Development and Therapy, 2011. 5: p. 185-210.

[255] Campieri, M., Ferguson, A., Doe, W., Persson, T., and Nilsson, L.G., Oral budesonide is as effective as oral prednisolone in active Crohn's disease. The Global Budesonide Study Group. Gut, 1997. 41(2): p. 209-14.

[256] Ardite, E., Panes, J., Miranda, M., Salas, A., Elizalde, J.I., et al., Effects of steroid treatment on activation of nuclear factor kappaB in patients with inflammatory bowel disease. British Journal of Pharmacology, 1998. 124(3): p. 431-3.

[257] Van Scoik, K.G., Johnson, C.A., and Porter, W.R., The pharmacology and metabolism of the thiopurine drugs 6-mercaptopurine and azathioprine. Drug Metabolism Reviews, 1985. 16(1-2): p. 157-74.

[258] Greenstein, R.J., Su, L., Haroutunian, V., Shahidi, A., and Brown, S.T., On the action of methotrexate and 6-mercaptopurine on *M. avium* subspecies *paratuberculosis*. PloS One, 2007. 2(1): p. e161.

[259] Hyoun, S.C., Obican, S.G., and Scialli, A.R., Teratogen update: methotrexate. Birth Defects Research. Part A, Clinical and Molecular Teratology, 2012. 94(4): p. 187-207.

[260] Schroder, H. and Campbell, D.E., Absorption, metabolism, and excretion of salicylazosulfapyridine in man. Clinical Pharmacology and Therapeutics, 1972. 13(4): p. 539-51.

[261] Peppercorn, M.A. and Goldman, P., Distribution studies of salicylazosulfapyridine and its metabolites. Gastroenterology, 1973. 64(2): p. 240-5.

[262] Dick, A.P., Grayson, M.J., Carpenter, R.G., and Petrie, A., Controlled Trial of Sulphasalazine in the Treatment of Ulcerative Colitis. Gut, 1964. 5: p. 437-42.

[263] Dew, M.J., Hughes, P., Harries, A.D., Williams, G., Evans, B.K., et al., Maintenance of remission in ulcerative colitis with oral preparation of 5-aminosalicylic acid. British Medical Journal, 1982. 285(6347): p. 1012.

[264] Azad Khan, A.K., Piris, J., and Truelove, S.C., An experiment to determine the active therapeutic moiety of sulphasalazine. Lancet, 1977. 2(8044): p. 892-5.

[265] Willoughby, C.P., Aronson, J.K., Agback, H., Bodin, N.O., and Truelove, S.C., Distribution and metabolism in healthy volunteers of disodium azodisalicylate, a potential therapeutic agent for ulcerative colitis. Gut, 1982. 23(12): p. 1081-7.

[266] Chan, R.P., Pope, D.J., Gilbert, A.P., Sacra, P.J., Baron, J.H., et al., Studies of two novel sulfasalazine analogs, ipsalazide and balsalazide. Digestive Diseases and Sciences, 1983. 28(7): p. 609-15.

[267] Ahnfelt-Ronne, I., Nielsen, O.H., Christensen, A., Langholz, E., Binder, V., et al., Clinical evidence supporting the radical scavenger mechanism of 5-aminosalicylic acid. Gastroenterology, 1990. 98(5 Pt 1): p. 1162-9.

[268] Kaiser, G.C., Yan, F., and Polk, D.B., Mesalamine blocks tumor necrosis factor growth inhibition and nuclear factor kappaB activation in mouse colonocytes. Gastroenterology, 1999. 116(3): p. 602-9.

[269] Mahida, Y.R., Lamming, C.E., Gallagher, A., Hawthorne, A.B., and Hawkey, C.J., 5-Aminosalicylic acid is a potent inhibitor of interleukin 1 beta production in organ culture of colonic biopsy specimens from patients with inflammatory bowel disease. Gut, 1991. 32(1): p. 50-4.

[270] Rhodes, J.M., Bartholomew, T.C., and Jewell, D.P., Inhibition of leucocyte motility by drugs used in ulcerative colitis. Gut, 1981. 22(8): p. 642-7.

[271] Swidsinski, A., Loening-Baucke, V., Bengmark, S., Lochs, H., and Dorffel, Y., Azathioprine and mesalazine-induced effects on the mucosal flora in patients with IBD colitis. Inflammatory Bowel Diseases, 2007. 13(1): p. 51-6.

[272] Greenstein, R.J., Su, L., Shahidi, A., and Brown, S.T., On the action of 5-amino-salicylic acid and sulfapyridine on *M. avium* including subspecies *paratuberculosis*. PloS One, 2007. 2(6): p. e516.

[273] Sandberg-Gertzen, H., Kjellander, J., Sundberg-Gilla, B., and Jarnerot, G., *In vitro* effects of sulphasalazine, azodisal sodium, and their metabolites on *Clostridium difficile* and some other faecal bacteria. Scandinavian Journal of Gastroenterology, 1985. 20(5): p. 607-12.

[274] Kaufman, J., Griffiths, T.A., Surette, M.G., Ness, S., and Rioux, K.P., Effects of mesalamine (5-aminosalicylic acid) on bacterial gene expression. Inflammatory Bowel Diseases, 2009. 15(7): p. 985-96.

[275] Braegger, C.P., Nicholls, S., Murch, S.H., Stephens, S., and MacDonald, T.T., Tumour necrosis factor alpha in stool as a marker of intestinal inflammation. Lancet, 1992. 339(8785): p. 89-91.

[276] Reinecker, H.C., Steffen, M., Witthoeft, T., Pflueger, I., Schreiber, S., et al., Enhanced secretion of tumour necrosis factor-alpha, IL-6, and IL-1 beta by isolated lamina propria mononuclear cells from patients with ulcerative colitis and Crohn's disease. Clinical and Experimental Immunology, 1993. 94(1): p. 174-81.

[277] Knight, D.M., Trinh, H., Le, J., Siegel, S., Shealy, D., et al., Construction and initial characterization of a mouse-human chimeric anti-TNF antibody. Molecular Immunology, 1993. 30(16): p. 1443-53.

[278] Ordas, I., Mould, D.R., Feagan, B.G., and Sandborn, W.J., Anti-TNF monoclonal antibodies in inflammatory bowel disease: pharmacokinetics-based dosing paradigms. Clinical Pharmacology and Therapeutics, 2012. 91(4): p. 635-46.

[279] Hanauer, S.B., Sandborn, W.J., Rutgeerts, P., Fedorak, R.N., Lukas, M., et al., Human anti-tumor necrosis factor monoclonal antibody (adalimumab) in Crohn's disease: the CLASSIC-I trial. Gastroenterology, 2006. 130(2): p. 323-33; quiz 591.

[280] Schreiber, S., Rutgeerts, P., Fedorak, R.N., Khaliq-Kareemi, M., Kamm, M.A., et al., A randomized, placebo-controlled trial of certolizumab pegol (CDP870) for treatment of Crohn's disease. Gastroenterology, 2005. 129(3): p. 807-18.

[281] Nesbitt, A., Fossati, G., Bergin, M., Stephens, P., Stephens, S., et al., Mechanism of action of certolizumab pegol (CDP870): *in vitro* comparison with other anti-tumor necrosis factor alpha agents. Inflammatory Bowel Diseases, 2007. 13(11): p. 1323-32.

[282] Scallon, B.J., Moore, M.A., Trinh, H., Knight, D.M., and Ghrayeb, J., Chimeric anti-TNF-alpha monoclonal antibody cA2 binds recombinant transmembrane TNF-alpha and activates immune effector functions. Cytokine, 1995. 7(3): p. 251-9.

[283] Vos, A.C., Wildenberg, M.E., Duijvestein, M., Verhaar, A.P., van den Brink, G.R., et al., Anti-tumor necrosis factor-alpha antibodies induce regulatory macrophages in an Fc region-dependent manner. Gastroenterology, 2011. 140(1): p. 221-30.

[284] Rawsthorne, P., Clara, I., Graff, L.A., Bernstein, K.I., Carr, R., et al., The Manitoba Inflammatory Bowel Disease Cohort Study: a prospective longitudinal evaluation of the use of complementary and alternative medicine services and products. Gut, 2012. 61(4): p. 521-7.

[285] Rahimi, R., Mozaffari, S., and Abdollahi, M., On the use of herbal medicines in management of inflammatory bowel diseases: a systematic review of animal and human studies. Digestive Diseases and Sciences, 2009. 54(3): p. 471-80.

[286] Quattropani, C., Ausfeld, B., Straumann, A., Heer, P., and Seibold, F., Complementary alternative medicine in patients with inflammatory bowel disease: use and attitudes. Scandinavian Journal of Gastroenterology, 2003. 38(3): p. 277-82.

[287] Ewaschuk, J.B. and Dieleman, L.A., Probiotics and prebiotics in chronic inflammatory bowel diseases. World Journal of Gastroenterology, 2006. 12(37): p. 5941-50.

[288] O'Hara, A.M. and Shanahan, F., Gut microbiota: mining for therapeutic potential. Clinical Gastroenterology and Hepatology, 2007. 5(3): p. 274-84.

[289] Guarner, F., Prebiotics, probiotics and helminths: the 'natural' solution? Digestive diseases, 2009. 27(3): p. 412-7.

[290] Guarner, F., Casellas, F., Borruel, N., Antolin, M., Videla, S., et al., Role of microecology in chronic inflammatory bowel diseases. European Journal of Clinical Nutrition, 2002. 56 Suppl 4: p. S34-8.

[291] Guarner, F., Prebiotics in inflammatory bowel diseases. The British Journal of Nutrition, 2007. 98 Suppl 1: p. S85-9.

[292] Chapman, T.M., Plosker, G.L., and Figgitt, D.P., Spotlight on VSL#3 probiotic mixture in chronic inflammatory bowel diseases. BioDrugs, 2007. 21(1): p. 61-3.

[293] Madsen, K., The use of probiotics in gastrointestinal disease. Canadian Journal of Gastroenterology, 2001. 15(12): p. 817-22.

[294] Esposito, E., Iacono, A., Bianco, G., Autore, G., Cuzzocrea, S., et al., Probiotics reduce the inflammatory response induced by a high-fat diet in the liver of young rats. The Journal of Nutrition, 2009. 139(5): p. 905-11.

[295] Ewaschuk, J., Endersby, R., Thiel, D., Diaz, H., Backer, J., et al., Probiotic bacteria prevent hepatic damage and maintain colonic barrier function in a mouse model of sepsis. Hepatology, 2007. 46(3): p. 841-50.

[296] Zwiers, A., Kraal, L., van de Pouw Kraan, T.C., Wurdinger, T., Bouma, G., et al., Cutting edge: a variant of the IL-23R gene associated with inflammatory bowel disease induces loss of microRNA regulation and enhanced protein production. Journal of immunology, 2012. 188(4): p. 1573-7.

[297] Gionchetti, P., Rizzello, F., Venturi, A., Brigidi, P., Matteuzzi, D., et al., Oral bacteriotherapy as maintenance treatment in patients with chronic pouchitis: a double-blind, placebo-controlled trial. Gastroenterology, 2000. 119(2): p. 305-9.

[298] Bibiloni, R., Fedorak, R.N., Tannock, G.W., Madsen, K.L., Gionchetti, P., et al., VSL#3 probiotic-mixture induces remission in patients with active ulcerative colitis. The American Journal of Gastroenterology, 2005. 100(7): p. 1539-46.

[299] Huynh, H.Q., deBruyn, J., Guan, L., Diaz, H., Li, M., et al., Probiotic preparation VSL#3 induces remission in children with mild to moderate acute ulcerative colitis: a pilot study. Inflammatory Bowel Diseases, 2009. 15(5): p. 760-8.

[300] Hoermannsperger, G., Clavel, T., Hoffmann, M., Reiff, C., Kelly, D., et al., Post-translational inhibition of IP-10 secretion in IEC by probiotic bacteria: impact on chronic inflammation. PloS One, 2009. 4(2): p. e4365.

[301] VSL#3 Frequently Asked Questions. Available from: http://www.vsl3.com/discover/faq.asp.

[302] Kruis, W., Schutz, E., Fric, P., Fixa, B., Judmaier, G., et al., Double-blind comparison of an oral *Escherichia coli* preparation and mesalazine in maintaining remission of ulcerative colitis. Alimentary Pharmacology & Therapeutics, 1997. 11(5): p. 853-8.

[303] Kruis, W., Fric, P., Pokrotnieks, J., Lukas, M., Fixa, B., et al., Maintaining remission of ulcerative colitis with the probiotic *Escherichia coli* Nissle 1917 is as effective as with standard mesalazine. Gut, 2004. 53(11): p. 1617-23.

[304] Rembacken, B.J., Snelling, A.M., Hawkey, P.M., Chalmers, D.M., and Axon, A.T., Non-pathogenic *Escherichia coli* versus mesalazine for the treatment of ulcerative colitis: a randomised trial. Lancet, 1999. 354(9179): p. 635-9.

[305] Jacobi, C.A., Grundler, S., Hsieh, C.J., Frick, J.S., Adam, P., et al., Quorum sensing in the probiotic bacterium *Escherichia coli* Nissle 1917 (Mutaflor) - evidence that furanosyl borate diester (AI-2) is influencing the cytokine expression in the DSS colitis mouse model. Gut Pathogens, 2012. 4(1): p. 8.

[306] Lodinova-Zadnikova, R. and Sonnenborn, U., Effect of preventive administration of a nonpathogenic *Escherichia coli* strain on the colonization of the intestine with microbial pathogens in newborn infants. Biology of the Neonate, 1997. 71(4): p. 224-32.

[307] Altenhoefer, A., Oswald, S., Sonnenborn, U., Enders, C., Schulze, J., et al., The probiotic *Escherichia coli strain* Nissle 1917 interferes with invasion of human intestinal epithelial cells by different enteroinvasive bacterial pathogens. FEMS Immunology and Medical Microbiology, 2004. 40(3): p. 223-9.

[308] Boudeau, J., Glasser, A.L., Julien, S., Colombel, J.F., and Darfeuille-Michaud, A., Inhibitory effect of probiotic *Escherichia coli* strain Nissle 1917 on adhesion to and invasion of intestinal epithelial cells by adherent-invasive *E. coli* strains isolated from patients with Crohn's disease. Alimentary Pharmacology & Therapeutics, 2003. 18(1): p. 45-56.

[309] Storm, D.W., Koff, S.A., Horvath, D.J., Jr., Li, B., and Justice, S.S., *In vitro* analysis of the bactericidal activity of *Escherichia coli* Nissle 1917 against pediatric uropathogens. The Journal of Urology, 2011. 186(4 Suppl): p. 1678-83.

[310] Why can't I buy Mutaflor in the US anymore? ; Available from: http://mutaflor.us/.

[311] Sauter, S.N., Allenspach, K., Gaschen, F., Grone, A., Ontsouka, E., et al., Cytokine expression in an *ex vivo* culture system of duodenal samples from dogs with chronic enteropathies: modulation by probiotic bacteria. Domestic Animal Endocrinology, 2005. 29(4): p. 605-22.

[312] Sauter, S.N., Benyacoub, J., Allenspach, K., Gaschen, F., Ontsouka, E., et al., Effects of probiotic bacteria in dogs with food responsive diarrhoea treated with an elimination diet. Journal of Animal Physiology and Animal Nutrition, 2006. 90(7-8): p. 269-77.

[313] Bybee, S.N., Scorza, A.V., and Lappin, M.R., Effect of the probiotic *Enterococcus faecium* SF68 on presence of diarrhea in cats and dogs housed in an animal shelter. Journal of Veterinary Internal Medicine, 2011. 25(4): p. 856-60.

[314] Hooda, S., Boler, B.M., Serao, M.C., Brulc, J.M., Staeger, M.A., et al., 454 pyrosequencing reveals a shift in fecal microbiota of healthy adult men consuming polydextrose or soluble corn fiber. The Journal of Nutrition, 2012. 142(7): p. 1259-65.

[315] Videla, S., Vilaseca, J., Antolin, M., Garcia-Lafuente, A., Guarner, F., et al., Dietary inulin improves distal colitis induced by dextran sodium sulfate in the rat. The American Journal of Gastroenterology, 2001. 96(5): p. 1486-93.

[316] Kanauchi, O., Suga, T., Tochihara, M., Hibi, T., Naganuma, M., et al., Treatment of ulcerative colitis by feeding with germinated barley foodstuff: first report of a multicenter open control trial. Journal of Gastroenterology, 2002. 37 Suppl 14: p. 67-72.

[317] Hanai, H., Kanauchi, O., Mitsuyama, K., Andoh, A., Takeuchi, K., et al., Germinated barley foodstuff prolongs remission in patients with ulcerative colitis. International Journal of Molecular Medicine, 2004. 13(5): p. 643-7.

[318] Faghfoori, Z., Navai, L., Shakerhosseini, R., Somi, M.H., Nikniaz, Z., et al., Effects of an oral supplementation of germinated barley foodstuff on serum tumour necrosis factor-alpha, interleukin-6 and -8 in patients with ulcerative colitis. Annals of Clinical Biochemistry, 2011. 48(Pt 3): p. 233-7.

[319] Lindsay, J.O., Whelan, K., Stagg, A.J., Gobin, P., Al-Hassi, H.O., et al., Clinical, microbiological, and immunological effects of fructo-oligosaccharide in patients with Crohn's disease. Gut, 2006. 55(3): p. 348-55.

[320] Sparkes, A.H., Papasouliotis, K., Sunvold, G., Werrett, G., Gruffydd-Jones, E.A., et al., Effect of dietary supplementation with fructo-oligosaccharides on fecal flora of healthy cats. American Journal of Veterinary Research, 1998. 59(4): p. 436-40.

[321] Sparkes, A.H., Papasouliotis, K., Sunvold, G., Werrett, G., Clarke, C., et al., Bacterial flora in the duodenum of healthy cats, and effect of dietary supplementation with fructo-oligosaccharides. American Journal of Veterinary Research, 1998. 59(4): p. 431-5.

[322] Willard, M.D., Simpson, R.B., Cohen, N.D., and Clancy, J.S., Effects of dietary fructooligosaccharide on selected bacterial populations in feces of dogs. American Journal of Veterinary Research, 2000. 61(7): p. 820-5.

[323] Mizoguchi, A., Animal models of inflammatory bowel disease. Progress in Molecular Biology and Translational Science, 2012. 105: p. 263-320.

[324] Solomon, L., Mansor, S., Mallon, P., Donnelly, E., Hoper, M., et al., The Dextran Sulfate Sodium (DSS) Model of Colitis: An Overview. Comparative Clinical Pathology, 2010. 19: p. 235-239.

[325] Mahler, M., Bristol, I.J., Leiter, E.H., Workman, A.E., Birkenmeier, E.H., et al., Differential susceptibility of inbred mouse strains to dextran sulfate sodium-induced colitis. The American Journal of Physiology, 1998. 274(3 Pt 1): p. G544-51.

[326] Okayasu, I., Hatakeyama, S., Yamada, M., Ohkusa, T., Inagaki, Y., et al., A novel method in the induction of reliable experimental acute and chronic ulcerative colitis in mice. Gastroenterology, 1990. 98(3): p. 694-702.

[327] Kitajima, S., Takuma, S., and Morimoto, M., Histological analysis of murine colitis induced by dextran sulfate sodium of different molecular weights. Experimental Animals / Japanese Association for Laboratory Animal Science, 2000. 49(1): p. 9-15.

[328] Bamba, S., Andoh, A., Ban, H., Imaeda, H., Aomatsu, T., et al., The severity of dextran sodium sulfate-induced colitis can differ between dextran sodium sulfate preparations of the same molecular weight range. Digestive Diseases and Sciences, 2012. 57(2): p. 327-34.

[329] Cooper, H.S., Murthy, S.N., Shah, R.S., and Sedergran, D.J., Clinicopathologic study of dextran sulfate sodium experimental murine colitis. Laboratory Investigation, 1993. 69(2): p. 238-49.

[330] Kitajima, S., Takuma, S., and Morimoto, M., Tissue distribution of dextran sulfate sodium (DSS) in the acute phase of murine DSS-induced colitis. The Journal of Veterinary Medical Science / The Japanese Society of Veterinary Science, 1999. 61(1): p. 67-70.

[331] Kitajima, S., Takuma, S., and Morimoto, M., Changes in colonic mucosal permeability in mouse colitis induced with dextran sulfate sodium. Experimental Animals / Japanese Association for Laboratory Animal Science, 1999. 48(3): p. 137-43.

[332] Ohkusa, T., Okayasu, I., Tokoi, S., Araki, A., and Ozaki, Y., Changes in bacterial phagocytosis of macrophages in experimental ulcerative colitis. Digestion, 1995. 56(2): p. 159-64.

[333] Araki, Y., Sugihara, H., and Hattori, T., *In vitro* effects of dextran sulfate sodium on a Caco-2 cell line and plausible mechanisms for dextran sulfate sodium-induced colitis. Oncology Reports, 2006. 16(6): p. 1357-62.

[334] Bylund-Fellenius, A.C., Landstrom, E., Axelsson, L.G., and Midtvedt, T., Experimental Colitis Induced by Dextran Sulphate in Normal and Germfree Mice. Microbial Ecology in Health and Disease 1994. 7: p. 207-215.

[335] Kitajima, S., Morimoto, M., Sagara, E., Shimizu, C., and Ikeda, Y., Dextran sodium sulfate-induced colitis in germ-free IQI/Jic mice. Experimental Animals / Japanese Association for Laboratory Animal Science, 2001. 50(5): p. 387-95.

[336] Neurath, M.F., Fuss, I., Kelsall, B.L., Presky, D.H., Waegell, W., et al., Experimental granulomatous colitis in mice is abrogated by induction of TGF-beta-mediated oral tolerance. The Journal of Experimental Medicine, 1996. 183(6): p. 2605-16.

[337] Kojima, R., Kuroda, S., Ohkishi, T., Nakamaru, K., and Hatakeyama, S., Oxazolone-induced colitis in BALB/C mice: a new method to evaluate the efficacy of therapeutic agents for ulcerative colitis. Journal of Pharmacological Sciences, 2004. 96(3): p. 307-13.

[338] Boirivant, M., Fuss, I.J., Chu, A., and Strober, W., Oxazolone colitis: A murine model of T helper cell type 2 colitis treatable with antibodies to interleukin 4. The Journal of Experimental Medicine, 1998. 188(10): p. 1929-39.

[339] NOTES, J. New IBD Model: C3Bir.129P2(B6)-Il10tm1cgn/Lt. 2006 Summer 2006 502].

[340] Rennick, D.M. and Fort, M.M., Lessons from genetically engineered animal models. XII. IL-10-deficient (IL-10(-/-) mice and intestinal inflammation. American journal of physiology. Gastrointestinal and liver physiology, 2000. 278(6): p. G829-33.

[341] Gomes-Santos, A.C., Moreira, T.G., Castro-Junior, A.B., Horta, B.C., Lemos, L., et al., New insights into the immunological changes in IL-10-deficient mice during the course of spontaneous inflammation in the gut mucosa. Clinical & developmental immunology, 2012. 2012: p. 560817.

[342] Berg, D.J., Davidson, N., Kuhn, R., Muller, W., Menon, S., et al., Enterocolitis and colon cancer in interleukin-10-deficient mice are associated with aberrant cytokine production and CD4(+) TH1-like responses. The Journal of clinical investigation, 1996. 98(4): p. 1010-20.

[343] Bristol, I.J., Farmer, M.A., Cong, Y., Zheng, X.X., Strom, T.B., et al., Heritable susceptibility for colitis in mice induced by IL-10 deficiency. Inflammatory bowel diseases, 2000. 6(4): p. 290-302.

[344] Mahler, M. and Leiter, E.H., Genetic and environmental context determines the course of colitis developing in IL-10-deficient mice. Inflammatory bowel diseases, 2002. 8(5): p. 347-55.

[345] Rennick, D.M., Fort, M.M., and Davidson, N.J., Studies with IL-10-/- mice: an overview. Journal of Leukocyte Biology, 1997. 61(4): p. 389-96.

[346] Sellon, R.K., Tonkonogy, S., Schultz, M., Dieleman, L.A., Grenther, W., et al., Resident enteric bacteria are necessary for development of spontaneous colitis and immune system activation in interleukin-10-deficient mice. Infection and immunity, 1998. 66(11): p. 5224-31.

[347] Madsen, K.L., Doyle, J.S., Tavernini, M.M., Jewell, L.D., Rennie, R.P., et al., Antibiotic therapy attenuates colitis in interleukin 10 gene-deficient mice. Gastroenterology, 2000. 118(6): p. 1094-105.

[348] Asseman, C., Mauze, S., Leach, M.W., Coffman, R.L., and Powrie, F., An essential role for interleukin 10 in the function of regulatory T cells that inhibit intestinal inflammation. The Journal of experimental medicine, 1999. 190(7): p. 995-1004.

[349] Davidson, N.J., Leach, M.W., Fort, M.M., Thompson-Snipes, L., Kuhn, R., et al., T helper cell 1-type CD4+ T cells, but not B cells, mediate colitis in interleukin 10-deficient mice. The Journal of Experimental Medicine, 1996. 184(1): p. 241-51.

[350] Spencer, D.M., Veldman, G.M., Banerjee, S., Willis, J., and Levine, A.D., Distinct inflammatory mechanisms mediate early versus late colitis in mice. Gastroenterology, 2002. 122(1): p. 94-105.

[351] Panwala, C.M., Jones, J.C., and Viney, J.L., A novel model of inflammatory bowel disease: mice deficient for the multiple drug resistance gene, *mdr1a,* spontaneously develop colitis. Journal of Immunology, 1998. 161(10): p. 5733-44.

[352] Maggio-Price, L., Shows, D., Waggie, K., Burich, A., Zeng, W., et al., *Helicobacter bilis* infection accelerates and *H. hepaticus* infection delays the development of colitis in multiple drug resistance-deficient (mdr1a-/-) mice. The American Journal of Pathology, 2002. 160(2): p. 739-51.

[353] Banner, K.H., Cattaneo, C., Le Net, J.L., Popovic, A., Collins, D., et al., Macroscopic, microscopic and biochemical characterisation of spontaneous colitis in a transgenic mouse, deficient in the multiple drug resistance 1a gene. British Journal of Pharmacology, 2004. 143(5): p. 590-8.

[354] Resta-Lenert, S., Smitham, J., and Barrett, K.E., Epithelial dysfunction associated with the development of colitis in conventionally housed mdr1a-/- mice. American Journal of Physiology. Gastrointestinal and Liver Physiology, 2005. 289(1): p. G153-62.

[355] Oostenbrug, L.E., Dijkstra, G., Nolte, I.M., van Dullemen, H.M., Oosterom, E., et al., Absence of association between the multidrug resistance (MDR1) gene and inflammatory bowel disease. Scandinavian Journal of Gastroenterology, 2006. 41(10): p. 1174-82.

[356] Ho, G.T., Soranzo, N., Nimmo, E.R., Tenesa, A., Goldstein, D.B., et al., ABCB1/MDR1 gene determines susceptibility and phenotype in ulcerative colitis: discrimination of critical variants using a gene-wide haplotype tagging approach. Human Molecular Genetics, 2006. 15(5): p. 797-805.

[357] Brant, S.R., Panhuysen, C.I., Nicolae, D., Reddy, D.M., Bonen, D.K., et al., MDR1 Ala893 polymorphism is associated with inflammatory bowel disease. American Journal of Human Genetics, 2003. 73(6): p. 1282-92.

[358] Potocnik, U., Ferkolj, I., Glavac, D., and Dean, M., Polymorphisms in multidrug resistance 1 (*MDR1*) gene are associated with refractory Crohn disease and ulcerative colitis. Genes and Immunity, 2004. 5(7): p. 530-9.

[359] Ehrhardt, R.O., Ludviksson, B.R., Gray, B., Neurath, M., and Strober, W., Induction and prevention of colonic inflammation in IL-2-deficient mice. Journal of Immunology, 1997. 158(2): p. 566-73.

[360] Garrett, W.S. and Glimcher, L.H., T-bet-/- RAG2-/- ulcerative colitis: the role of T-bet as a peacekeeper of host-commensal relationships. Cytokine, 2009. 48(1-2): p. 144-7.

[361] Garrett, W.S., Gallini, C.A., Yatsunenko, T., Michaud, M., DuBois, A., et al., *Enterobacteriaceae* act in concert with the gut microbiota to induce spontaneous and maternally transmitted colitis. Cell Host & Microbe, 2010. 8(3): p. 292-300.

[362] Powrie, F., Leach, M.W., Mauze, S., Menon, S., Caddle, L.B., et al., Inhibition of Th1 responses prevents inflammatory bowel disease in scid mice reconstituted with CD45RBhi CD4+ T cells. Immunity, 1994. 1(7): p. 553-62.

[363] Leach, M.W., Bean, A.G., Mauze, S., Coffman, R.L., and Powrie, F., Inflammatory bowel disease in C.B-17 scid mice reconstituted with the CD45RBhigh subset of CD4+ T cells. The American Journal of Pathology, 1996. 148(5): p. 1503-15.

[364] Aranda, R., Sydora, B.C., McAllister, P.L., Binder, S.W., Yang, H.Y., et al., Analysis of intestinal lymphocytes in mouse colitis mediated by transfer of CD4+, CD45RBhigh T cells to SCID recipients. Journal of Immunology, 1997. 158(7): p. 3464-73.

[365] Podolsky, D.K., Inflammatory bowel disease (1). The New England Journal of Medicine, 1991. 325(13): p. 928-37.

[366] Liu, Z., Ramer-Tait, A.E., Henderson, A.L., Demirkale, C.Y., Nettleton, D., et al., *Helicobacter bilis* colonization enhances susceptibility to typhlocolitis following an inflammatory trigger. Digestive Diseases and Sciences, 2011. 56(10): p. 2838-48.

[367] Jergens, A.E., Dorn, A., Wilson, J., Dingbaum, K., Henderson, A., et al., Induction of differential immune reactivity to members of the flora of gnotobiotic mice following colonization with *Helicobacter bilis* or *Brachyspira hyodysenteriae*. Microbes and Infection 2006. 8(6): p. 1602-10.

[368] Jergens, A.E., Wilson-Welder, J.H., Dorn, A., Henderson, A., Liu, Z., et al., *Helicobacter bilis* triggers persistent immune reactivity to antigens derived from the commensal bacteria in gnotobiotic C3H/HeN mice. Gut, 2007. 56(7): p. 934-40.

[369] Liu, Z., Henderson, A.L., Nettleton, D., Wilson-Welder, J.H., Hostetter, J.M., et al., Mucosal gene expression profiles following the colonization of immunocompetent defined-flora C3H mice with *Helicobacter bilis*: a prelude to typhlocolitis. Microbes and Infection 2009. 11(3): p. 374-83.

[370] Myles, M.H., Livingston, R.S., Livingston, B.A., Criley, J.M., and Franklin, C.L., Analysis of gene expression in ceca of *Helicobacter hepaticus*-infected A/JCr mice before and after development of typhlitis. Infection and Immunity, 2003. 71(7): p. 3885-93.

[371] Livingston, R.S., Myles, M.H., Livingston, B.A., Criley, J.M., and Franklin, C.L., Sex influence on chronic intestinal inflammation in *Helicobacter hepaticus*-infected A/JCr mice. Comparative Medicine, 2004. 54(3): p. 301-8.

[372] Maggio-Price, L., Bielefeldt-Ohmann, H., Treuting, P., Iritani, B.M., Zeng, W., et al., Dual infection with *Helicobacter bilis* and *Helicobacter hepaticus* in p-glycoprotein-deficient mdr1a-/- mice results in colitis that progresses to dysplasia. The American Journal of Pathology, 2005. 166(6): p. 1793-806.

[373] Kullberg, M.C., Ward, J.M., Gorelick, P.L., Caspar, P., Hieny, S., et al., *Helicobacter hepaticus* triggers colitis in specific-pathogen-free interleukin-10 (IL-10)-deficient mice through an IL-12- and gamma interferon-dependent mechanism. Infection and Immunity, 1998. 66(11): p. 5157-66.

[374] Burich, A., Hershberg, R., Waggie, K., Zeng, W., Brabb, T., et al., *Helicobacter*-induced inflammatory bowel disease in IL-10- and T cell-deficient mice. American Journal of Physiology, 2001. 281(3): p. G764-78.

[375] Taylor, D.J. and Alexander, T.J., The production of dysentery in swine by feeding cultures containing a spirochaete. The British Veterinary Journal, 1971. 127(11): p. 58-61.

[376] Hutto, D.L. and Wannemuehler, M.J., A comparison of the morphologic effects of Serpulina hyodysenteriae or its beta-hemolysin on the murine cecal mucosa. Veterinary Pathology, 1999. 36(5): p. 412-22.

[377] Brandenburg, A.C., Miniats, O.P., Geissinger, H.D., and Ewert, E., Swine dysentery: inoculation of gnotobiotic pigs with *Treponema hyodysenteriae* and *Vibrio coli* and a *Peptostreptococcus*. Canadian Journal of Comparative Medicine, 1977. 41(3): p. 294-301.

[378] Harris, D.L., Alexander, T.J., Whipp, S.C., Robinson, I.M., Glock, R.D., et al., Swine dysentery: studies of gnotobiotic pigs inoculated with Treponema hyodysenteriae, Bacteroides vulgatus, and Fusobacterium necrophorum. Journal of the American Veterinary Medical Association, 1978. 172(4): p. 468-71.

[379] Whipp, S.C., Robinson, I.M., Harris, D.L., Glock, R.D., Matthews, P.J., et al., Pathogenic synergism between Treponema hyodysenteriae and other selected anaerobes in gnotobiotic pigs. Infection and immunity, 1979. 26(3): p. 1042-7.

[380] Sacco, R.E., Hutto, D.L., Waters, W.R., Xiasong, L., Kehrli, M.E., Jr., et al., Reduction in inflammation following blockade of CD18 or CD29 adhesive pathways during the acute phase of a spirochetal-induced colitis in mice. Microbial pathogenesis, 2000. 29(5): p. 289-99.

[381] Liu, Z., Wilson-Welder, J.H., Hostetter, J.M., Jergens, A.E., and Wannemuehler, M.J., Prophylactic treatment with *Hypoxis hemerocallidea corm* (African potato) methanolic extract ameliorates *Brachyspira hyodysenteriae*-induced murine typhlocolitis. Experimental Biology and Medicine, 2010. 235(2): p. 222-30.

[382] Taconic. Animal Health Standards. 2011.

[383] Kim, S.C., Tonkonogy, S.L., Albright, C.A., Tsang, J., Balish, E.J., et al., Variable phenotypes of enterocolitis in interleukin 10-deficient mice monoassociated with two different commensal bacteria. Gastroenterology, 2005. 128(4): p. 891-906.

[384] Balish, E. and Warner, T., *Enterococcus faecalis* induces inflammatory bowel disease in interleukin-10 knockout mice. The American Journal of Pathology, 2002. 160(6): p. 2253-7.

[385] Dieleman, L.A., Arends, A., Tonkonogy, S.L., Goerres, M.S., Craft, D.W., et al., *Helicobacter hepaticus* does not induce or potentiate colitis in interleukin-10-deficient mice. Infection and Immunity, 2000. 68(9): p. 5107-13.

[386] Sydora, B.C., Tavernini, M.M., Doyle, J.S., and Fedorak, R.N., Association with selected bacteria does not cause enterocolitis in IL-10 gene-deficient mice despite a systemic immune response. Digestive Diseases and Sciences, 2005. 50(5): p. 905-13.

[387] Moran, J.P., Walter, J., Tannock, G.W., Tonkonogy, S.L., and Sartor, R.B., *Bifidobacterium animalis* causes extensive duodenitis and mild colonic inflammation in monoassociated interleukin-10-deficient mice. Inflammatory Bowel Diseases, 2009. 15(7): p. 1022-31.

[388] Trexler, P.C. and Reynolds, L.I., Flexible film apparatus for the rearing and use of germfree animals. Applied Microbiology, 1957. 5(6): p. 406-12.

[389] Orcutt, R.P., Application of Gnotobiotic Techniques for Contamination Control, in 50 years of Laboratory Animal Science 1950-2000, W. Charles, Editor 1999, AALAS. p. 125-128.

[390] Dewhirst, F.E., Chien, C.C., Paster, B.J., Ericson, R.L., Orcutt, R.P., et al., Phylogeny of the defined murine microbiota: Altered Schaedler flora. Applied and Environmental Microbiology, 1999. 65(8): p. 3287-3292.

[391] Sarma-Rupavtarm, R.B., Ge, Z.M., Schauer, D.B., Fox, J.G., and Polz, M.F., Spatial distribution and stability of the eight microbial species of the altered Schaedler flora in the mouse gastrointestinal tract. Applied and Environmental Microbiology, 2004. 70(5): p. 2791-2800.

[392] Stehr, M., Greweling, M.C., Tischer, S., Singh, M., Blocker, H., et al., Charles River altered Schaedler flora (CRASF) remained stable for four years in a mouse colony housed in individually ventilated cages. Laboratoy Animals, 2009. 43(4): p. 362-70.

[393] Ge, Z., Feng, Y., Taylor, N.S., Ohtani, M., Polz, M.F., et al., Colonization dynamics of altered Schaedler flora is influenced by gender, aging, and *Helicobacter hepaticus* infection in the intestines of Swiss Webster mice. Applied and Environmental Microbiology, 2006. 72(7): p. 5100-3.

[394] Alexander, A.D., Orcutt, R.P., Henry, J.C., Baker, J., Bissahoyo, A.C., et al., Quantitative PCR assays for mouse enteric flora reveal strain-dependent differences in composition that are influenced by the microenvironment. Mammalian Genome, 2006. 17(11): p. 1093-1104.

[395] Norin, E. and Midtvedt, T., Intestinal microflora functions in laboratory mice claimed to harbor a "normal" intestinal microflora. Is the SPF concept running out of date? Anaerobe, 2010. 16(3): p. 311-3.

[396] Benno, P., Bark, J., Collinder, E., Hellstrom, P.M., Midtvedt, T., et al., Major alterations in metabolic activity of intestinal microflora in Crohn's disease. Scandinavian Journal of Gastroenterology, 2012. 47(2): p. 251-2.

[397] Faith, J.J., McNulty, N.P., Rey, F.E., and Gordon, J.I., Predicting a human gut microbiota's response to diet in gnotobiotic mice. Science, 2011. 333(6038): p. 101-4.

[398] Denou, E., Rezzonico, E., Panoff, J.M., Arigoni, F., and Brussow, H., A Mesocosm of *Lactobacillus johnsonii, Bifidobacterium longum, and Escherichia coli* in the mouse gut. DNA and Cell Biology, 2009. 28(8): p. 413-22.

[399] Mahowald, M.A., Rey, F.E., Seedorf, H., Turnbaugh, P.J., Fulton, R.S., et al., Characterizing a model human gut microbiota composed of members of its two dominant bacterial phyla. Proceedings of the National Academy of Sciences of the United States of America, 2009. 106(14): p. 5859-64.

[400] Faith, J.J., Rey, F.E., O'Donnell, D., Karlsson, M., McNulty, N.P., et al., Creating and characterizing communities of human gut microbes in gnotobiotic mice. The ISME journal, 2010. 4(9): p. 1094-8.

[401] Pena, J.A., Li, S.Y., Wilson, P.H., Thibodeau, S.A., Szary, A.J., et al., Genotypic and phenotypic studies of murine intestinal lactobacilli: species differences in mice with and without colitis. Applied and Environmental Microbiology, 2004. 70(1): p. 558-68.

[402] Robertson, B.R., O'Rourke, J.L., Neilan, B.A., Vandamme, P., On, S.L., et al., *Mucispirillum schaedleri* gen. nov., sp. nov., a spiral-shaped bacterium colonizing the mucus layer of the gastrointestinal tract of laboratory rodents. International Journal of Systematic and Evolutionary Microbiology, 2005. 55(Pt 3): p. 1199-204.

[403] Wilkins, T.D., Fulghum, R.S., and Wilkins, J.H., *Eubacterium plexicaudatum* sp. nov., an anaerobic bacterium with a subpolar tuft of flagella, isolated from a mouse cecum. International Journal of Systemic Bacteriology, 1974. 24(4): p. 408-411.

[404] Sakamoto, M. and Benno, Y., Reclassification of *Bacteroides distasonis, Bacteroides goldsteinii* and *Bacteroides merdae* as *Parabacteroides distasonis* gen. nov., comb. nov., *Parabacteroides goldsteinii* comb. nov. and *Parabacteroides merdae* comb. nov. International Journal of Systematic and Evolutionary Microbiology, 2006. 56(Pt 7): p. 1599-605.

[405] Song, Y., Liu, C., Lee, J., Bolanos, M., Vaisanen, M.L., et al., "*Bacteroides goldsteinii* sp. nov." isolated from clinical specimens of human intestinal origin. Journal of Clinical Microbiology, 2005. 43(9): p. 4522-7.

Chapter 4

Fibrosis in Crohn's Disease

Lauri Diehl

Additional information is available at the end of the chapter

http://dx.doi.org/10.5772/46222

1. Introduction

The objectives of this chapter are to review clinical and pathophysiologic aspects of fibrosis in inflammatory bowel disease, particularly in Crohn's disease. Potential therapeutic strategies and the current status of preclinical animal models to evaluate these therapeutic strategies will also be discussed.

2. Clinical considerations

Crohn's disease (CD) and ulcerative colitis (UC) are chronic, relapsing inflammatory gastrointestinal diseases which often onset in young adulthood. Unlike in UC, where inflammation is limited to the mucosa, CD patients frequently develop transmural disease which can extend to involve the muscularis and serosa. While inflammatory disease accounts for much of the symptomatology associated with CD, significant morbidity results from fibrotic lesions and their resulting complications.

CD can be broadly categorized as having three major clinical subtypes: stricturing, penetrating or inflammatory (nonstricturing nonpenetrating) disease [1]. This categorization is reflected by the inclusion of disease behavior (stricturing, penetrating or inflammatory) as one of three variables elected for inclusion in the Vienna classification in 1998 [2]. Review of natural history data from shows that the majority of patients undergo progression from inflammatory disease to development of complications including stricture [3]. Even though most patients present with inflammatory disease only and later progress to a more complicated disease phenotype, a subset of patients will present with stricturing or penetrating disease. In population-based studies, 19-36% of patients newly diagnosed with CD present with disease complications such as strictures, fistulas or abscesses [4-6].

Intestinal stricture is a common and serious complication of long term CD. Critical intestinal stricture formation will occur in at least one-third of CD patients within 10 years of onset [7-9]. By contrast, fibrosis associated with UC is generally limited to the mucosa and stricture formation is rare although rectal strictures, when they occur, can be problematic to manage [10]. Advances in CD treatment have yet to make significant impact on the incidence of strictures and the associated morbidity [11].

While surgical resection is a highly effective short term treatment, remission after surgical resection in CD is only temporary. The disease course in CD patients postsurgery is relatively consistent and has allowed development of a postoperative recurrence model [12, 13]. In this model, a focal inflammatory infiltrate forms in the ileum above the anastomosis followed by aphthous ulcers which are endoscopically visible in two-thirds of patients within 3 months after surgery. These patients go on to develop extensive superficial and deep ulcers that precede the development of a new stricture. Postoperative reoccurrence is very common with fewer than 5% of patients having normal endoscopy results 10 years after surgery. Symptoms occur on average 2-3 years after lesions are observed.

In patients with a fibrostenotic disease behavior, symptomatic strictures tend to return despite medical therapy and this leads to repeated bowel resections and eventually to short bowel syndrome [14-16]. Endoscopic balloon dilation can provide a treatment option for patients with fibrostenotic strictures 7 cm or less in length although there is some risk of perforation [17, 18]. Strictureplasty can be a useful bowel-preserving surgical option for stenosing small bowel CD in patients with multiple obstructions and in those vulnerable to short bowel syndrome [19]. The incidence of postoperative recurrence is very similar between strictureplasty and resection [11].

Strictures can arise due to either inflammatory or fibrotic processes. There is evidence that direct steroid injection can provide symptom relief in some CD patients with anastomotic strictures, presumably in patients with active inflammation and relatively little fibromuscular proliferation at the anastomotic site [18]. Given the risk of multiple bowel resection surgeries and the possibility of short bowel syndrome, the ability to differentiate between inflammatory or fibrotic strictures could be used to drive treatment decisions. Endoscopy-based techniques such as colonoscopy, small intestinal endoscopy, and capsule endoscopy have high clinical utility but only visualize the mucosal surface. Cross-sectional imaging techniques can be used to visualize deep layers of the intestinal wall and assess for strictures. Computed tomography enterography (CTE) has become the most widely used cross-sectional imaging technology for CD although concern about cumulative radiation exposure, particularly in young patients, has led to interest in alternative imaging modalities [20, 21].

Imaging methods such as magnetic resonance (MR) enterography or ultrasonography are effective in determining the anatomic location and length of affected intestinal segments and these techniques, as well as CTE, have shown a good correlation with endoscopy [22-24]. However, distinguishing stricture composition remains a challenge. In 2006, the European Crohn's and Colitis Organization (ECCO) stated in their consensus report on treatment of CD that current techniques are insufficiently accurate to differentiate between inflammatory and fibrostenotic strictures [25]. A recent study confirms that, while the combination of MR-enterography and ultrasound as well as the combination of ^{18}FDG-PET/CT and ultrasound are highly efficient in detecting CD strictures, no current imaging techniques shows sufficient sensitivity or specificity to reliably differentiate inflamed from fibrotic strictures [26]. The clinical need for this for such differentiation remains high and may require both technologic advancement and establishment of criteria for grading or distinguishing strictures which contain both fibrotic and inflammatory components [27]. [25]. In clinical practice, a variety of diagnostic tools including imaging techniques and inflammatory biomarkers are often applied in an effort to obtain sufficient evidence to inform treatment decisions [28].

Therapeutic strategies have evolved over the past decade and having the ability to predict disease outcomes could guide the clinician's choice of therapy. The goals of CD treatment should include 1.) steroid-free sustained clinical remission; 2.) mucosal healing; 3.) potential induction and maintenance of radiological healing; 4.) prevention of surgery; 5.) maintenance of normal gastrointestinal function; and 6.) prevention of disability [6]. There are a number of therapeutic options available for the treatment of inflammation in CD patients, however none of these have been demonstrated to be effective in preventing preventing or treating fibrostenosis thereby failing to achieve at least 2 of the 6 major treatment goals in patients with fibrostenotic disease. There have been some reports of regression of strictures and of overall benefit following infliximab treatment in a subset of patients with small bowel stricturing disease [18, 29, 30]. This data is largely anecdotal and remains controversial as large controlled trials have not yet been performed.

In CD, disease location (ileal vs. colonic) remains relatively stable but clinical behavior can alter significantly over time [8, 31, 32]. During the first few years of disease, inflammatory forms predominate, whereas, after 40 years, most patients have experienced complications and are classified as having penetrating or stricturing disease[33]. However, the rate at which disease behavior evolves can vary widely between CD patients and those differences would determine therapeutic strategies if rapidly progressing patients could be identified. For example, initiation of more aggressive treatment early in the course of disease has the potential to result in better outcomes, however, these therapies can also lead to greater risk of toxicity and adverse effects [34, 35]. Decisions on whether to use a conservative or an aggressive treatment strategy in newly diagnosed patients could be informed by the ability to identify patients at higher risk for developing disabling or complicated disease.

3. Fibrosis risk factors

A number of retrospective studies have identified specific disease characteristics that may be of use in predicting risk for individual CD patients. These include an initial CD diagnosis under age 40, need for steroid therapy at diagnosis, and perianal fistulizing disease [31, 36]. Localization of inflammation to the small bowel has also been identified as predictive of progression to more complicated disease and higher rate of surgery [37]. However, all of these clinical features tend to correlate with the presence of small intestinal disease and do not necessarily identify which patients with small bowel disease are at greatest risk of developing fibrostenosing disease.

Genetic polymorphisms play an important role in susceptibility to CD so the use of genetic markers to provide risk stratification and drive clinical decisions is very attractive. The observation that some CD patients are susceptible to stricture development early and often in their clinical course while others never develop a stenosing phenotype argues for the existence of a genetic background which predisposes to stricturing behavior in CD.

One of the genes linked with susceptibility to CD is the CARD15/NOD2 gene which encodes a protein involved in bacterial recognition and activation of nuclear factor kB. Carriers of two mutant alleles have 17 to 42 times the risk while carriers of one mutation have 1.5 to 3 times the risk of developing CD [38, 39]. There is a significant body of evidence suggesting that the main NOD2/CARD15 variants (Arg702Trp, Gly908Arg, and Leu1007insC) are associated with risk for developing stenotic disease and increased need for surgery [40-44]. However, this finding is not reproducible in every CD cohort evaluated [45, 46]. One large meta-analysis of the NOD2/CARD15 literature indicated that carrying at least one NOD2/CARD15 variant increased the risk of both small intestinal disease and of the stenosing phenotype [47]. The discrepancy between studies may be due to differences in definitions of disease behavior between studies and, perhaps, to the particular genetic epidemiological analyses used. At present, understanding whether the relationship between the NOD2/CARD15 variants and a stenosing phenotype is a true association or whether it instead reflects aspects of disease duration and ileal localization remains a matter of controversy.

Other gene polymorphisms have been described as associated with a fibrostenotic phenotype although the existing data is much less extensive than that available for NOD2/CARD15. The ATG16L1 gene encodes for a protein involved in autophagy and mutations in this gene have been associated with stricturing disease as well as perianal involvement in CD [48]. CX3CR1, the receptor of CX3CL1 (fractalkine), is involved in regulation of inflammatory response and the V249I polymorphism has been reported to be associated with intestinal strictures [49]. A recent study linked the receptor for advanced glycation endproducts (RAGE) -374T/A polymorphism to protection from stricturing phenotype in CD. The polymorphism increases RAGE gene transcription which may provide protection by increasing levels of soluble RAGE leading to neutralization of proinflammatory mediators [50]. Some fibrostenosis-related polymorphisms have been observed in combination with NOD2/CARD15. CXCL16 is a chemokine involved in bacterial defense mechanisms. CD patients with at least one CXCL16 p.Ala181Val allele and one CARD15/NOD2 variant had a higher incidence of stricturing and penetrating phenotype as well as stenosis as patients with the NOD2 variant alone [51].

Despite their potential, genetic markers may never fully be able to predict the clinical course of CD. The low frequency, incomplete penetrance, and interplay with other genetic polymorphisms greatly complicate interpretation of genetic markers. In addition, environmental factors can modulate disease history and impact phenotypic features. It is probable that genetic markers will need to be integrated with other clinical and serologic information in order to be useful predictors of disease course and to inform treatment decisions.

4. Serologic biomarkers

Serologic markers may identify CD patients at higher risk of developing disease-related complications. Some of the best characterized serologic markers associated with CD are directed against microbial peptides. Most of the available data is from cross sectional studies in which the patient samples analyzed have been collected at various times in the disease course allowing for comparison of serum from before, concomitant with, and after diagnosis or treatment of bowel stricture.

Disease progression from non-complicated CD to stricturing and/or penetrating phenotypes has been significantly associated with the presence and magnitude of serologic response to microbial antigens. This concept was initially triggered by the observation that high anti-Saccharomyces cerevisiae antibody (ASCA) levels were found to be associated with fibrostenosing and penetrating disease and with the need for surgery [52]. This observation was repeated in another cross sectional study where ASCA positive patients were more likely to undergo surgery within 3 years of diagnosis than ASCA negative patients [53]. Time to first complication was shown to be shorter in ASCA positive pediatric CD patients than in ASCA negative patients [54]. In addition, anti-I2 (an antibody directed against *Pseudomonas* fluorescens), anti-OmpC (the outer membrane porin protein of *Escherichia* coli) and anti-CBir1 (anti-flagellin) levels have also been shown to associated with fibrostenotic disease [55-60]. A multi-center study evaluated the association of ASCA, anti-I2, anti-OmpC, and anti-CBir1 reactivity with disease course in a large cohort of pediatric CD patients and found that the frequency of fibrostenotic or penetrating disease increased in parallel with the number of antigens recognized [61]. Combining anti-microbial antibody titers and evaluation of NOD2 variants or other gene polymorphisms may improve detection of patients at higher risk of developing fibrostenotic disease [62].

The predictive value of other serologic markers for fibrostenotic disease has been evaluated on a much more limited basis than the anti-microbial antibodies. C-reactive protein (CRP) is widely used to monitor inflammatory disease activity and one prospective study found a significant association between CRP levels and subsequent risk of intestinal resection in patients with ileal disease [63]. Despite the prominent place of extracellular matrix proteins in composition of fibrostenotic lesions, little association has been found with levels of these molecules in the circulation [64]. However, one study did find that higher levels of plasma fibronectin were associated with stricture formation in CD patients [65]. Growth factors have also been evaluated in a limited fashion. Serum levels of YKL-40, a mammalian glycoprotein member of the chitinase family, has been reported as increased in CD patients with stricturing disease compared to those without strictures [66]. Another study found serum levels of basic fibroblast growth factor, a cytokine promoting fibroblast activation and proliferation, were higher in CD patients with intestinal strictures compared to patients with fistulizing or inflammatory phenotypes [67]. Prospective studies will be required to determine which, if any, of these serologic tests may have potential as a clinically useful biomarker of fibrostenotic disease.

5. Histologic features

Stricture due to fibrostenotic change resulting in chronic obstruction is a major pathologic event in chronic CD. Histologically, CD strictures are characterized by hyperplasia of the intestinal muscle layers which is typically manifest as islands of smooth muscle cells in the submucosa surrounded by dense collagen deposits. These regions of smooth muscle proliferation may become so extensive that they obliterate the submucosa [68]. Transmission electron microscopy studies show alteration of muscle cells of the muscularis propria, especially the inner muscle layer, including hypertrophy, synthesis and deposition of collagen, and focal cellular necrosis [69].

Despite the general categorization of strictures as inflammatory, fibrostenotic or both, fibrosis is often well correlated with inflammation and the majority of strictures contain some degree of both processes [70]. When histologic tissue inflammation and fibrosis were compared in a relatively small cohort of patients undergoing surgical resection, the authors found that all specimens which were significantly fibrotic were also significantly inflamed [71]. This may accurately reflect the reality of stricturing disease in many patients, however, this has not yet been confirmed in studies of larger patient cohorts and the results may be skewed because histologic evaluation is only possible in patients undergoing surgical resection. This excludes stricture patients who either respond to aggressive medical therapy or who undergo bowel-sparing procedures which may inadvertently exclude many patients who fall on either end of the inflammation/fibrosis spectrum.

Further consideration of the relationship between histologic categorization and disease behavior is needed and new histologic scoring systems may be required which consider cellular composition or other features in order to more effectively categorize strictures. One retrospective study has been published where biopsies were evaluated to determine if certain histologic characteristics correspond to eventual development of complicated CD [72]. The authors report that severe lymphoid infiltration of the lamina propria with crypt atrophy and absence of intraepithelial lymphocytes correlates with non-stricturing/non-penetrating disease while these features were absent in 80% of CD patients with stricturing disease. Once again, these findings were based on a small cohort size and need further evaluation but do accord with the larger concept of inflammatory vs. fibrostenotic stricture processes.

Other studies comparing histologic features with biologic behavior are limited. At least two studies have noted an association of mast cells in the submucosa and especially in the muscularis propria with stricture formation in CD patients [73, 74]. When compared to normal bowel or non-strictured CD bowel, mast cell numbers were significantly higher in the thickened muscularis propria of CD strictures. No increase in mast cells was associated with ulcerative colitis or other intestinal inflammatory conditions. Also, epitheliold granulomas have been implicated as a risk factor for progression to complicated disease behavior. Epitheliod granulomas are one of the most characteristic histologic features in biopsies or resected tissue from patients with CD although only about 15-25% of patients present with this lesion. Several studies have shown an association between the occurrence of epitheliod granulomas, especially at presentation, and a more aggressive disease course [75].

6. Pathophysiology of fibrosis

Tissue injury or inflammation triggers a cascade of wound healing activities in the surrounding cell populations. Normal wound healing is a tightly regulated and coordinated series of events triggered by secretion of mediators from activated immune and mesenchymal cells which induce cell proliferation, migration, and extracelluar matrix (ECM) production. Wound healing activity is followed by resolution of inflammation and tissue remodeling. A balance must be achieved between processes involved in ECM production and degradation and those involved in cellular hyperplasia (proliferation and cell death). In the intestinal tract, tissue repair and regeneration are of great importance in mucosal homeostasis and intestinal barrier function. Rapid wound healing and restitution of an intact mucosal barrier is crucial for controlling mucosal inflammation. However, excessive wound healing response can result in fibrosis and stricture formation while insufficient tissue repair can result in fistula formation.

The classic model of wound healing has 4 phases: hemostasis, inflammation, proliferation, and remodeling [76, 77]. In the hemostasis phase, platelet degranulation and fibrin formation provide both hemostasis and a provisional matrix for subsequent healing events to take place. Cytokine and chemokine expression, initially by the innate immune system and later including the adaptive immune system, drives the inflammatory phase. During the proliferative phase, activated fibroblasts and myofibroblasts secrete collagen and other matrix molecules which provide a granulation tissue scaffold on which tissue structure repair can commence. During the proliferative phase, cytokines and growth factors regulate reconstitution of the mucosal epithelium allowing closing of the epithelial defect. Angiogenesis and lymphangiogenesis also take place during this phase and there is expansion of the fibroblast/myofibroblast population with concomitant ECM production. Finally, in the remodeling phase, myofibroblasts produce matrix-modifying molecules which assist in the restoring anatomic structural integrity and completing the transition from wound to normal or near normal intestine architecture.

When severe mucosal tissue damage occurs, myofibroblasts migrate to the edges of the tissue defect. The ability of myofibroblasts to migrate to the wound area and synthesize ECM proteins is critical in proliferative phase of intestinal wound healing [78]. Migration of subepithelial myofibroblasts can be mediated by a variety of soluble factors such as transforming growth factor –β (TGFβ), insulin-like growth factor (IGF-1), platelet-derived growth factor-AB (PDGF-AB), and epidermal growth factor (EGF) [79]. Fibronectin, synthesized by myofibroblasts, is essential and is largely responsible for autocrine induction of intestinal myfibroblast migration [80].

Wound healing and myofibroblast migration can be affected by chronic inflammation [79]. Subepithelial myofibroblasts isolated from CD patients show a significant reduction in migration response when compared to cells from control patients [81]. Similar reduction in fibroblast migration can be induced by treatment with tumor necrosis factor (TNF) or gamma interferon (IFN-g) suggesting that an inflammatory environment can induce changes in myofibroblast function [82]. However, environmental impact on fibroblast migration is complex. For example, fibroblasts from lung tissue with dense fibrosis show higher PDGF-driven migratory potential than do fibroblasts from tissues at an early stage of fibrosis [83]. A recent paper compared migratory potential in colonic fibroblasts isolated from CD patients with either fistulizing (penetrating) or fibrotic (stricturing) disease [81]. These authors showed that, while migratory potential is reduced in CD patients with fistulizing disease, there is in an increase in fibroblast migratory potential in patients with fibrotic disease.

Fibrosis in CD is thought to result from an excessive wound healing response. For reasons that are not wholly understood, the wound repair process in a subset of CD patients continues to progress rather than reaching a termination and allowing for tissue remodeling. Ultimately, the fibrotic process leads to thickening of the intestinal wall and luminal narrowing which can result in bowel obstruction. There are three hallmark pathological features which characterize intestinal stricutres in CD: proliferation of mesenchymal cells including myofibroblasts, smooth muscle cells and fibroblasts; hypertrophy of smooth muscle cells and myofibroblasts ; and accumulation of excess extracellular matrix proteins [84].

Mesenchymal cells in the intestine can be broadly classed as fibroblasts, smooth muscle cells or myofibroblasts on the basis of immunostaining properties with antibodies to vimentin (V) and smooth muscle actin (A) [85, 86]. Fibroblasts are typically V+/A- and are present in the intestinal submucosal and serosa. Subepithelial myofibroblasts (SEMF) are found adjacent to intestinal epithelial cells and are V+/A+. Intestinal smooth muscle cells of the muscularis mucosa and muscularis propria are normally V-/A+. All of these mesenchymal cell types have been implicated in collagen production in CD patients [69, 87, 88].

Activated fibroblasts or myofibroblasts in tissues undergoing a fibrotic process may be derived from a variety of sources. There are three general mechanisms which allow for tissue accumulation of these cells: proliferation of existing tissue fibroblasts, recruitment of fibroblast precursor cells from bone marrow, and transformation either of epithelial cells via epithelial to mesenchymal transistion (EMT), or of endothelial cells by endothelial to mesenchymal transition (EndoMT) [89, 90]. Proliferation and activation of tissue fibroblasts occurs in response to profibrotic signals from infiltrating inflammatory cells or from colonic epithelial cells exposed to proinflammatory cytokines [91]. Soluble inflammatory mediators also drive recruitment of fibroblast precursor cells (fibrocytes) from bone marrow. These fibrocytes migrate from the bloodstream into tissues undergoing pathologic fibrosis in response to specific chemokine gradients [89]. EMT and EndoMT are induced by TGFβ [92]. The relative significance of each of mechanisms discussed above to activated fibroblast/myofibroblast accumulation at the site of injury in CD is not yet fully understood

Smooth muscle hyperplasia surrounded by collagen deposits is the major histologic feature of fibrostenotic CD. This smooth muscle proliferation expands and disrupts the muscularis mucosa. Thickening of the muscular layer is associated with an increase in the number of vimentin-positive cells [93, 94]. In severely affected tissue, even histologically normal muscularis mucosa is populated largely by V+/A- and V+/A+ cells rather than the V-/A+ smooth muscle cells seen in normal muscularis mucosa from non-CD patients. This suggests a transition from an enteric smooth muscle cell phenotype toward a fibroblast or myofibroblast phenotype.

Mesenchymal cells including myofibroblasts as well as smooth muscle cells of the muscularis mucosa and muscularis propria are the main producers of ECM proteins in the intestine. These ECM proteins include structural proteins such as collagen, matricellular proteins such as osteopontin and thrombospondin, and other specialized proteins such as vitronectin and fibronectin. Collagen is the major ECM component associated with intestinal fibrosis. The most common collagen subtypes in normal intestine are type I, type III, and type V in order of abundance. In intestinal fibrosis, there is an increase in total collagen as well as specific and relative increases in collagen types III and V [95-97].

Fibronectin and vitronectin are ligands for the $\alpha V\beta 3$ integrin and, in the presence of fibronectin, smooth muscle IGF-1-stimulated IGF-1 receptor activation is augmented [98]. This suggests that increased production of these proteins by smooth muscle cells at sites of intestinal stricture could activate $\alpha V\beta 3$ integrin and further increase secretion of collagen as well as promote cellular proliferation creating a positive feedback loop which could further subvert the normal healing process. Fibronectin is also an important mediator in focal adhesion kinase (FAK) signaling pathways involved in cell migration [99]. Myofibroblasts synthesize abundant fibronectin which is largely responsible for the autocrine induction of intestinal myofibroblast migration [100].

The balance between formation and breakdown of ECM proteins determines the net deposition in tissues. In intestinal fibrosis, mechanisms to degrade ECM fail to keep pace with deposition. Matrix metalloproteinases (MMPs), a large family of proteolytic enzymes, are responsible for the breakdown of ECM components. The proteolytic activity of MMPs is controlled by tissue inhibitors of metalloproteinases (TIMPs) and an imbalance between MMP and TIMP activity can result in excessive deposition of ECM proteins with subsequent fibrosis [101]. Higher levels of constitutive TIMP-1 expression have been shown in intestinal myofibroblast culture derived from fibrotic CD patients than those from normal individuals [102].

Transforming growth factor –β (TGFβ) is a pleotrophic cytokine and one of the most influential factors in fibrotic processes. It is a component of Th17 as well as regulatory T cell type immune responses as well as a profibrotic mediator. TGFβ exerts profibrotic effects through its ability to regulate collagen expression and extracellular matrix dynamics. There are three isoforms of TGFβ: TGFβ1, TGFβ2, and TGFβ3. TGFβ1 activates the canonical Smad signaling cascade leading to translocation of the Smad receptor complex into the nucleus and regulation of gene transcription including ECM genes such as collagen I, collagen III, and fibronectin [103]. TGFβ also induces EMT in organ-fibrosis inducing diseases [104] and can to induce EndoMT in vitro via a "noncanonical" signaling pathway [105]. In CD patients, TGFβ1 and TGFβ3 are increased in in smooth muscle, fibroblasts and myofibroblasts from the strictured region when compared to normal intestine [102, 106].

TGFβ family proteins are important in regulating the synthesis and breakdown of ECM proteins [107]. TGFβ1 downregulates MMP expression and enhances the expression of TIMP-1 [101]. Characterization of the role of TGFβ expression in disease has been done using myofibroblast cultures. Myofibroblasts from normal intestine predominantly express TGFβ3 while those patients with fibrotic CD had significantly lower expression of TGFβ3 and higher levels of TGFβ1 and TGFβ2 [102, 108].

Insulin-like growth factor has also been implicated in the pathogenesis of stricture formation [109]. Intestinal smooth muscle cells express IGF-1 which activates the IGF-1 receptor thereby regulating smooth muscle cell hyperplasia by simultaneously stimulating proliferation and inhibiting apoptosis [110, 111]. Studies using CD tissue from patients undergoing intestinal resection show increased expression of both IGF-1 as well as synergistic IGF binding protein 5 (IGFBP-5) in lesional tissue [112]. Localization studies show IGF-1 is upregulated in smooth muscle cells in regions of stricture when compared to tissue from surgical margins.

7. Preclinical models

A major challenge facing scientists interested in developing treatments for CD-associated fibrotic disease is the need for a robust animal model which develops morphologic features and utilizes pathogenic processes similar to those characterized for the human disease. Preclinical models should provide a consistent environment for testing intervention strategies and quantifying outcomes. At present, no animal model exists which reproduces the unique histologic features associated with CD intestinal strictures. There are several models which address some aspects of CD stricture pathogenesis and those are reviewed below.

Intestinal inflammation and fibrosis can be induced in rats by injection of peptidoglycan-polysaccharide (PG-PS) into the intestinal wall or by repeated rounds of trinitrobenzene sulfonic acid (TNBS) treatment [113, 114]. PG-PS injection causes acute inflammation which peaks by 2 days followed by remission. Spontaneous reactivation of inflammation occurs in genetically susceptible rat strains by 12-17 days and is characterized by progressive transmural granulomatous enterocolitis [115]. Multiple cycles of intrarectal injection of TNBS in ethanol also induces a granulomatous transmural inflammatory response which becomes dominated by chronic inflammation and fibrosis after cycle 4[113, 116]. This model features transmural collagen deposition which is most prominent in the submucosa. Smooth muscle proliferation and expansion into the submucosal space is not a feature of these models.

Given that no existing preclinical model completely mimics changes found in human CD fibrostenosis, assessment of the value of models should be based on the presence of pathways of interest as well as tractability in testing potential therapeutic entities. These rat models show transmural inflammation associated with transmural fibrosis as well as overexpression of TGFβ and/or IGF-1 in a manner consistent with human disease [116-119]. However, given the availability of reagents and other research tools, mouse models of intestinal fibrosis are more desirable to the research community.

http://dx.doi.org/10.5772/46222

While many murine models of inflammatory colitis or enteritis exist, these models are generally not suitable for study the pathogenesis of stricture formation or for testing intervention strategies because they generate very little intestinal fibrosis. Fibrotic models have been challenging to develop given the inherent resistance of mice when compared to other species in development of fibrotic disease [94]. However, progress is being made in this area.

Ileocecal resection is a common surgical intervention in CD and is associated with high rates of disease recurrence[120]. After surgery, recurrence of inflammation and/or fibrosis typically occurs at the anastomosis and in the small intestine immediately upstream of the anastomosis. A model of ileocecal resection in IL-10 gene knockout mice has been described which develops inflammation and fibrosis both at the anastomosis site and in other regions of the small intestine [121]. This approach is attractive because it models a major clinical feature of CD fibrostenotic disease and is highly relevant to future clinical trials where therapeutics targeting CD fibrosis will likely be evaluated for prevention of postsurgical recurrence. However, IL-10 null mice do not spontaneously develop small intestinal inflammation and this surgical approach may need to be combined with one of the existing murine ileitis models to achieve the most relevant preclinical model.

Chronic TNBS treatment has been used to induce colitis in mice as well as rats. In the mouse, TNBS with concomitant administration of ethanol as an epithelial barrier disrupter induces intestinal ulceration and inflammation. This model is widely used to investigate acute inflammation in the gut. Chronic TNBS treatment has been tested in an effort to develop a more robust intestinal fibrosis model in mouse [122]. This model has been reported to have some common features with CD including transmural inflammation and stricturing with proximal dilation and fibrosis. Affected animals have increased expression of MMP-1 and collagen type 1. Fibrosis in this model can be enhanced by treatment with indomethacin, a cyclooxygenase (COX) inhibitor which can block the anti-fibrotic effects of COX-2 [123].

Dextran sulfate sodium added to drinking water is frequently used to induce epithelial injury and acute colitis in mice. Fibrosis with associated increase in collagen, TGFβ, and matrix metalloproteinase expression has been described in C57BL6 mice following a single 5 day cycle of DSS exposure [124]. The authors were also able to show an increase in fibroblasts (V+/A-) and myofibroblasts (V+/A+) cells in the mucosa and submucosa. While this likely reflects a primary intestinal wound healing response rather than the chronic fibrotic process suggested by the authors, it is worth considering if this could be a useful pathway model which might allow rapid testing the effect of therapeutic candidates on specific elements of the wound healing/fibrotic response. Other groups have investigated the effect of multiple cycles of DSS exposure on fibrotic response in FVB-N and C57BL6 mice [125]. A single cycle of DSS exposure in C57BL6 mice does result in ECM deposition followed by mucosal repair and normalized mucosal architecture. Multiple cycles of DSS exposure did not result in enhanced fibrosis in FVB-N mice, however, it did result in prolongation of a fibrotic response in C57BL6 mice as measured by procollagen $\alpha 1$(I) promoter-GFP reporter transgene reporter activity. Further characterization will be needed to determine the utility of this model.

Salmonella species are facultative intracellular gram negative bacteria which cause a range of illnesses including, but not limited to, enterocolitis [126]. *Salmonella enterica* serovar Typhimurium is an enteric bacterial pathogen which normally causes little intestinal pathology in mice but instead mimics human typhoid. However, a model which utilizes oral streptomycin pretreatment has been developed which allows study of *S.* Typhimurium-induced cecal inflammation [127]. This work has been extended by utilizing attenuated *S.* Typhimurium strains or by infecting resistant mouse strains which carry a functional nramp1 gene to induce chronic infection which results in intestinal fibrosis characterized by transmural collagen deposition and accumulation of fibroblasts in the intestinal submucosa [128]. While increase in collagen deposition is observed throughout the colon, the most intense lesions are present in the cecum. The *Salmonella* model of intestinal fibrosis is unique in that it is induced by bacterial colitis. It results in a relatively long term fibrotic process where fibrosis can be observed in the cecal submucosa at least to day 40 post infection. Similar to human CD, increased TGFβ and IGF-1 are associated with fibrosis in this model.

8. Prevention or treatment of CD fibrosis

While considerable progress has been made, the pathophysiology of fibrostenotic disease in CD patients is incompletely understood. The drug development challenges this creates are greatly compounded by the absence of a well defined and widely accepted preclinical animal model of intestinal fibrosis. Recognition of the unmet need for medical interventions which can effectively prevent or treat CD fibrostenotic disease drives ongoing research in both areas. Despite the challenges, a number of potential therapeutic agents or pathways have undergone preliminary testing. A few of these results are summarized below. The data available for all of these agents is quite limited.

Prostaglandins (PGE1 and 2) are known to inhibit smooth muscle proliferation as well as fibroblast proliferation induced by proinflammatory cytokines [129, 130]. Reduced PGE2 levels are associated with development of fibrosis in idiopathic pulmonary fibrosis (IPF) [131] and indomethacin treatment, which inhibits PGE2, increases fibrosis in the chronic murine TNBS model of colon fibrosis. However, mice deficient in prostaglandin endoperoxide synthase (Ptgs) 2, an enzyme involved in prostaglandin production, showed deficient wound healing following full-thickness colonic biopsy so the effects of prostaglandins may be complex and, perhaps, dependent on the stage of wound healing [132]. Phosphatidyl choline, a polyunsaturated fatty acid which is a precursor to PGE2, has been shown to decrease stricture formation in the rat TNBS intestinal fibrosis model [133]. These data suggest a role for PGE2 in intestinal wound healing and fibrosis but the potential for a therapeutic role requires further investigation.

The steroid hormone retinoic acid (RA) is another potential agent for modification of fibrosis in CD. RA has been shown to have effects on human fibroblast proliferation in cells isolated from IPF lungs [134] and to protect against bleomycin-induced pulmonary fibrosis in mice [135]. More recently, RA has been shown to reduce intestinal fibrosis in the chronic TNBS mouse model of intestinal fibrosis [123]. Much more research will be needed to determine if RA has promise as a fibrosis modifying agent in CD.

Resveratrol (trans-3,5,4'-trihydroxystilbene) is a phytoalexin found in a variety of plant products including berries, peanuts, grapes and red wine. It has been shown to reduce inflammation in rat colitis [136]. Resveratrol has also been shown to reduce activation of NF-kB in TNBS colitis [137]. A recent paper reports that resveratrol exposure results in decreased collagen synthesis as well as apoptosis in rat intestinal smooth muscle cells [138]. While the data on resveratrol is quite preliminary, the data is of interest because it targets smooth muscle rather than the fibroblasts or myofibroblasts.

Anti-inflammatory and anti-fibrotic effects of the cholesterol lowering 3-hydroxy-3-methyl-glutaryl-CoA reductase inhibitors (statins) have been reported. Statins may play an anti-fibrotic role through inhibition of the activation and proliferation of fibroblasts and by inducing apoptosis of activated fibroblasts [139]. Angiotensin type 1 receptor blockers [140] and the angiotensin-converting enzyme inhibitor captopril [141] have also been proposed as fibrosis inhibitors.

Fibrosis has traditionally been considered an irreversible process. Further testing of these and other agents which have potential to block initiation or inhibit progression of fibrosis may also reveal if medical treatment has the potential to reverse existing fibrotic lesions. Research to further characterize the underlying pathophysiologic processes involved in fibrostenotic disease and to test potential therapeutic approaches remains important to the goal of fully meeting CD therapeutic needs.

Author details

Lauri Diehl

Department of Pathology, Genentech, USA

References

[1] Greenstein, A.J., et al., *Perforating and non-perforating indications for repeated operations in Crohn's disease: evidence for two clinical forms.* Gut, 1988. 29: p. 588-592.

[2] Gasche, C., et al., *A simple classification of Crohn's disease: Report of the working party for the World Congresses of Gastroenterology, Vienna 1998.* Inflammatory Bowel Diseases, 2000. 6(1): p. 8-15.

[3] Peyrin-Biroulet, L., et al., *The Natural History of Adult Crohn ' s Disease in Population-Based Cohorts.* American Journal of Gastroenterology, 2010. 105: p. 289–297.

[4] D'Haens, G.R., et al., *Endpoints for Clinical Trials Evaluating Disease Modification and Structural Damage in Adults with Crohn's Disease.* inflammatory Bowel Disease Monitor, 2009. 15(10): p. 1599–1604.

[5] Romberg-Camps, M.J.L., et al., *Influence of Phenotype at Diagnosis and of Other Potential Prognostic Factors on the Course of Inflammatory Bowel Disease.* American Journal of Gastroenterology, 2009. 104: p. 371–383.

[6] Ordas, I., B.G. Feagan, and W.J. Sandborn, *Early use of immunosuppressives or TNF antagonists for the treatment of Crohn's disease: time for a change.* Gut, 2011. 60: p. 1754-1763.

[7] Cosnes, J., et al., *Long-term evolution of disease behavior of Crohn's disease.* Inflammatory Bowel Diseases, 2002. 8(4): p. 244-250.

[8] Louis, E., et al., *Behaviour of Crohn's disease according to the Vienna classification: changing pattern over the course of the disease.* Gut, 2001. 49: p. 777-782.

[9] Assche, G.V., K. Goboes, and P. Rutgeerts, *Medical therapy for Crohn's disease strictures.* Inflammatory Bowel Diseases, 2004. 10: p. 55-60.

[10] Yamagata, M., et al., *Submucosal fibrosis and basic-fibroblast growth factor-positive neutrophils correlate with colonic stenosis in cases of ulcerative colitis.* Digestion, 2011. 84: p. 12-21.

[11] Broering, D.C., et al., *Quality of Life after Surgical Therapy of Small Bowel Stenosis in Crohn's Disease.* Digestive Surgery, 2001. 18: p. 124-130.

[12] Olaison, G., K. Smedh, and R. Sjödahl, *Natural course of Crohn's disease after ileocolic resection: endoscopically visualised ileal ulcers preceding symptoms.* Gut, 1992. 33: p. 331-335.

[13] Rutgeerts, P., et al., *Predictability of the postoperative course of Crohn's disease.* Gastroenterology, 1990. 99(4): p. 956-963.

[14] Bernell, O., A. Lapidus, and G. Hellers, *Risk Factors for Surgery and Postoperative Recurrence in Crohn's Disease.* Annals of Surgery, 2000. 231(1): p. 38-45.

[15] Heimann, T.M., et al., *Comparison of Primary and Reoperative Surgery in Patients With Crohns Disease.* Annals of Surgery, 1998. 227(4): p. 492-495.

[16] Wettergren, A. and J. Christiansen, *Risk of Recurrence and Reoperation after Resection for Ileocolic Crohn's Disease.* Scandinavian Journal of Gastroenterology, 1991. 26(12): p. 1319-1322.

[17] Felleya, C., et al., *Appropriate therapy for fistulizing and fibrostenotic Crohn's disease: Results of a multidisciplinary expert panel — EPACT II.* Journal of Crohn's and Colitis, 2009. 3(4): p. 250–256.

[18] Swaminath, A. and S. Lichtiger, *Dilation of colonic strictures by intralesional injection of infliximab in patients with Crohn's colitis.* Inflammatory Bowel Diseases, 2008. 14(2): p. 213-216.

[19] Ozuner, G., et al., *How safe is strictureplasty in the management of Crohn's disease?* The American Journal of Surgery, 1996. 171(1): p. 57–61.

[20] Brenner, D.J. and E.J. Hall, *Computed Tomography — An Increasing Source of Radiation Exposure.* The New England Journal of Medicine, 2007. 357: p. 2277-2284.

[21] Kroeker, K.I., et al., *Patients With IBD are Exposed to High Levels of Ionizing Radiation Through CT Scan Diagnostic Imaging. A Five-year Study.* Journal of Clinical Gastroenterology, 2011. 45: p. 34–39.

[22] Ripolles, T., et al., *Effectiveness of contrast-enhanced ultrasound for characterisation of intestinal inflammation in Crohn's disease: A comparison with surgical histopathology analysis.* Journal of Crohn's and Colitis, 2012.

[23] Martin, D.R., et al., *Magnetic resonance enterography in Crohn's disease: techniques, interpretation, and utilization for clinical management.* Diagnostic and Interventional Radiology, 2012. 18: p. 374-386.

[24] Panés, J., et al., *Systematic review: the use of ultrasonography, computed tomography and magnetic resonance imaging for the diagnosis, assessment of activity and abdominal complications of Crohn's disease.* Alimentary Pharmacology and Therapeutics, 2011. 34(2): p. 125-145.

[25] Stange, E.F., et al., *European evidence based consensus on the diagnosis and management of Crohn's disease: definitions and diagnosis.* Gut, 2006. 55(SUPPL. 1): p. i1-i15.

[26] Lenze, F., et al., *Detection and differentiation of inflammatory versus fibromatous Crohn's disease strictures: Prospective comparison of ^{18}F-FDG-PET/CT, MR-enteroclysis, and transabdominal ultrasound versus endoscopic/histologic evaluation.* Inflammatory Bowel Diseases, 2012.

[27] Jacene, H.A., et al., *Prediction of the need for surgical intervention in obstructive Crohn's disease by ^{18}F-FDG PET/CT.* Journal of Nuclear Medicine, 2009. 50: p. 1751-1759.

[28] Rogler, G., *Is this stricture inflammatory?* Digestion, 2011. 83: p. 261-262.

[29] Bouguen, G., et al., *Long-term outcome of non-fistulizing (ulcers, stricture) perianal Crohn's disease in patients treated with infliximab.* Alimentary Pharmacology and Therapeutics, 2009. 30(7): p. 749-756.

[30] Pelletier, A.-L., et al., *Infliximab treatment for symptomatic Crohn's disease strictures.* Alimentary Pharmacology and Therapeutics, 2009. 29(3): p. 279-285.

[31] Tarrant, K.M., et al., *Perianal Disease Predicts Changes in Crohn's Disease Phenotype—Results of a Population-Based Study of Inflammatory Bowel Disease Phenotype.* The American Journal of Gastroenterology, 2008. 103: p. 3082–3093.

[32] Lakatos, P.L., et al., *Perianal disease, small bowel disease, smoking, prior steroid or early azathioprine/biological therapy are predictors of disease behavior change in patients with Crohn's disease.* World Journal of Gastroenterology, 2009. 15(28): p. 3504-3510.

[33] Louis, E., et al., *Behaviour of Crohn's disease according to the Vienna classification: changing pattern over the course of the disease.* Gut, 2001. 49: p. 777-782

[34] Hommes, D., et al., *Changing Crohn's disease management: Need for new goals and indices to prevent disability and improve quality of life.* Journal of Crohn's and Colitis, 2012. 6S2: p. S224-S234.

[35] Lichtenstein, G.R., et al., *A Pooled Analysis of Infections, Malignancy, and Mortality in Infliximab- and Immunomodulator-Treated Adult Patients With Inflammatory Bowel Disease.* The American Journal of Gastroenterology, 2012. 107: p. 1051–1063.

[36] Lichtenstein, G.R., et al., *Factors Associated with the Development of Intestinal Strictures or Obstructions in Patients with Crohn's Disease.* American Journal of Gastroenterology, 2006. 101: p. 1030–1038.

[37] Beaugerie, L. and H. Sokol, *Clinical, serological and genetic predictors of inflammatory bowel disease course.* World Journal of Gastroenterology, 2012. 18(29): p. 3806-3813.

[38] Ogura, Y., et al., *A frameshift mutation in Nod2 associated with susceptibility to Crohn's disease.* Nature, 2001. 411: p. 603–606.

[39] Hugot, J.-P., et al., *Association of NOD2 leucine-rich repeat variants with susceptibility to Crohn's disease.* Nature, 2001. 411: p. 599-603.

[40] Ahmad, T., et al., *The molecular classification of the clinical manifestations of Crohn's disease.* Gastroenterology, 2002. 122(4): p. 854-866.

[41] Lesage, S., et al., *CARD15/NOD2 Mutational Analysis and Genotype-Phenotype Correlation in 612 Patients with Inflammatory Bowel Disease.* The American Journal of Human Genetics, 2002. 70(4): p. 845–857.

[42] Abreu, M.T., et al., *Mutations in NOD2 are associated with fibrostenosing disease in patients with Crohn's disease.* Gastroenterology, 2002. 123: p. 679-688.

[43] Alvarez-Lobos, M., et al., *Crohn's Disease Patients Carrying Nod2/CARD15 Gene Variants Have an Increased and Early Need for First Surgery due to Stricturing Disease and Higher Rate of Surgical Recurrence.* Annals of Surgery, 2005. 242(5): p. 693-700.

[44] Brant, S.R., et al., *Defining complex contributions of NOD2/CARD15 gene mutations, age at onset, and tobacco use on Crohn's disease phenotypes.* Inflammatory Bowel Diseases, 2009. 9(5): p. 281-289.

[45] Shaoul, R., et al., *Disease Behavior in Children with Crohn's Disease: The Effect of Disease Duration, Ethnicity, Genotype, and Phenotype.* Digestive Diseases and Sciences, 2009. 54: p. 142–150.

[46] Teimoori-Toolabi, L., et al., *Three common CARD15 mutations are not responsible for the pathogenesis of Crohn's disease in Iranians.* Hepatogastroenterology, 2010. 57(98): p. 275-82.

[47] Economou, M., et al., *Differential Effects of NOD2 Variants on Crohn's Disease Risk and Phenotype in Diverse Populations: A Metaanalysis.* The American Journal of Gastroenterology, 2004. 99: p. 2393–2404.

[48] Weersma, R.K., et al., *Molecular prediction of disease risk and severity in a large Dutch Crohn's disease cohort.* Gut, 2009. 58: p. 388-395.

[49] Sabate, J.-M., et al., *The V249I polymorphism of the CX3CR1 gene is associated with fibrostenotic disease behavior in patients with Crohn's disease.* European Journal of Gastroenterology & Hepatology, 2008. 20(8): p. 748-755.

[50] Däbritz, J., et al., *The functional -374T/A polymorphism of the receptor for advanced glycation end products may modulate Crohn's disease.* American Journal of Physiology - Gastrointestinal and Liver Physiology, 2011. 300: p. G823–G832,.

[51] Seiderer, J., et al., *Genotype–phenotype analysis of the CXCL16 p.Ala181Val polymorphism in inflammatory bowel disease.* Clinical Immunology, 2008. 127: p. 49-55.

[52] Vasiliauskas, E.A., et al., *Marker antibody expression stratifies Crohn's disease into immunologically homogeneous subgroups with distinct clinical characteristics.* Gut, 2000. 47: p. 487-496.

[53] Forcione, D.G., et al., *Anti-Saccharomyces cerevisiae antibody (ASCA) positivity is associated with increased risk for early surgery in Crohn's disease.* Gut, 2004. 53: p. 1117-1122.

[54] Amre, D.K., et al., *Utility of serological markers in predicting the early occurrence of complications and surgery in pediatric Crohn's disease patients.* American Journal of Gastroenterology, 2006. 101: p. 645-652.

[55] Mow, W.S., et al., *Association of antibody responses to microbial antigens and complications of small bowel Crohn's disease.* Gastroenterology, 2004. 126: p. 414-424.

[56] Arnott, I.D., et al., *Sero-reactivity to microbial components in Crohn's disease is associated with disease severity and progression, but not NOD2/CARD15 genotype.* American Journal of Gastroenterology, 2004. 99: p. 2376-2384.

[57] Targan, S.R., et al., *Antibodies to CBir1 flagellin define a unique response that is associated independently with complicated Crohn's disease.* Gastroenterology, 2005. 128: p. 2020-2028.

[58] Xue S, S.J., Elkadri AA, Greenberg GR, Walters and G.A. TD, Steinhart H, Silverberg MS., *Serological markers are associated with severity of disease and need for surgery in IBD patients.* Gastroenterology, 2006. 130: p. S1303.

[59] Ferrante, M., et al., *New serological markers in inflammatory bowel disease are associated with complicated disease behaviour.* Gut, 2007. 56: p. 1394–1403.

[60] Papp, M., et al., *New Serological Markers for Inflammatory Bowel Disease Are Associated With Earlier Age at Onset, Complicated Disease Behavior, Risk for Surgery, and NOD2/ CARD15 Genotype in a Hungarian IBD Cohort.* American Journal of Gastroenterology, 2008. 103: p. 665–681.

[61] Dubinsky, M.C., et al., *Increased immune reactivity predicts aggressive complicating Crohn's disease in children.* Clinical Gastroenterology and Hepatology 2008. 6: p. 1105-1111.

[62] Ippoliti, A., et al., *Combination of Innate and Adaptive Immune Alterations Increased the Likelihood of Fibrostenosis in Crohn's Disease.* inflammatory Bowel Diseases, 2010. 16: p. 1279–1285.

[63] Henriksen, M., et al., *C-reactive protein: a predictive factor and marker of inflammation in inflammatory bowel disease. Results from a prospective population-based study.* Gut, 2008. 57: p. 1518-1523.

[64] Koutroubakis, I.E., et al., *Serum laminin and collagen IV in inflammatory bowel disease.* Journal of Clinical Pathology, 2003. 56: p. 817-820.

[65] Allan, A., et al., *Plasma fibronectin in Crohn's disease.* Gut, 1989. 30: p. 627-633.

[66] Koutroubakis, I.E., et al., *Increased serum levels of YKL-40 in patients with inflammatory bowel disease.* International Journal of Colorectal Disease, 2003. 18: p. 254–259.

[67] DiSabatino, A., et al., *Serum bFGF and VEGF Correlate Respectively with Bowel Wall Thickness and Intramural Blood Flow in Crohn's Disease.* Inflammatory Bowel Diseases, 2004. 10: p. 573–577.

[68] Koukoulis, G., et al., *Obliterative muscularization of the small bowel submucosa in Crohn disease.* Archives of Pathology & Laboratory Medicine, 2001. 125: p. 1331-1334.

[69] Dvorak, A.M., et al., *Crohn's disease: Transmission electron microscopic studies **: III. Target tissues. Proliferation of and injury to smooth muscle and the autonomic nervous system.* Human Pathology, 1980. 11(6): p. 620–634.

[70] Zappa, M., et al., *Which magnetic resonance imaging findings accurately evaluate inflammation in small bowel Crohn's disease? A retrospective comparison with surgical pathologic analysis.* Inflammatory Bowel Diseases, 2011. 17: p. 984-993.

[71] Adler, J., et al., *Computed Tomography Enterography Findings Correlate with Tissue Inflammation, Not Fibrosis in Resected Small Bowel Crohn's Disease.* inflammatory Bowel Diseases, 2012. 18: p. 849–856.

[72] Bataille, F., et al., *Histopathological parameters as predictors for the course of Crohn's disease.* Virchows Archives, 2003. 443: p. 501-507.

[73] Dvorak, A.M., et al., *Crohn's disease: Transmission electron microscopic studies **: II. Immunologic inflammatory response. Alterations of mast cells, basophils, eosinophils, and the microvasculature.* Human Pathology, 1980. 11(6): p. 606–619.

[74] Gelbmann, C.M., et al., *Strictures in Crohn's disease are characterised by accumulation of mast cells colocalised with laminin but not with fibronectin or vitronectin.* Gut, 1999. 45: p. 210-217.

[75] Heresbach, D., et al., *Frequency and significance of granulomas in a cohort of incident cases of Crohn's disease.* Gut, 2005. 54: p. 215–222.

[76] Rieder, F., et al., *Wound healing and fibrosis in intestinal disease.* Gut, 2007. 56: p. 130-139.

[77] Diegelmann, R.F. and M.C. Evans, *Wound healing: an overview of acute, fibrotic and delayed healing.* Frontiers in bioscience : a journal and virtual library, 2004. 9: p. 283-289.

[78] Tarnawski, A.S., *Cellular and Molecular Mechanisms of Gastrointestinal Ulcer Healing.* Digestive Diseases and Sciences 2005. 50(1 (supplement)): p. S24-S33.

[79] Leeb, S.N., et al., *Regulation of Migration of Human Colonic Myofibroblasts.* Growth Factors, 2002. 20(2): p. 81-91.

[80] Dignass, A.U., *Mechanisms and modulation of intestinal epithelial repair.* Inflammatory Bowel Disease Monitor, 2001. 7(1): p. 68-77.

[81] Meier, J.K.-H., et al., *Specific Differences in Migratory Function of Myofibroblasts Isolated from Crohn's Disease Fistulae and Strictures.* Inflammatory Bowel Disease Monitor, 2011. 17(1): p. 202-212.

[82] Leeb, S.N., et al., *Reduced migration of fibroblasts in inflammatory bowel disease: role of inflammatory mediators and focal adhesion kinase.* Gastroenterology, 2003. 125(5): p. 1341–1354.

[83] Suganuma, H., et al., *Enhanced migration of fibroblasts derived from lungs with fibrotic lesions.* Thorax, 1995. 50: p. 984-989.

[84] Bien, A.C. and J.F. Kuemmerle, *Fibrosis in Crohn's Disease.* Inflammatory Bowel Disease Monitor, 2012. 12(3): p. 102-109.

[85] Powell, D.W., et al., *Myofibroblasts. II. Intestinal subepithelial myofibroblasts.* American Journal of Physiology - Cell Physiology, 1999. 277(2): p. C183-C201.

[86] Powell, D.W., et al., *Mesenchymal cells of the intestinal lamina propria.* Annual Review of Physiology, 2011. 73: p. 213-237.

[87] Graham, M.F., *Pathogenesis of intestinal strictures in Crohn's disease - an update.* inflammatory Bowel Diseases, 1995. 1: p. 220-227.

[88] Pucilowska, J.B., et al., *IGF-I and procollagen $\alpha 1(I)$ are coexpressed in a subset of mesenchymal cells in active Crohn's disease.* American Journal of Physiology - Gastrointestinal and Liver Physiology, 2000. 6: p. G1307-G1322.

[89] Bellini, A. and S. Mattoli, *The role of the fibrocyte, a bone marrow-derived mesenchymal progenitor, in reactive and reparative fibroses.* Laboratory Investigation, 2007. 87: p. 858–870.

[90] Postlethwaite, A.E., H. Shigemitsu, and S. Kanangat, *Cellular origins of fibroblasts: possible implications for organ fibrosis in systemic sclerosis.* Current Opinion in Rheumatology, 2004. 16: p. 733–738.

[91] Drygiannakis, I., et al., *Proinflammatory cytokines induce crosstalk between colonic epithelial cells and subepithelial myofibroblasts: Implication in intestinal fibrosis.* Journal of Crohn's and Colitis, 2012.

[92] Piera-Velazquez, S., Z. Li, and S.A. Jimenez, *Role of endothelial-mesenchymal transition (EndoMT) in the pathogenesis of fibrotic disorders.* The American Journal of Pathology, 2011. 179(3): p. 1074-1080.

[93] Burke, J.P., et al., *Fibrogenesis in Crohn's Disease.* The American Journal of Gastroenterology, 2007. 102: p. 439–448.

[94] Pucilowska, J.B., K.L. Williams, and P.K. Lund, *Fibrogenesis IV. Fibrosis and inflammatory bowel disease: Cellular mediators and animal models.* American Journal of Physiology - Gastrointestinal and Liver Physiology 2000. 279(4): p. G653-G659.

[95] Graham, M.F., et al., *Collagen content and types in the intestinal strictures of Crohn's disease.* Gastroenterology, 1988. 94: p. 257-265.

[96] Stallmach, A., et al., *Increased collagen type III synthesis by fibroblasts isolated from strictures of patients with Crohn's disease.* Gastroenterology, 1992. 102(6): p. 1920-1929.

[97] Matthes, H., et al., *Cellular localization of procollagen gene transcripts in inflammatory bowel diseases.* Gastroenterology, 1992. 102(2): p. 431-442.

[98] Kuemmerle, J.F., *Occupation of* $a_V b_3$*-integrin by endogenous ligands modulates IGF-1 receptor activation and proliferation of human intestinal smooth muscle.* American Journal of Physiology Gastrointestinal and Liver Physiology, 2006. 290: p. G1194-G1202.

[99] Meng, X.N., et al., *Characterisation of fibronectin-mediated FAK signalling pathways in lung cancer cell migration and invasion.* British Journal of Cancer, 2009. 101: p. 327–334.

[100] Leeb, S.N., et al., *Autocrine Fibronectin-Induced Migration of Human Colonic Fibroblasts.* The American Journal of Gastroenterology, 2004. 99: p. 335–340.

[101] Gomez, D.E., et al., *Tissue inhibitors of metalloproteinases: structure, regulation and biological functions.* European Journal of Cell Biology, 1997. 74(2): p. 111-122.

[102] McKaig, B.C., et al., *Expression and Regulation of Tissue Inhibitor of Metalloproteinase-1 and Matrix Metalloproteinases by Intestinal Myofibroblasts in Inflammatory Bowel Disease* American Journal of Pathology, 2003. 162(4): p. 1355-1360.

[103] Yan, X., Z. Liu, and Y. Chen, *Regulation of TGF-β signaling by Smad7.* Acta Biochimica et Biophysica Sinica, 2009. 41(4): p. 263–272.

[104] Willis, B.C. and Z. Borok, *TGF-β-induced EMT: mechanisms and implications for fibrotic lung disease.* American Journal of Physiology - Lung Cellular and Molecular Physiology, 2007. 293(3): p. L525-L534.

[105] Piera-Velazquez, S., Z. Li, and S.A. Jimenez, *Role of Endothelial-Mesenchymal Transition (EndoMT) in the Pathogenesis of Fibrotic Disorders.* American Journal of Pathology, 2011. 179(3): p. 1074-1080.

[106] Burke, J.P., et al., *Transcriptomic analysis of intestinal fibrosis-associated gene expression in response to medical therapy in Crohn's disease.* Inflammatory Bowel Disease Monitor, 2008. 14(9): p. 1197-1204.

[107] Border, W.A. and N.A. Noble, *Transforming growth factor beta in tissue fibrosis.* The New England Journal of Medicine, 1994. 331: p. 1286-1292.

[108] McKaig, B.C., et al., *Differential expression of TGF-β isoforms by normal and inflammatory bowel disease intestinal myofibroblasts.* American Journal of Physiology - Cell Physiology, 2002. 282: p. C172–C182.

[109] Flynn, R.S., et al., *Endogenous IGFBP-3 Regulates excell collagen expression in intestinal smooth muscle cells of Crohn's disease strictures.* Inflammatory Bowel Diseases, 2011. 17(1): p. 193-201.

[110] Kuemmerle, J.F., *Endogenous IGF-1 protects human intestinal smooth muscle cells from apoptosis by regulation of GSK-3 b activity.* American Journal of Physiology Gastrointestinal and Liver Physiology, 2004. 288: p. G101-G110.

[111] Kuemmerle, J.F., *IGF-I elicits growth of human intestinal smooth muscle cells by activation of PI3K, PDK-1, and p70S6 kinase.* American Journal of Physiology Gastrointestinal and Liver Physiology, 2003. 284: p. G411-G422.

[112] Zimmermann, E.M., et al., *Insulin-like growth factor 1 and insulin-like growth factor binding protein 5 in Crohn's disease.* American Journal of Physiology Gastrointestinal and Liver Physiology, 2001. 280: p. G1022-G1029.

[113] Morris, G.P., et al., *Hapten-induced model of chronic inflammation and ulceration in the rat colon.* Gastroenterology, 1989. 96(3): p. 795-803.

[114] Rahal, K., et al., *Resveratrol has antiinflammatory and antifibrotic effects in the peptidoglycan-polysaccharide rat model of Crohn's disease.* Inflammatory Bowel Disease Monitor, 2012. 18(4): p. 613-623.

[115] Sartor, R.B., *Current concepts of the etiology and pathogenesis of ulcerative colitis and Crohn's disease.* Gastroenterology Clinics of North America, 1995. 24: p. 475-507.

[116] Zhu, M.Y., et al., *Dynamic progress of 2,4,6-trinitrobenzene sulfonic acid induced chronic colitis and fibrosis in rat model.* Journal of Digestive Diseases, 2012. 13: p. 42--429.

[117] Zeeh, J.M., et al., *Differential Expression and Localization of IGF-I and IGF Binding Proteins in Inflamed Rat Colon.* Journal of Receptors and Signal Transduction, 1998. 18(4-6): p. 265-280.

[118] Zimmermann, E.M., et al., *Insulinlike growth factor I and interleukin 1 beta messenger RNA in a rat model of granulomatous enterocolitis and hepatitis.* Gastroenterology, 1993. 105(2): p. 399-409.

[119] Latella, G., et al., *Prevention of colonic fibrosis by Boswellia and Scutellaria extracts in rats with colitis induced by 2,4,5-trinitrobenzene sulphonic acid.* European Journal of Clinical Investigation, 2008. 38(6): p. 410-420.

[120] Penner, R.M., K.L. Madsen, and R.N. Fedorak, *Postoperative Crohn's disease.* inflammatory Bowel Diseases, 2005. 11: p. 765-777.

[121] Rigby, R.J., et al., *A new animal model of postsurgical bowel inflammation and fibrosis: the effect of commensal microflora.* Gut, 2009. 58: p. 1104-1112.

[122] Lawrance, I.C., et al., *A Murine Model of Chronic Inflammation–Induced Intestinal Fibrosis Down-Regulated by Antisense NF-kB.* Gastroenterology, 2003. 125: p. 1750-1761.

[123] Klopcic, B., et al., *Indomethacin and Retinoic Acid Modify Mouse Intestinal Inflammation and Fibrosis: A Role for SPARC.* Digestive Diseases and Sciences, 2008. 53: p. 1553-1563.

[124] Suzuki, K., et al., *Analysis of intestinal fibrosis in chronic colitis in mice induced by dextran sulfate sodium.* Pathology International, 2011. 61(4): p. 228-238.

[125] Ding, S., et al., *Mucosal Healing and Fibrosis after Acute or Chronic Inflammation in Wild Type FVB-N Mice and C57BL6 Procollagen α1(I)-Promoter-GFP Reporter Mice.* PLOS one, 2012. 7(8).

[126] Santos, R.L., et al., *Animal models of Salmonella infections: enteritis versus typhoid fever.* Microbes and Infection, 2001. 3(14-15): p. 1335–1344.

[127] Barthel, M., et al., *Pretreatment of Mice with Streptomycin Provides a Salmonella enterica Serovar Typhimurium Colitis Model That Allows Analysis of Both Pathogen and Host.* Infection and Immunity, 2003. 71(5): p. 2839-2858.

[128] Grassl, G.A., et al., *Chronic Enteric Salmonella Infection in Mice Leads to Severe and Persistent Intestinal Fibrosis* Gastroenterology, 2008. 134(3): p. 768–780.

[129] Corcoran, M.L., et al., *Interleukin 4 inhibition of prostaglandin E2 synthesis blocks interstitial collagenase and 92-kDa type IV collagenase/gelatinase production by human monocyes.* Journal of Biological Chemistry, 1992. 267: p. 515-519.

[130] Johnson, P.R., et al., *Heparin and PGE2 inhibit DNA synthesis in human airway smooth muscle cells in culture.* American Journal of Physiology - Molecular Physiology, 1995. 269: p. L514-L519.

[131] Wilborn, J., et al., *Cultured lung fibroblasts isolated from patients with idiopathic pulmonary fibrosis have a diminished capacity to synthesize prostaglandin E2 and to express cyclooxygenase-2.* Journal of Clinical Investigation, 1995. 95(4): p. 1861-1868.

[132] Manieri, N.A., et al., *Igf2bp1 is required for full induction of Ptgs2 mRNA in colonic mesenchymal stem cells in mice.* Gastroenterology, 2012. 143: p. 110-121.

[133] Mourelle, M., F. Guarner, and J.-R. Malagelada, *Polyunsaturated phosphatidylcholine prevents stricture formation in a rat model of colitis.* Gastroenterology, 1996. 110(4): p. 1093-1097.

[134] Torry, D.J., et al., *Modulation of the anchorage-independent phenotype of human lung fibroblasts obtained from fibrotic tissue following culture with retinoid and corticosteroid.* Experimental Lung Research, 1996. 22: p. 231-244.

[135] Tabata, C., et al., *All-trans-retinoic acid prevents radiation- or bleomycin-induced pulmonary fibrosis.* American Journal of Respiratory and Critical Care Medicine 2006. 174(12): p. 1352-1360.

[136] Larrosa, M., et al., *Effecct of a low dose of dietary resveratrol on colon microbiota, inflammation and tissue damage in a DSS-induced colitis rat model.* Journal of Agricultural and Food Chemistry, 2009. 2009: p. 2211-2220.

[137] Martin, A.R., et al., *The effects of resveratrol, a phytoalexin derived from red wines, on chronic inflammation induced in an experimentally induced colitis model.* British Journal of Pharmacology, 2006. 147: p. 873-885.

[138] Garcia, P., et al., *Resveratrol causes cell cycle arrest, decreased collagen synthesis, and apoptosis in rat intestinal smooth muscle cells.* American Journal of Physiology - Gastrointestinal and Liver Physiology, 2012. 302: p. G326-335.

[139] Yang, J.I., et al., *Synergistic antifibrotic efficacy of statin and proteinkinase C inhibitor in hepatic fibrosis.* American Journal of Physiology - Gastrointestinal and Liver Physiology, 2010. 298: p. G126-G132.

[140] Moreno, M., et al., *Reduction of advanced liver fibrosis by short-term targeted delivery of an angiotensin receptor blocker to hepatic stellate cells in rats.* Hepatology, 2010. 51: p. 942-952.

[141] Wengrower, D., et al., *Prevention of fibrosis in experimental colitis by captopril: the role of TGF-beta1.* inflammatory Bowel Diseases, 2004. 10: p. 536-545.

Section 2

Management of Disease

Chapter 5

The Imaging of Inflammatory Bowel Disease: Current Concepts and Future Directions

Rahul A. Sheth and Michael S. Gee

Additional information is available at the end of the chapter

http://dx.doi.org/10.5772/53025

1. Introduction

Radiologic techniques play an integral role in the diagnosis and management of patients with inflammatory bowel disease (IBD). Imaging has long been utilized to evaluate segments of the digestive tract that are inaccessible to conventional endoscopy. While endoscopy offers unparalleled visualization of the large bowel lumen and biopsy capabilities, the small bowel remains essentially wholly inaccessible by conventional endoscopic techniques [1]. Thus, one important role that imaging plays in the care of patients with IBD is the evaluation of the small bowel.

With the advancement of cross-sectional imaging techniques such as computed tomography (CT) and magnetic resonance imaging (MRI), the role of imaging in IBD has greatly expanded to include the mucosal, transmural, extraluminal, and extra-intestinal manifestations of these diseases. Imaging now not only assists in making the diagnosis of IBD, including helping to discriminate between ulcerative colitis and Crohn's disease, but also is a critical component in the determination of active versus indolent disease. Imaging assessment of IBD activity is increasingly being utilized by surgeons and gastroenterologists for treatment planning and as a biomarker of treatment response/resistance. Urgent and emergent complications of IBD including abscesses, fistulae, perforations, obstructing strictures, and toxic megacolon are also best detected by cross-sectional imaging techniques over endoscopic methods [2]. Imaging is pivotal in the identification of extra-intestinal involvement of IBD, processes that both provide important adjunctive data in the diagnosis of IBD as well as contribute significantly to the morbidity and mortality of IBD. Techniques such as MRI that provide superior soft tissue contrast allow for both the improved visualization of the perianal disease manifestations of Crohn's disease such as fistulae and abscesses, as well as the precise anatomic localization for treatment planning [3]. Moreover, as our understanding of the pathophysiologic underpinnings of IBD continually expands, novel molecular imaging approaches have been applied to highlight the specific intra-cellular perturbations occurring within the bowel and thus identify areas of pathology with unparalleled resolution and specificity.

Multiple radiologic modalities, including fluoroscopy, CT, MRI, ultrasound, and nuclear medicine/molecular imaging techniques, have been applied towards imaging IBD. In this chapter, we will discuss technical considerations, appropriate indications, and key imaging findings for the most common imaging modalities currently applied in the care of patients with IBD. We will also discuss the risks attendant to the use of ionizing radiation, imaging findings of the extra-intestinal manifestations of IBD, and the potential role that molecular imaging may play in the future for patients with IBD.

2. Fluoroscopic imaging

2.1. Indications

Fluoroscopic imaging historically has been considered as the "gold standard" approach to imaging the small bowel. Despite the promotion of newer endoscopic technologies such as video capsule endoscopy and double balloon endoscopy, as well as the development of cross-sectional methods such as CT and MR enterography, fluoroscopy remains a staple tool for the identification of small bowel pathology, particularly pathology involving the terminal ileum. The benefits of fluoroscopic imaging include the ability to visualize peristaltic loops of small bowel in real time, a feature that allows for the discrimination between true abnormalities and transient changes in configuration related to motion. Additionally, with optimal contrast opacification, inspection of the mucosal surface of the entire length of the small bowel in relief is feasible. The examination may be performed as either a small bowel follow through, in which oral contrast is administered, or as a small bowel enteroclysis, in which the patient undergoes nasojejunal intubation followed by catheter instillation of both positive and negative contrast agents at a controlled rate. Advantages of the latter include more uniform distention and opacification of the entire small bowel leading to enhanced detection of segmental strictures and mucosal disease from double contrast opacification. Enteroclysis is particularly useful in patients with intermittent symptoms of IBD, as the complete distention of the small bowel can provoke correlative imaging findings which may otherwise go undetected with a standard oral contrast preparation in a small bowel follow through. Significant disadvantages of enteroclysis are invasiveness and patient discomfort. Though fluoroscopic examination of the small bowel is still widely used, trans- and extramural disease are poorly detected with this technique. Moreover, the exposure of patients to ionizing radiation with this modality should be taken into consideration, particularly in patients who are likely to undergo frequent imaging examinations.

2.2. Technical considerations

In fluoroscopic imaging, conventional two-dimensional radiographs are obtained with the patient lying on an examination table. The patient is kept nil per os (NPO) for several hours prior to the examination; a bowel cleansing regimen is rarely employed. Bowel visualization

http://dx.doi.org/10.5772/53025

is achieved following the administration of radio-opaque contrast agents, a large class of solutions that generally contain varying concentrations of barium. The benefits of fluoroscopic imaging include the ability to visualize peristaltic loops of small bowel in real time, a feature that allows for the discrimination between true abnormalities and transient changes in configuration related to motion. Additionally, with optimal contrast opacification, inspection of the mucosal surface along the entire length of the small bowel in relief is feasible. The patient's position can be adjusted by the fluoroscopist to any desirable obliquity with respect to the X-ray source so that the outline of every loop of small bowel is visualized. The fluoroscopist also employs compressive maneuvers using paddles, balloons, and gloves to spread out the loops of bowel so that they are individually visible.

In a small bowel follow through, the patient is asked to drink approximately 500cc of a barium containing oral contrast solution. Serial spot radiographs are obtained until the bolus has passed the terminal ileum into the cecum; this takes approximately 45-60 minutes, though pro-peristaltic agents such as metoclopramide may be administered to accelerate the process. Fluoroscopy with compression is then performed to identify areas of pathology.

In enteroclysis, a naso-jejunal catheter is placed such that the tip of the catheter terminates in the proximal jejunum, distal to the ligament of Treitz. A barium-containing solution is then infused at a uniform rate through the catheter. One variation is to infuse methylcellulose after a small amount of barium; this "double contrast" technique offers an improved inspection of the mucosal surface pattern [4]. Advantages of naso-jejunal intubation include bypassing the regulatory mechanisms of the pylorus and a more uniform distention and opacification of the entire small bowel, particularly in patients who are unable to drink an adequate volume of contrast by their own volition. Enteroclysis is particularly effective in provoking radiographic evidence of low-grade partial obstructions in patients with intermittent symptoms, findings that may have been undetectable by small bowel follow through. The process of naso-jejunal intubation and infusion of contrast, however, can be very uncomfortable, and in some cases intolerable, for patients; some institutions provide conscious sedation for that reason.

2.3. Interpretation of imaging findings

Much of the fluoroscopic imaging of UC, which predominantly involves the large bowel, has been replaced by colonoscopy. However, approximately 20% of patients with severe UC have associated "backwash" ileitis. Fluoroscopy demonstrates a patulous, incompetent ileocecal valve with a granulated mucosal relief pattern of the terminal ileum. This finding is in contrast to Crohn's disease, which is characterized by a stenotic ileocecal valve with luminal narrowing and ulceration of the terminal ileum. Backwash ileitis usually resolves following total colectomy [5].

Crohn's disease can affect the digestive tract anywhere from the mouth to the anus; approximately 80% of these patients have small bowel involvement (Figure 1). Unlike UC, "skip areas" of uninvolved bowel may be interspersed between segments of affected bowel. However, Crohn's disease has a predilection for affecting the terminal ileum. The earliest radiographic sign of Crohn's disease is aphthous ulcers, which appear as shallow collections of contrast with surrounding radiolucent haloes due to adjacent mucosal edema. Aphthous ulcers are not specific to Crohn's disease and may be seen in a number of diseases. However, as Crohn's disease progresses, the ulcers coalesce to form linear, curvilinear, or spiculated areas of ulceration along the mesenteric border of the small bowel. There is resultant retraction of the bowel wall, leading to pseudodiverticula and pseudosacculation of the anti-mesenteric bowel wall. These active inflammatory changes can lead to intermittent small bowel obstruction, which is best diagnosed by enteroclysis technique. Severe disease produces a classic "cobblestone" appearance, with deep transverse and longitudinal ulcerations bordered by areas of edema creating a checkered mucosal relief pattern. Chronic Crohn's disease leads to circumferential bowel wall thickening and irreversible stricture formation.

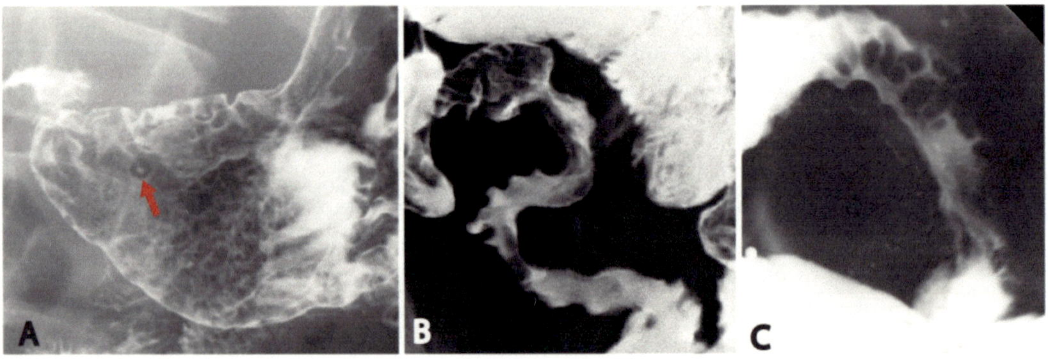

Figure 1. Fluoroscopic imaging findings in Crohn's disease. A, Aphthous ulcers, which appear as focal collections of contrast with surrounding haloes of mucosal edema, are present in early Crohn's disease (red arrow). B, Progressive disease results in longitudinal ulcerations on the mesenteric bowel surface with pseudosacculation formation on the anti-mesenteric surface. C, Severe disease can have a "cobblestone" mucosal relief pattern due to intersecting transverse and longitudinal ulcers.

Though fluoroscopic examination of the small bowel is still widely used, trans- and extramural disease are poorly detected with this technique. Moreover, the exposure of patients to ionizing radiation with this modality should be taken into consideration, particularly in patients who are likely to undergo frequent imaging examinations.

3. Computed tomographic imaging

3.1. Indications

Computed tomography remains the work-horse imaging modality for IBD and its complications in the United States. As a high-resolution cross-sectional technique, CT can visualize not only the bowel lumen, but also the bowel wall, visceral fat, intra-abdominal lymph nodes, and mesenteric vasculature supplying the bowel. Extraintestinal disease manifestations such as nephrolithiasis, sacroiliitis, and primary sclerosing cholangitis can readily be evaluated. Computed tomography can additionally be performed rapidly, and CT scanners are present in most emergency rooms, rendering it an ideal choice in the urgent or emergent setting. As such, CT is an appropriate imaging examination for the diagnosis of IBD, the evaluation of response to intervention including post-surgical changes, and the detection of urgent and emergent complications such as abscess formation and acute bowel obstruction. However, since subtle mucosal ulcerations are not well visualized by CT, this modality should not be used as a first line approach for the detection of suspected mild disease.

3.2. Technical considerations

The past two decades have witnessed a revolution in the technology of CT scanners. The introduction of the helical CT scanner has permitted the acquisition of volumetric data sets in a continuous, uninterrupted manner. The source data are obtained with sub-millimeter slice thickness, so that images may be be reconstructed from the source axial plane into standard coronal or sagittal planes, or any other plane desired by the radiologist. Also, the advent of multidetector row scanners, initially with 4-slice devices in 1998, followed by 8-, 16-, 64-, and most recently 320-slice devices, has had a dramatic effect on reducing scanning time. This, in turn, has shortened the requisite breath hold for the patient, making the examination more comfortable and less often degraded by respiratory motion artifact [6].

There exist a variety of CT protocols for abdominal indications. With regards to IBD, a common reason to pursue imaging is for the assessment of small bowel pathology. CT enterography is usually the imaging protocol of choice, which combines large volume enteral contrast distention of small bowel with intravenous contrast administration. For this imaging examination, patients are kept NPO for several hours prior; similar to fluoroscopy, a bowel cleansing regimen is not routinely required. Intravenous contrast is always used when possible. Enteral contrast is an indispensible component of the technique. Initial CT enterography relied on "positive" enteral contrast agents, usually barium containing solutions whose higher attenuation characteristics opacify the bowel lumen. However, differentiating the thin line of mucosal enhancement due to intravenous contrast from the opaque enteral contrast in the bowel lumen can be challenging. Therefore, a more popular approach is to use "neutral" enteral contrast agents that distend but do not opacify the bowel lumen. In this manner, mucosal enhancement patterns are better seen, as are areas of non-distensibility such as strictures. Water is a commonly used neutral enteral agent, but since this has the disadvantage of being absorbed by the body, commercially available preparations that are isodense to water on CT imaging but are non-absorbable are also prevalent [7]. Essentially all current CT enterography protocols utilize neutral enteral contrast.

The volume of enteral contrast administered to the patient and the duration over which they are asked to ingest contrast vary by institution. However, the overall goal is to maximize uniform distention of the small bowel, which typically requires 1000-1500 mL of contrast. Patients are first instructed to drink the enteral contrast, generally over approximately 45 to 60 minutes. They then lie down on the CT scanner; intravenous contrast is administered; originally CT enterography studies were scanned at 55-60 seconds post-contrast (enterographic phase) coinciding with peak superior mesenteric artery enhancement. However, many institutions now perform scanning during portal venous phase (~70 seconds) for optimal visceral organ evaluation.

The CT analog to fluoroscopic enteroclysis, known at CT enteroclysis, is also used as a method to achieve optimal luminal filling. A naso-jejunal tube is required and is usually inserted in a fluoroscopy suite. Contrast is administered under fluoroscopic guidance, after which the patient is transported to the CT scanner. Unlike fluoroscopy, though, a real-time assessment of bowel distensibility cannot be made by CT, as the patients are usually only imaged after the contrast has been fully administered. The disadvantage of patient discomfort caused by naso-jejunal intubation is no different.

For patients suspected of bowel obstruction or perforation, oral contrast is frequently contraindicated and traditional CT imaging with IV contrast only is recommended.

An important concern with CT is the use of ionizing radiation. Recent studies suggest that CT exams account for the vast majority of ionizing radiation exposure to IBD patients from imaging, especially among patients diagnosed at an early age. An informed analysis of the associated risks, especially for the pediatric patient, should be performed prior to each examination.

3.3. Interpretation of imaging findings – Crohn's disease

A principal clinical question for which CT is utilized in IBD is the determination of active versus inactive disease in the small bowel. This distinction is of high clinical significance: patients with active inflammation are treated medically with immuno-modulatory therapy, while symptomatic patients with inactive, fibrosed strictures often require surgical intervention. Areas of actively inflamed bowel on CT most commonly demonstrate pathologic bowel thickening, which is defined as bowel wall greater than 3mm in thickness. A 3mm cutoff was selected by consensus as the best compromise between sensitivity and specificity and is for the most part used universally for all cross-sectional modalities including MRI and ultrasound. Another differentiating characteristic of active disease is mucosal hyperenhancement, which appears as a pencil-thin line outlining the luminal surface of the bowel wall and reflects the hyperemia of inflammation (Figure 2A). This finding is considered the most sensitive for active disease, and the degree of hyperenhancement may correlate with the degree of underlying inflammation. Active inflammation also results in submucosal edema, which manifests on CT examination as a lower attenuation submucosal layer interposed between mucosal and serosal layers. This mural stratification is also referred to as the "target sign" due to its characteristic appearance (Figure 2C). The most specific feature for active Crohn's disease is engorgement of the vasa recta adjacent to an inflamed loop of bowel, a finding known as the "comb sign" (Figure 2B). Secondary signs for active inflammation include mesenteric fat stranding, focal ascites adjacent to bowel, and lymphadenopathy. Of note, while mucosal hyperenhancement and abnormal bowel thickening are frequent features of active Crohn's disease, they are not specific and may be seen in infectious enteritis or mesenteric ischemia. Similarly, mural stratification can be seen in UC as well as bowel ischemia. On the other hand, the "comb sign" is considered fairly specific for Crohn's disease [2, 7].

http://dx.doi.org/10.5772/53025

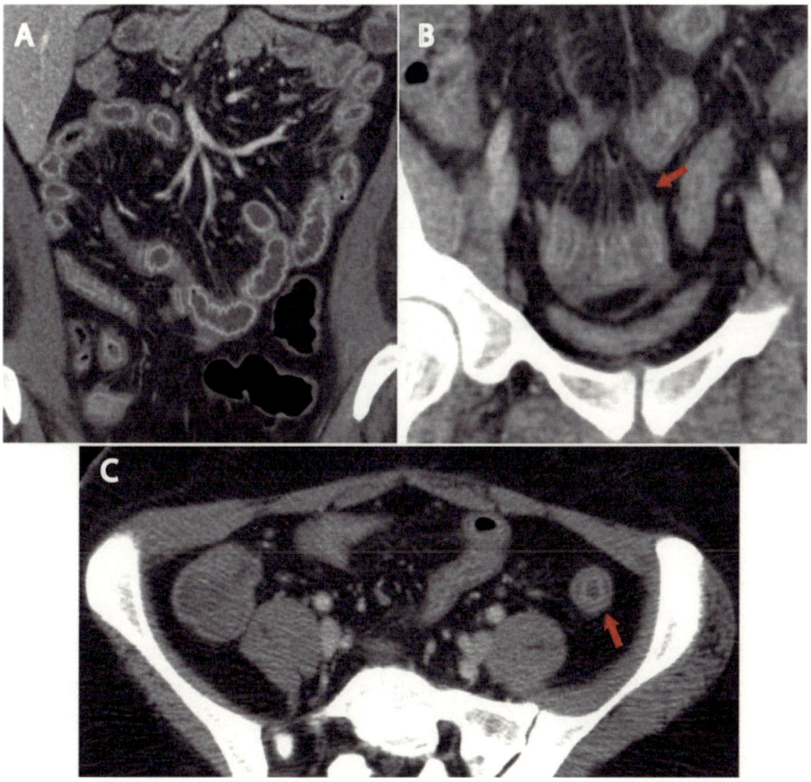

Figure 2. CT findings in acute Crohn's disease. A, Active inflammation causes mucosal hyperenhancement and bowel wall thickening greater than 3mm. B, Engorgement of the vasa recta adjacent to an inflamed loop of bowel is a specific finding in active Crohn's disease and has been coined the "comb sign." C, Submucosal edema yields a characteristic "target sign."

The presence of mucosal hyperenhancement, abnormal bowel wall thickening, mural stratification, and prominent adjacent vasa recta in an area of poorly distensible bowel suggests that the stricture is due to active inflammation and is thus potentially reversible by medical interventions. The strictures of chronic Crohn's disease, in contrast, are fibrotic, irreversible, and do not demonstrate the features of active disease described above. The presence of luminal narrowing with proximal bowel dilation is suggestive of fibrosis. Long-standing inflammation leads to fat deposition within the submucosa of the bowel wall; this apparent mural stratification should not be confused with the "target sign" of active disease and can be differentiated based on the Hounsfield attenuation characteristics of fat, which is less than 0 Housfield units (Figure 3A). Secondly, the fibrotic retraction preferentially affects the mesenteric bowel wall, leading to the pseudosacculation appearance on the anti-mesenteric side that can also be seen by fluoroscopy. Finally, chronic transmural Crohn's disease, possibly due to chronic inflammatory stimulation, produces a fibrofatty proliferation of the mesenteric fat, also known on CT examinations as the "creeping fat sign" (Figure 3B).

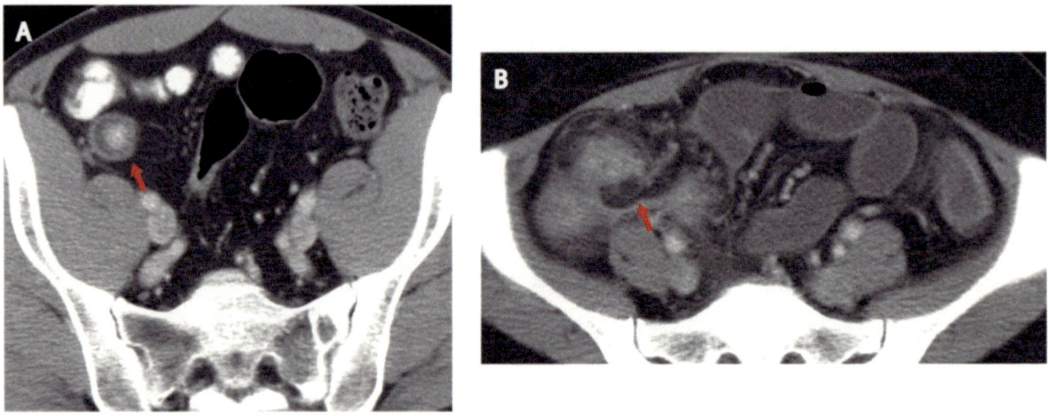

Figure 3. CT findings in chronic Crohn's disease. A, Fatty depositions in the submucosal layer may mimic the "target sign" of active disease (red arrow). B, Fibrofatty proliferation of the mesenteric fat, or "creeping fat," (red arrow) is seen in chronic, transmural disease.

The extra-mural complications of Crohn's disease are excellently depicted by CT. Penetrating disease is present in approximately 20% with Crohn's disease, with fistulas representing the most common pathology in this category [3]. Fistulous tracts may form between any two epithelially lined viscera in the abdomen, such as other loops of bowel (entero-enteric), the bladder (entero-vesicular), and the skin (entero-cutaneous). A communicating tract that fills with enteral contrast is diagnostic (Figure 4A). Evaluation with CT is highly sensitive for the detection of fistulae, though certain anatomic locations such as the perianal region are better imaged by MRI, as discussed below.

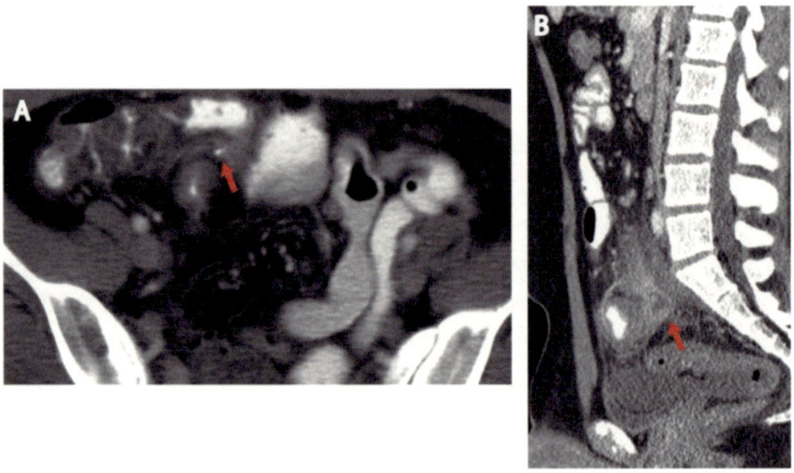

Figure 4. Complications of Crohn's disease on CT. A, A fistula between two loops of small bowel is well depicted by CT as a thin tract of oral contrast connecting the lumens of the two loops. B, An intra-abdominal abscess posterior to the distal large bowel, likely due to a microperforation, was identified in this patient.

http://dx.doi.org/10.5772/53025

Intra-abdominal abscesses are extra-luminal fluid collections that do not communicate with the bowel (Figure 4B). The discontinuity of the abscess collection with the bowel lumen is important to verify but can occasionally be challenging, as neural enteral contrast within the bowel mimics the attenuation characteristics of the infected fluid within the abscess cavity. For this reason, positive enteral contrast is often preferred to neutral contrast in patients with suspected abscess.

3.4. Interpretation of imaging findings – Ulcerative colitis

As discussed previously, colonoscopy remains the primary approach for diagnosing and determining extent of disease in UC. However, severe complications of UC such as toxic megacolon are an important indication for imaging, with CT representing the mainstay modality in these unstable patients. CT findings include thinning of the colonic wall, luminal distension, and pneumatosis; severe cases can lead to perforation and free intraperitoneal gas.

4. Magnetic resonance imaging

4.1. Indications

Magnetic resonance imaging enjoys many inherent advantages over other cross sectional imaging modalities. These include the ability to acquire images in any imaging plane, the lack of ionizing radiation, and excellent soft tissue resolution. Because of the lack of ionizing radiation, imaging may be performed at multiple time points during an examination, for example at different phases of contrast enhancement, providing a multiparametric assessment of any particular pathology. Additionally, "cine" images can be obtained sequentially over time, in an MRI analog to fluoroscopy.

The strengths of MRI when applied towards IBD are best suited for investigating the small bowel and the perianal region, anatomic locations towards which Crohn's disease demonstrates a tropism. Magnetic resonance imaging of the large bowel, an examination that would have increased relevance in UC, is not routinely performed. The intrinsic spatial resolution of MRI is inferior to that of CT. An MRI examination also takes longer to complete than a CT exam. However, the widespread adoption of new, faster MRI pulse sequences, described in the subsequent section, has significantly reduced scanning time and opened the door for small bowel imaging. For specific clinical scenarios, such as perianal disease, MRI is the recognized gold standard non-invasive technique.

4.2. Technical considerations

As with CT, multiple different MRI protocols exist for examining the abdomen. In the realm of IBD, one very useful MR examination is magnetic resonance enterography (MRE). Although an in-depth discussion of the various pulse sequences used in abdominal MRI imaging is beyond the scope of this text, a familiarity with the commonly used sequences is valuable in understanding the applicability of MRE. Sequences with T2 weighting are the best for evaluating the bowel wall. Intravenous contrast enhancement appears bright on T1 weighted sequences; however, as feces can occasionally be bright on T1 imaging too, pre-contrast T1 image sets are obtained to help identify true enhancement. Conventional spin echo pulse sequences do not afford the requisite temporal resolution to image the abdomen during a single breath hold; as such, the resulting images are often degraded by respiratory motion artifact. Beyond that, high temporal resolution is made all the more critical when investigating a moving target as the bowel. For these reasons, MRE capitalizes on customized MR pulse sequences that offer improved temporal resolution and are able to image the entire abdomen during a single breath hold. For example, single-shot turbo spin echo (e.g. SSFSE or HASTE) sequences produce high quality, motion-free T2 weighted images of the entire bowel [8]. Balanced steady state free precession sequences (e.g. FIESTA or TrueFISP) are T1 and T2 intermediate-weighted sequences that that are rapid and demonstrate increased conspicuity of the mesentery for detection of inflammatory changes or fistula formation [9]. These sequences, due to their rapidity, can be performed as thick slab cinematic acquisitions to evaluate bowel peristalsis, known as MR fluoroscopy. Fat suppression is routinely employed during both T2-weighted and T1-weighted post-contrast sequences, to highlight areas of bowel wall edema and enhancement. The post-contrast T1 fat-suppressed sequences are performed using 3-D techniques to accelerate image acquisition and enable dynamic evaluation of bowel enhancement at multiple timepoints post-contrast. An average imaging time for MRE, exclusive of the time required for enteral contrast administration, is approximately 30-45 minutes.

Diffusion weighted imaging (DWI) is an MRI technique that has been used with tremendous success in neurological imaging and has shown promise in gastrointestinal imaging. Diffusion imaging provides quantitative maps of the ability of water molecules in tissue to randomly move in a process known as Brownian motion. In areas of inflammation, hypercellularity, or ischemia, the free movement of water molecules is restricted; this characteristic manifests as a low apparent diffusion coefficient (ADC) value when MRI sequences sensitive to diffusion are obtained. Diffusion weighted imaging is at present an experimental technique in IBD imaging (Figure 5), but initial reports have suggested that this method may not only improve disease detection but also provide a quantitative metric for assessing interval changes in bowel wall inflammation [10].

There is no specific bowel preparation prior to MRE, but patients generally are kept NPO for several hours prior to the exam. Anti-peristaltic agents such as glucagon may help improve image quality and are often administered just prior to imaging. Intravenous contrast with a gadolinium-chelate containing agent is standardly administered. There are several options in enteral contrast, which can be categorized by their MRI signal characteristics. "Negative" agents are intrinsically T1 and T2 dark compounds that usually contain superparamagnetic iron oxide particles. Their principal advantage is that they emphasize mucosal enhancement and bowel wall edema. "Positive" agents are intrinsically T1 and T2 bright compounds; these, similar to positive CT contrast agents, may obscure mucosal enhancement findings and thus are infrequently used. The most commonly used class of MR enteral contrast agents is the "biphasic" type, which are T1 dark and T2 bright (e.g. dilute barium with sorbi-

http://dx.doi.org/10.5772/53025

tol, polyethylene glycol). With these agents, one can readily assess the pattern of bowel wall folds on T2 weighted images without losing mucosal enhancement data on T1 weighted images [11]. Contrast agents are often hyperosmolar to maximize luminal distention; an important side effect for patients to be aware of is diarrhea. It is critically important that patients ingest adequate enteric contrast for MR enterography. Unlike CT in which underdistended bowel loops can still be evaluated, the relative diminished spatial resolution of MRI renders collapsed bowel difficult to assess for disease. In addition, enteric contrast is needed to displace intraluminal air that can produce significant susceptibility artifact on dynamic post-contrast MRI sequences.

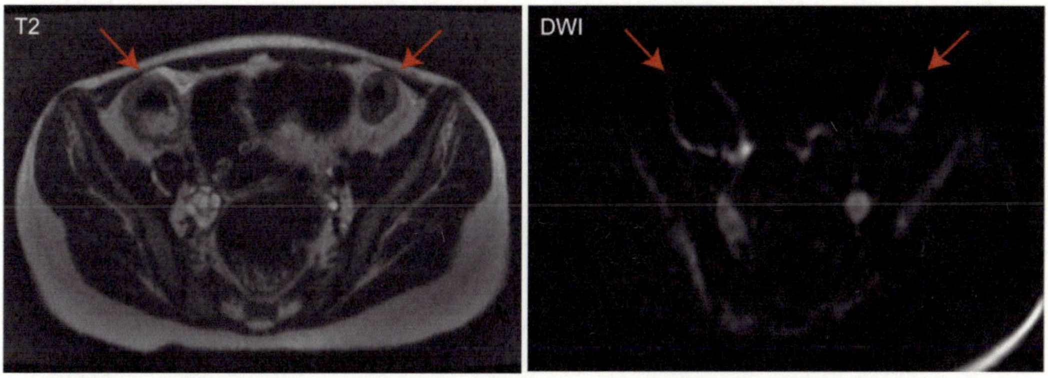

Figure 5. Representative T2 (left) and diffusion weighted (right) images from an MR enterography of a child with Crohn's disease. Images demonstrate two colonic loops (red arrows) exhibiting bowel edema and restricted water diffusion, consistent with active inflammation.

Enteral contrast is primarily administered orally, though MR enteroclysis is also an option. The attendant patient discomfort and added radiation from the fluoroscopy-guided placement of the naso-jejunal tube are identical to the CT analog. However, one benefit of MR enteroclysis is the ability to perform MR fluoroscopy during the instillation of enteral contrast, a technique that provides dynamic information regarding bowel distensibility.

Patients may be imaged in the supine or prone position; the latter orientation is preferred at some institutions as the patient's own weight is used to spread out loops of small bowel; the compression in the anterior-posterior dimension also reduces imaging volume.

4.3. Interpretation of imaging findings – Crohn's disease

Magnetic resonance imaging is an excellent tool for the detection of active Crohn's disease, with a sensitivity of > 90% [12]. Many of the imaging characteristics of active Crohn's disease on MRI, as one may expect, are morphologically identical to those appreciated on CT. For example, bowel wall thickening greater than 3mm is considered abnormal and evidence of active inflammation. Active disease with intramural edema manifests as T2 hyperintensity between the mucosa and muscularis propria (Figure 6A) [13]. Mucosal hyperenhancement is also an important marker of active disease. Diffuse, avid, homogeneous mucosal enhancement is suggestive of active disease (Figure 6B). Alternatively, low-level, heterogeneous mural enhancement without a mucosal component with upstream dilatation favors the diagnosis of mural fibrosis due to irreversible collagen deposition in the bowel wall (Figure 6C). Ulceration may be difficult to identify without proper bowel distention; ulcers appear as thin lines of high signal intensity within thickening loops of bowel. Both MRI and CT are insensitive for early aphthous ulcers, for which fluoroscopy or endoscopy should be considered as more sensitive.

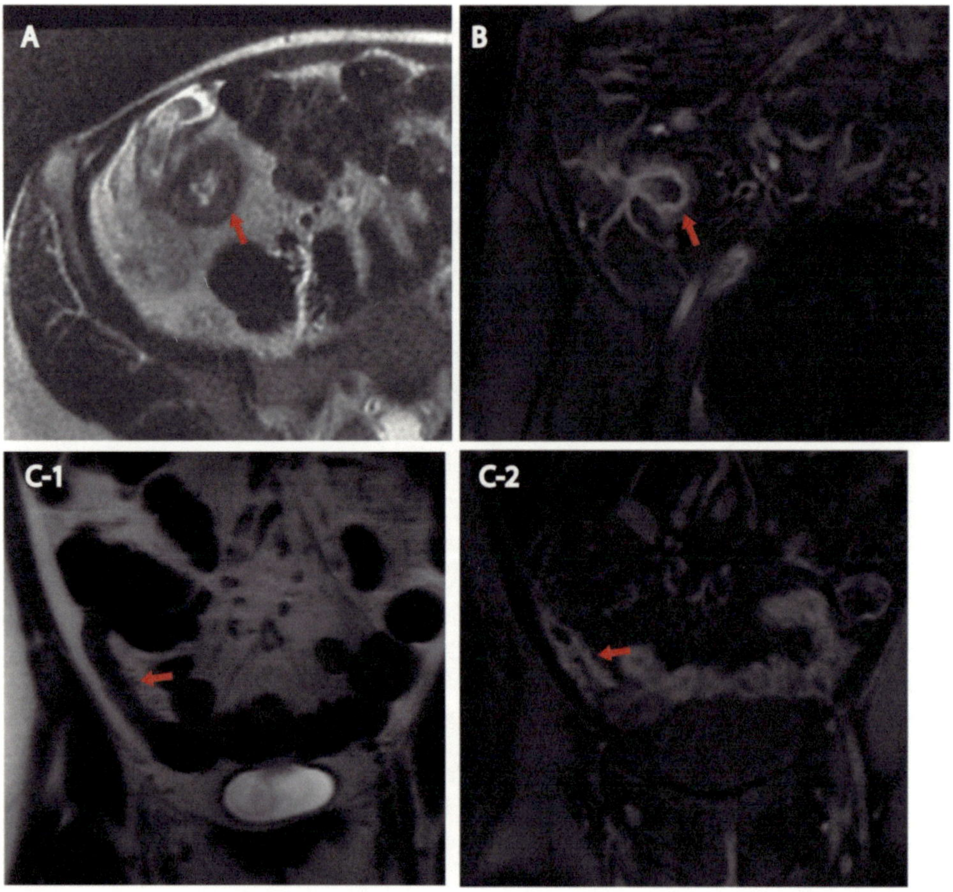

Figure 6. Findings of Crohn's disease by MR enterography. A) Submucosal edema appears as T2 hyperintensity interposed between the mucosa and muscularis propria (red arrow). B) Homogeneous, avid mucosal enhancement on T1-weighted imaging is suggestive of active disease (red arrow). C) Conversely, fixed lumimal narrowing on a T2 weighted image (red arrow, C-1) that demonstrates delayed mural enhancement on a post contrast T1 weighted image (red arrow, C-2) without a mucosal component is seen in chronic fibrosis.

Additional evidence of active disease such as the "comb sign," in which there is engorgement of the mesenteric vessels adjacent to an inflamed loop of bowel, are well identified by MRI. Strictures appear as a focal narrowing in the bowel lumen and are considered signifi-

http://dx.doi.org/10.5772/53025

cant if there is a pre-stenotic dilation of the proximal bowel. The so-called "creeping fat sign" occurs in chronic, transmural inflammation, in which hypertrophy of the mesenteric fat produces mass effect and surrounds viscera; this sign is specific for Crohn's disease. Another sign of chronic fibrosis is T2 hypointensity of the bowel wall relative to muscle.

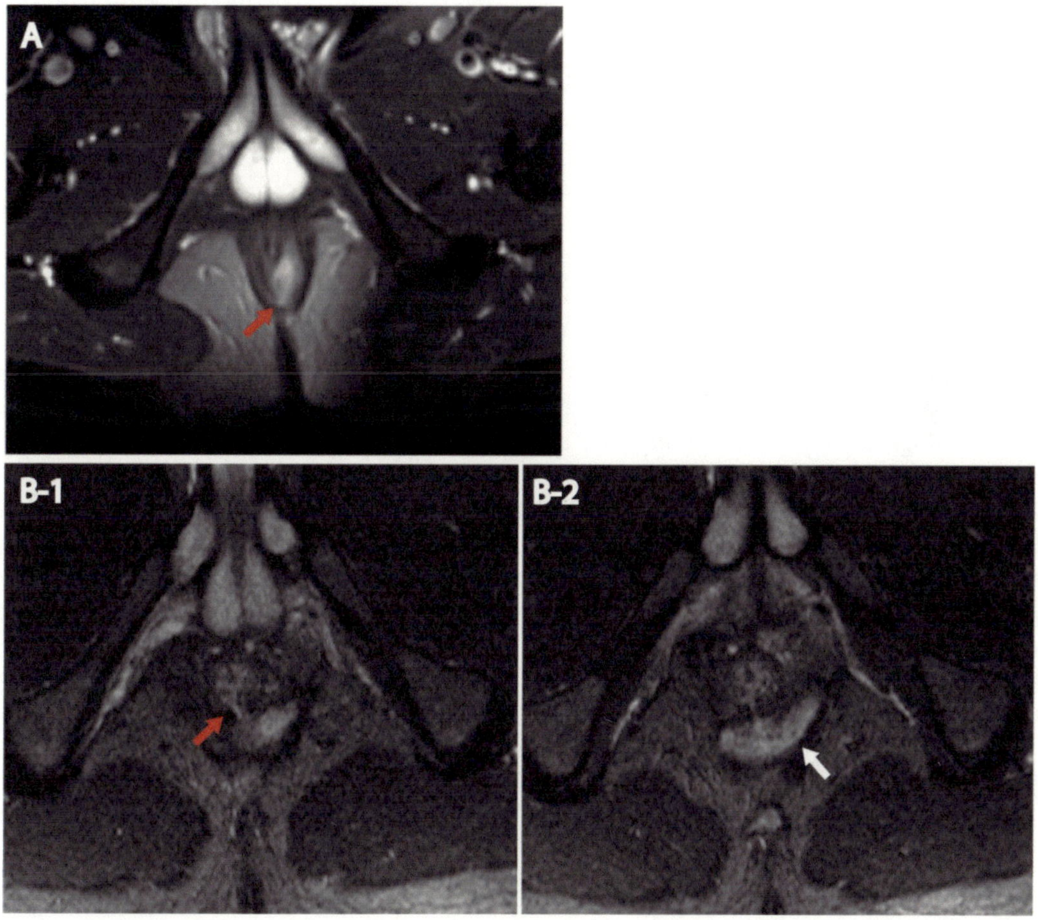

Figure 7. MRI findings of anorectal fistulae. A, T2 hyperintensity that extends between the external and internal sphincter complexes is diagnostic of an intersphincteric fistula (red arrow). B, Two sequential T2 weighted images demonstrate a linear hyperintense focus traversing through the internal and external sphincter complexes consist with a transsphincteric fistula (red arrow, B-1). The subsequent image demonstrates an associated fluid collection extending into the left ischioanal fossa (white arrow, B-2).

Extramural disease is as conspicuous, if not more so, on MRI as it is on CT. Fistulae appear as T2 hyperintense tracts that avidly enhance and extend from bowel to a second epithelial lined organ such as another segment of bowel, the skin, or the bladder. Sinuses are blind-ending tracts that extend from bowel and typically terminate within the mesentery. Both fistulae and sinuses cause translocation of gut flora out of the bowel and can be associated with abscess formation.

In addition to evaluating the small bowel with enterography, MRI is a powerful tool in the investigation of perianal Crohn's disease because of its superior soft tissue contrast for delineation of the anal sphincter complex. The lifetime risk of developing fistulous disease in Crohn's disease is approximately 20-40%. Anorectal fistulae are common and are classified based on their location relative to the anal sphincter complex and pelvic floor musculature, as anatomic location impacts upon treatment options. The most common type of anorectal fistula is the intersphincteric fistula (Figure 7A), followed by the transphincteric fistula (Figure 7B). The accuracy of MRI for diagnosing and classifying anorectal fistulae is comparable to exam under anesthesia [3].

5. Ultrasound

5.1. Indications

Ultrasound is a cross-sectional imaging technique that has been used extensively in the imaging of IBD. As with other technologies, ultrasound has its own unique set of advantages, such as low relative cost, lack of ionizing radiation, and real-time imaging capability. Disadvantages include the inability to visualize portions of small bowel, rectum, and sigmoid, difficulty tracing long bowel segments, as well as operator dependence, with the quality of the examination contingent on the technical skill of the ultrasonographer. Ultrasound has been shown to possibly be as accurate in the diagnosis of IBD as CT and MRI based on detection of wall thickening and hypervascularity by Doppler. However, a high sensitivity is likely achievable only in the hands of an expert ultrasonographer, a resource that is not widely available or easy to standardize. Ultrasound is particularly relevant in pediatric imaging: the smaller body habitus in this patient population allows for a more complete examination, and the lack of ionizing radiation is likely safer compared to CT. The most common indication for ultrasound is evaluation for active inflammation in a symptomatic IBD patient whose anatomic distribution of bowel inflammation is known.

5.2. Technical considerations

Similar to the previously described modalities, minimal patient preparation is required in ultrasound. Since luminal gas can cause acoustic shadowing artifacts that obscure underlying structures, non-effervescent liquid may be administered to displace bowel gas distally and provide some luminal distension. The choice of ultrasound transducer is predicated by the patient's body size. Higher frequency transducers produce higher resolution images but have poorer tissue penetration compared to lower frequency transducers. Practically, an ultrasonographer will begin the examination with the highest frequency transducer available, which is usually a 15 megahertz transducer; if there are structures that are not well seen, the ultrasonographer change to a lower frequency one.

The approach to handling the ultrasound transducer and physically tracing it across the abdomen is of paramount importance. A key technique in imaging the bowel is known as "graded compression." Increasing pressure is applied with the transducer head as it is swept across the surface of the abdomen. This has the effect of displacing bowel gas and overlying bowel loops so that the area of interest can be inspected with the greatest possible clarity [14].

5.3. Interpretation of imaging findings

A normal segment of bowel on ultrasound exhibits five discrete layers. The inner-most layer is a thin hyperechoic line that demarcates the interface between the lumen and the mucosa. The next layer is a hypoechoic line at the interface between the mucosa and submucosa. The third layer is a hyperechoic line between submucosa and the muscularis propria; this is the most commonly involved layer in IBD. The fourth layer is the muscularis propria itself and is hypoechoic. The fifth and final layer is hyperechoic and represents the serosa [15].

Inflammatory bowel disease is manifested on ultrasound as abnormal bowel wall thickening, defined as greater than 3mm, and loss of definition of the discrete bowel wall layers. Both UC and Crohn's disease result in bowel wall thickening. However, in UC the bowel wall layers are preserved, as opposed to Crohn's disease; this distinction though may not be sufficiently accurate to differentiate the two diseases by US alone. Intra-mural edema appears as generalized hypoechogenicity within the bowel wall. Conversely, fibrostenoic disease exhibits hyperechogenicity of the submucosal layer. Superficial ulcers may be detected as hypoechoic interruptions within the innermost bowel wall layer.

Doppler ultrasound can provide useful adjunct data to the structural information from conventional ultrasound. Normal bowel wall, as well as fibrostenotic bowel wall, does not usually demonstrate detectable Doppler blood flow. Therefore, the presence of intramural blood flow is suggestive of the hyperemia of active disease.

6. Nuclear medicine/Molecular imaging

As molecule-targeted therapies become increasingly prevalent in the treatment of IBD, it is likely that imaging their downstream effects directly via molecular imaging techniques will play a pivotal role in the management of patients with IBD. Molecular imaging with radionuclides in IBD has been thoroughly investigated. Analogous to conventional fluoroscopy, planar scintigraphic imaging was the predominant method of nuclear imaging for IBD in the past, but recently tomographic techniques such as single photon emission computed tomography (SPECT) and positron emission tomography (PET) have supplanted this two-dimensional modality. As novel, targeted imaging agents become clinically available, it is reasonable to expect that molecular imaging will be critical in directly tracking the efficacy of therapies in patients with IBD in a manner that far precedes anatomic changes detectable by conventional imaging methods.

The pathophysiology of IBD involves infiltration of gut mucosa with activated lymphocytes and macrophages. By radiolabeling autologous white blood cells (WBCs) and re-injecting the cells into the patient, non-invasive imaging of WBC migration into areas of inflammation can be achieved. The radionuclide Tc-99m has been used in such a paradigm to label WBCs, and Tc-99m-labeled WBCs have been thoroughly investigated as a highly sensitive and specific instrument for diagnosing IBD. Radiolabeled WBCs may also be helpful to prognosticate response to therapy within only a few days of its initiation [16, 17].

Beyond WBCs, multiple radio-labeled probes targeting inflammation have been studied, including interleukins such as IL-2 and IL-8. Additionally, Annexin V, a molecular probe specific for apoptosis, has been shown to function as an early marker of response to therapy in patients with IBD being treated with infliximab.

The advent of positron-emitting radionuclides has paved the way for the introduction of PET imaging into clinical practice, a modality that enjoys far greater spatial resolution than single photon techniques. The most widely used PET imaging agent is 2-deoxy-2[^{18}F]fluoro-d-glucose (FDG), a radiolabeled glucose molecule that accumulates in areas of increased glycolysis. Imaging with FDG-PET has a reported sensitivity and specificity for colonic mucosal inflammation on par with endoscopy.

With the recent introduction of whole-body PET-MRI scanners, combined PET imaging with MR enterography offers the benefits of MRI morphological assessment of diseased areas with PET quantitation of inflammatory activity. The exquisite soft tissue differentiation of MRI coupled with the molecular sensitivity of PET has the potential to provide unparalleled structure-function correlation. The simultaneous acquisition of the two data sets that can be performed with new hybrid PET-MRI systems allows for true co-registration of PET and MR images (Figure 8); this feature is particularly relevant for abdominal imaging, as peristalsis can result in significant changes in bowel positioning.

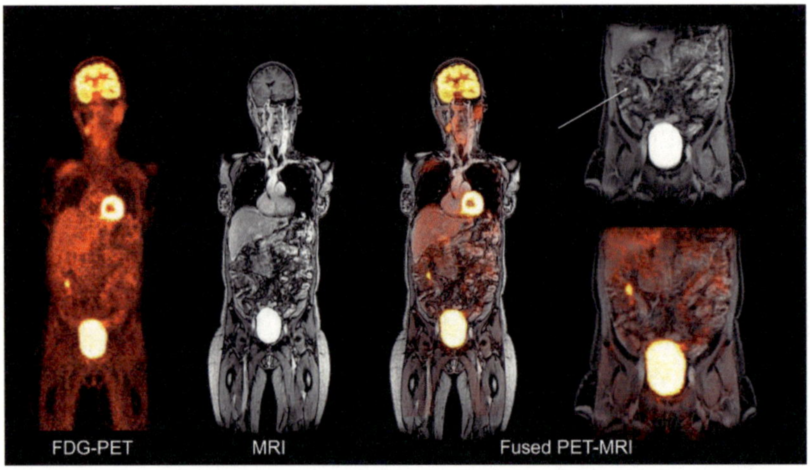

Figure 8. PET-MRI of patient with cecal inflammation. Fused imaging demonstrates small area of active inflammatory changes in the cecum that would be difficult to diagnose on either FDG-PET or MR imaging independently. Images generously provided by Drs. Alex Guimaraes, Ciprian Catana, Bruce Rosen, and David Berger (Massachusetts General Hospital, Boston, MA).

http://dx.doi.org/10.5772/53025

7. Special considerations in the pediatric population

Performing diagnostic imaging examinations on pediatric patients requires consideration of several important factors. For example, pediatric patients may not be able to tolerate prolonged examinations such as MR enterography, necessitating the use of sedation to obtain satisfactory images. Moreover, not only are pediatric patients with IBD committed to a lifetime of imaging studies, but also their increased percentage of actively dividing tissue and relatively smaller body habitus render them inherently more sensitive to radiation injury and mutagenesis compared an adult. When these risks are coupled with their baseline increased risk of malignancy due to IBD, the importance of radiation dose reduction becomes apparent.

The association between diagnostic radiation and cancer risk is controversial. Directly studying the effects of ionizing radiation on malignancy risk is extremely challenging. Frequently cited epidemiologic data are based on atomic bomb survivors and nuclear power plant workers who were exposed to radiation levels that exceed those in diagnostic imaging. Moreover, the deleterious effects of radiation likely have a prolonged incubation time, perhaps on the order of decades, before they are clinically apparent. A recent large retrospective study of CT scans performed on pediatric patients suggests a measurable but small increase in the risk of malignancy [18]. It should be noted that the radiation doses associated with CT scans included in that study are significantly higher than current CT technique. Nonetheless, there is little doubt that every effort should be made to reduce the radiation exposure in pediatric patients to minimize any potential risk.

Estimating the magnitude of absorbed radiation during a CT examination can be made through the use of phantoms. Though no patient, and especially no pediatric patient, is identical to the standard, adult-sized body phantom, this approach remains the most quantitative means of estimating radiation levels within the body during a CT exam. However, extrapolating malignancy risk from these data is difficult, as different organs exhibit unique susceptibilities to radiation exposure. For example, the gonads are far more radio-sensitive than muscle tissue. For this reason, the concept of "effective dose" was introduced. This term, measured in millisieverts (mSv), reflects an attempt to create a standard metric that quantifies the impact of the absorbed radiation [19]. Effective dose is calculated by multiplying the absorbed radiation dose by a conversion factor for the body segment that was imaged; this conversion factor varies based upon the radiosensitivity of the exposed organs.

The choice of imaging modality for IBD over the past two decades has trended towards an increase in the use of CT. Pediatric patients may undergo multiple CT examinations over their lifetime, and the cumulative effective dose they receive may exceed 75 mSv, a level beyond which radiation-induced malignancy is felt to become an increasing concern. Patients with Crohn's disease are imaged far more frequently than those with UC. Also, patients who require immunosuppressive therapy or surgery are also at a higher risk of frequent imaging. Additional risk factors include stricturing or penetrating disease [20].

The most important avenue for reducing radiation dose is the eradication of unnecessary examinations. Minimizing exposure time during fluoroscopy should be standard practice.

Multiple techniques for reducing radiation dose in CT examinations have been developed and should be implemented when imaging pediatric patients. Finally, substituting non-ionizing radiation imaging modalities such as MRI and ultrasound should be considered when appropriate.

8. Conclusions and recommendations

The modalities described in this chapter each demonstrate their own unique set of advantageous and disadvantageous features. While fluoroscopy may show superficial mucosal disease better than any cross-sectional technique, extra-luminal disease is poorly visualized. The high spatial and temporal resolution of CT has driven its rise in popularity over the past two decades; however, this examination requires the use of ionizing radiation, and an appreciation of the possible associated risks is paramount prior to selecting this modality. While MRI is more costly and time consuming, it may be the best choice in a clinical situation where minimizing radiation dose is important or when soft tissue characterization is required.

For imaging symptomatic patients with suspected IBD, we recommend fluoroscopic upper GI and small bowel series because of its high sensitivity for early IBD as well as its accuracy for diagnosing other disease entities (e.g. sprue, infectious enteritides) that can mimic IBD. For initial imaging evaluation of newly diagnosed Crohn's disease, as well as evaluation of symptomatic exacerbation of known Crohn's disease in adult patients, CT enterography is recommended because of its superior ability to detect active bowel inflammation as well as extraluminal and extraintestinal disease manifestations. Urgent and emergent complications such as abscess formation and acute bowel obstruction are best imaged with traditional CT using intravenous and no enteric contrast. Crohn's disease patients with perianal symptoms should be investigated with pelvic MRI. MR enteroraphy is becoming the preferred primary imaging modality for pediatric patients, as well as adult patients who previously have undergone multiple prior CT exams, because of its lack of ionizing radiation. In patients with longstanding IBD with persistent obstructive symptoms, MR enterography is the best imaging modality for distinguishing inflammatory from fibrotic stricture [21], which has important therapeutic implications. Enteroclysis techniques should generally be reserved for those patients with remitting-relapsing obstructive symptoms despite normal enterography studies, as a provocative examination to detect short strictures. There is likely to be an increasing role for ultrasound in surveillance imaging in the future given its low cost and lack of requirement of sedation or oral contrast preparation.

Acknowledgements

We gratefully acknowledge the generosity of Drs. Alex Guimaraes, Ciprian Catana, Bruce Rosen, and David Berger (Massachusetts General Hospital, Boston, MA) for providing the PET-MRI images shown in Figure 8.

http://dx.doi.org/10.5772/53025

Author details

Rahul A. Sheth and Michael S. Gee

Massachusetts General Hospital, Harvard Medical School, Boston, Massachusetts, USA

References

[1] Maglinte DDT. Small bowel imaging-- a rapidly changing field and a challenge to radiology. European Radiology 2006; 16(5): 967-971.

[2] Elsayes KM, Al-Hawary MM, Jagdish J, Ganesh HS, Platt JF. CT enterography: principles, trends, and interpretation of findings. Radiographics : a review publication of the Radiological Society of North America, Inc 2010; 30(7): 1955-1970.

[3] Schreyer AG, Seitz J, Feuerbach S, Rogler G, Herfarth H. Modern imaging using computer tomography and magnetic resonance imaging for inflammatory bowel disease (IBD) AU1. Inflammatory bowel diseases 2004; 10(1): 45-54.

[4] Maglinte DD, Lappas JC, Kelvin FM, Rex D, Chernish SM. Small bowel radiography: how, when, and why? Radiology 1987; 163(2): 297-305.

[5] Carucci LR, Levine MS. Radiographic imaging of inflammatory bowel disease. Gastroenterology Clinics of North America 2002; 31(1): 93-117, ix.

[6] Kalra MK, Maher MM, D'Souza R, Saini S. Multidetector computed tomography technology: current status and emerging developments. Journal of computer assisted tomography 2004; 28 Suppl 1S2-6.

[7] Horsthuis K, Stokkers PCF, Stoker J. Detection of inflammatory bowel disease: diagnostic performance of cross-sectional imaging modalities. Abdominal imaging 2008; 33(4): 407-416.

[8] Fidler J. MR imaging of the small bowel. Radiologic clinics of North America 2007; 45(2): 317-331.

[9] Chalian M, Ozturk A, Oliva-Hemker M, Pryde S, Huisman TAGM. MR Enterography Findings of Inflammatory Bowel Disease in Pediatric Patients. American Journal of Roentgenology 2011; 196(6): W810-816.

[10] Maccioni F, Patak MA, Signore A, Laghi A. New frontiers of MRI in Crohn's disease: motility imaging, diffusion-weighted imaging, perfusion MRI, MR spectroscopy, molecular imaging, and hybrid imaging (PET/MRI). Abdominal imaging 2012.

[11] Tolan DJM, Greenhalgh R, Zealley IA, Halligan S, Taylor SA. MR enterographic manifestations of small bowel Crohn disease. Radiographics : a review publication of the Radiological Society of North America, Inc 2010; 30(2): 367-384.

[12] Masselli G, Gualdi G. MR Imaging of the Small Bowel. Radiology 2012; 264(2): 333-348.

[13] Sinha R, Murphy P, Hawker P, et al. Role of MRI in Crohn's disease. Clinical Radiology 2009; 64(4): 341-352.

[14] Darge K, Anupindi S, Keener H, Rompel O. Ultrasound of the bowel in children: how we do it. Pediatric radiology 2010; 40(4): 528-536.

[15] Migaleddu V, Quaia E, Scano D, Virgilio G. Inflammatory activity in Crohn disease: ultrasound findings. Abdominal imaging 2008; 33(5): 589-597.

[16] Gotthardt M, Bleeker-Rovers CP, Boerman OC, Oyen WJG. Imaging of inflammation by PET, conventional scintigraphy, and other imaging techniques. Journal of nuclear medicine : official publication, Society of Nuclear Medicine 2010; 51(12): 1937-1949.

[17] McBride HJ. Nuclear imaging of autoimmunity: focus on IBD and RA. Autoimmunity 2010; 43(7): 539-549.

[18] Pearce MS, Salotti JA, Little MP, et al. Radiation exposure from CT scans in childhood and subsequent risk of leukaemia and brain tumours: a retrospective cohort study. Lancet 2012; 380(9840): 499-505.

[19] Peloquin JM, Pardi DS, Sandborn WJ, et al. Diagnostic ionizing radiation exposure in a population-based cohort of patients with inflammatory bowel disease. The American Journal of Gastroenterology 2008; 103(8): 2015-2022.

[20] Desmond AN, O'Regan K, Curran C, et al. Crohn's disease: factors associated with exposure to high levels of diagnostic radiation. Gut 2008; 57(11): 1524-1529.

[21] Gee MS, Nimkin K, Hsu M, et al. Prospective evaluation of MR enterography as the primary imaging modality for pediatric Crohn disease assessment. AJR Am J Roentgenol; 197(1): 224-231.

Chapter 6

An Update to Surgical Management of Inflammatory Bowel Diseases

V. Surlin, C. Copaescu and A. Saftoiu

Additional information is available at the end of the chapter

http://dx.doi.org/10.5772/53057

1. Introduction

Surgery still has its place in the treatment of inflammatory bowel diseases (IBD) but it is reserved generally to cases in which medical treatment is unsuccessful in relieving symptoms, preventing disease progression and complications. As the medical treatment has added new drugs (especially newly targeted therapy) and surgical advance in technology has gain in more complex procedures with less morbidity and mortality and minimal invasivity there is a need for periodic update.

2. Perioperative care of patients with IBD

Good perioperative care always ensures better surgical results. Patients undergoing surgery for IBD must be prepared psychologically and medically.

Psychological preparation should start by explaining the patient the need for surgery. In this approach the surgeon must be aided by the gastroenterologist that has managed the patient for a long time in most of the cases. After acceptance of surgery, the patient must be explained the objectives, the advantages and disadvantages of each surgical intervention and the decision must be taken in common. People that will be submitted to stomas should also get a consultation from stomatherapist.

Medical preparation of the patients includes correction of hemoglobin, volemia, electrolytes and acid-base levels, coagulopathy, liver function. Total parenteral nutrition may be necessary in patients with nutritional deficits. Coexisting diseases should also be addressed. Any corticosteroid and immunosuppressive therapy should be discontinued before surgery, but corticosteroids need to be tapered immediately after surgery.

2.1. Prevention of infection

Adequate antibiotic prophylaxis or antibiotic therapy should be given, especially in cases with prolonged corticosteroid or infliximab therapy. Anyway, antibiotic prophylaxis pre and intraoperative is mandatory in colon surgery, but we think that may be continued several days after surgery especially in patient treated by corticosteroids and immunosupressive and immunomodulator therapy because of higher risk of infection on a reduced immune host defense.

The mechanical bowel preparation in elective cases is no longer mandatory in colon surgery and is contraindicated in patients with an acute abdomen or obstruction [1]

2.2. Prophylaxis for venous thrombosis

Patients with IBD are at increased risk for thromboembolic venous and arterial complications [2, 3]. Thus, intermittent pneumatic compression and/or low dose heparin should be used prophylactically.

3. Indications for surgery in ulceative colitis (UC)

Approximately 30–40% of patients with ulcerative colitis will require surgical treatment.

Indications for surgery are:

- intractable chronic disease,
- lack of response to high-dose corticosteroid therapy
- recurrence of symptoms upon stop of corticosteroid therapy,
- disease progression under maximal medical therapy,
- significant treatment-related complications such as severe steroid or infliximab side effects,
- dysplasia or cancer in patients with long-standing colitis during endoscopic surveillance,
- colonic strictures,
- acute exacerbation of the disease not responsive to rescue therapy such as intravenous steroids, cyclosporine, or infliximab,
- acute complications: hemorrhage, toxic megacolon, perforation, fulminant colitis,
- extracolonic manifestations.

3.1. Elective procedures

The development of restorative procedures such as the ileal pouch anal-canal anastomosis has made surgery a more attractive option in patients in whom medical therapy has been unsuccessful or undesirable.

3.2. Refractory colitis

The treatment of choice for acute severe steroid refractory ulcerative colitis is controversial [4]. Gastroenterologists sustain infliximab [5], while surgeons plead for colectomy [6].

3.3. Intractable chronic disease

The most common indication for elective surgery is disease activity that has been intractable to medical therapy. However, "intractable" is kind of blurry. Some authors have suggested that disease should be considered intractable when it or its treatment is associated with severe and persistent impairment in the quality of life [7]. However, these parameters are difficult to measure and are variable among individual patients.

3.4. Refractory Acute Severe Ulcerative Colitis (RASUC)

Refractory acute severe ulcerative colitis (RASUC), is defined by greater than six bloody stools per day and one of the following: heart rate more that 90 beat/min, erythrocyte sedimentation rate more than 30mm/h, temperature more than 37.8°C, and hemoglobin less than 10.5 g/dl. The appropriate time to initiate surgical intervention during the treatment of RASUC has been a topic of investigation, because patients are usually severely malnourished, immunocompromised, and weakened by side-effects of immunomodulating drugs. [8].

3.5. Emergency surgery

Advances in medical therapy (including use of infliximab) have reduced the need for emergency surgery due to catastrophic complications such as massive hemorrhage, perforation, fulminant colitis, and acute colonic obstruction [9].

A longer duration of in-hospital ineffective medical therapy (8 versus 5 days) that delays surgical therapy in patients with acute severe ulcerative colitis is associated with an increased risk of postoperative complications [10].

Biologic agents were introduced with the intent to help avoid operative intervention in patients with moderately to severely active IBD who have demonstrated an inadequate response to conventional therapies. Ananthakrishnan et al. analyzing a large number of cases hospitalized for IBD found that the use of biologic agents decreases the incidence of emergency surgery in patients with mild disease, but not in those with severe forms. [11]

For Ousslan et al, failure to respond to infliximab determined the decision for colectomy in 19% of the patients. Predicting factors for colectomy were C-reactive protein > 10mg/l before treatment with infliximab, hemoglobin less than 9.4 g/dl, episodic use of infliximab, and previous treatment with cyclosporin. [12]

In the study of Gustavsson et al, with 3-year follow-up, infliximab significantly reduced the need for surgery at 3 month compared to placebo (29% vs 67%), for patients with corticosteroid refractory UC. At 3 years, 50% of patients in the infliximab group and 76% of patients in placebo group needed colectomy. [13]

In a spanish multicenter experience, patients in whom corticosteroids and ciclosporin failed to control the disease, were submitted to infliximab. A 40 years patient, operated because of infliximab failure died after surgery from nosocomial pneumonia. Authors stated that salvage therapy with infliximab after failed corticosteroids and ciclosporin may be associated with risk for morbidity and mortality and therefore should be used in selected patients. [14]

Adalimumab emerged as an indication in the cases in which there is partial or no response to infliximab. In a study from Taxonera et al at 48 weeks of follow-up only 20% of the patients needed surgery. Therefore, application of this new therapy may diminish the indications for surgery in the group of patient non-responders to infliximab therapy.

3.6. Suspicion of cancer

The risk of malignancy is directly proportional to the duration of disease. The risk during the first decade of disease is low, but increases substantially after that. After 30 years of disease the risk is about 50 %. [8] Patients with more than 10 years of disease should undergo a colonoscopy each year. Most of the gastroenterologists consider discovery of moderate to severe dysplasia an indication for surgery.

3.7. Extraintestinal manifestations

Surgical indication is seldom for extracolonic manifestations of IBD. Benefits from surgery will be in the rare cases of massive hemolytic anemia unresponsive to treatment. In those cases splenectomy should be associated to colectomy [7]. Another extracolonic indication for colectomy is thromboembolic complications. Erythema nodosum and arthralgia of the small and large joints appear to benefit the most from proctocolectomy [15]. In cases of pyoderma gangrenosum, ankylosing spondylitis and arthritis, sclerosing cholangitis surgery may not be so profitable.

Surgical options for ulcerative colitis are:

- Proctocolectomy with permanent ileostomy (Brooke ileostomy)
- Proctocolectomy with continent ileostomy (Kock pouch)
- Abdominal colectomy with ileorectal anastomosis
- Colectomy, mucosal proctectomy, and ileal pouch-anal canal anastomosis (IPAA)
- Colectomy and stapled ileal pouch distal rectal anastomosis (IPDRA)

3.8. Elective procedures

- Curative procedure - Proctocolectomy with permanent ileostomy.

- Avoiding of ileostomy - IPAA. Patients under infliximab - three stages IPAA

In the elective surgical population, the standard operation performed is a total proctocolectomy with ileal pouch anal anastomosis. Described by Parks and Nichols in 1978, the procedure involves excision of the abdominal colon, pelvic dissection to remove the rectum, creation of an ileal reservoir, and anastomosis of the pouch to the anus. A variety of pouch designs can be used. The most commonlyof thrm is the J-pouch. Preference for the J-pouch lies in its limited use of bowel, reliable emptying, and ease of construction. [8]

Mortality is low - 0.2–0.4%; however, the risk of pelvic sepsis can be as high as 23% from leaks from the ileoanal anastomosis. To prevent this complication, the operation could be performed in multiple stage (two or three), to allow anastomoses to heal without important consequences [16,17].

3.9. In emergency situations

Toxic megacolon – the procedure of choice is open colectomy with ileostomy and closure of the rectum or distal colostomy. The rectum may be resected afterwards with ileal pouch-anal anastomosis. IPAA from the beginning should not be performed because of risk of complications.

Hemmorhage – Proctocolectomy, suture of a bleeding ulcer or Hartmann-type colectomy leaving a small stump of distal rectum.

3.10. Other options for restorative proctocolectomy

Ileal pouch distal rectum anastomosis (IPDRA) – anastomosis between ileal pouch and distal rectum – easier to perform, better anal sensation and continence especially at night.

Main disadvantage – leaving rectal mucosa behind, that should be avoided in patients with cancer or severe dysplasia in colorectal mucosa, severe extraintestinal manifestations.

Advantage – older patients, lack of adequate mobilisation for tension-free anastomosis – ileorectal anastomosis (IRA)

Indications

- Patients not suitable for IPAA
- Refusal of ileostomy
- Medical conditions in which a stoma is relatively contraindicated (eg, portal hypertension or ascites),
- Women of childbearing age because of the risk of infertility,
- Patients in whom Crohn's disease cannot be excluded,
- Patients with colitis complicated by advanced colonic malignancy,

Functional results after IRA

A retrospective analysis of the functional results after IRA for ulcerative colitis or indeterminant colitis in 86 patients found that the rectum was eventually resected in 17% of cases, rectal dysplasia occurred in 17%, rectal cancer 8% and refractory proctitis 28%. The cumulative probability of developing rectal dysplasia at 5, 10, 15, and 20 years was 7, 9, 20, and 25 percent, respectively. The cumulative probability of developing rectal cancer at 5, 10, 15, and 20 years was 0, 2, 5, and 14 percent, respectively. The cumulative probability of having a functioning IRA at 10 and 20 years was 74 and 46 percent, respectively. [18]

Satisfactory rectal function varies greatly depending upon the selections of patients and length of follow-up. The risk of cancer in the residual rectum has been reported to be 6 % at 20 years and 15 % at 30 years. The risk is significant considering that most patients are young and have many years to live.

Farouk et al noted that in 1386 patients with restorative proctocolectomy and over 8-year follow-up, 80% reported complete diurnal continence, with 50% requiring medications to slow intestinal transit. [19]

4. Surgical options for Crohn's disease

Crohn's disease is not curable by surgery. Therefore, this is actualy reserved for complications or to symptoms refractory to medical therapy [20].

Surgical decision making in Crohn's disease is driven by anatomic distribution and inflammatory subtype of disease. Forty percent of patients have ileal disease with segments of colonic involvement, with 20–25% of patients exhibiting isolated colonic disease and 5–10% with isolated anorectal disease [21]. Surgical intervention is primarily performed for the complications of Crohn's disease: stricture and obstruction, fistula, or medically refractory disease. Approximately 70% of Crohn's disease patients ultimately require surgery, often multiple, making minimally invasive options appealing

Indications for surgery are:

- obstruction,
- perforation in small intestinal Crohn's disease,
- failure to respond to medical therapy in patients with colonic involvement,
- strictures,
- fistula

Surgery should to adress only to segments causing obstruction, bleeding, or perforation. Resection is performed when there is an abscess or fistula to an adjacent organ. The disease-free margins are established by gross inspection, microscopic disease at the margins will not be associated with recurrence. Therefore we should avoid large margins, in the idea of preserving as much as possible of small bowel capital because the patients may need another resection in the future and thus preventing the short bowel syndrome.

Ileocolic resections should be followed by a side-to-side anastomosis. A meta-analysis of eight comparative studies found that a side-to-side anastomosis was associated with fewer anastomotic leaks and postoperative complications, a shorter hospital stay and a lower peri-anastomotic recurrence rates compared to end-to-end anastomosis [22]. However, the authors suggested that further randomized controlled trials are needed to confirm these associations.

4.1. Duodenal disease

Duodenal Crohn's disease very rarely requires surgery. The major indications for surgery are obstruction and less often perforation or fistula formation. Gastrojejunostomy rather than resection is typically performed. Strictureplasty, duodenojejunostomy, and endoscopic balloon dilation have also been described [23].

4.2. Intra-abdominal abscess, peritonitis

- Intraperitoneal abscesses were classically drain by open surgery and were followed by surgical resection of the diseased segment of the bowel.
- Progress of interventional radiology, new biologic agents and progress of laparoscopy changed this classic approach [24,25].
- Percutaneous drainage guided by CT or abdominal ultrasound has a low rate of complications and a high rate of success - approximately 70% of attempted cases. Complete drainage of the abscess may necessitate repeated punctures. This attitude allows the patient to be prepared for an elective resection of the bowel after the sepsis resides, after improving nutritional status and decreasing corticosteroids. Controversy exists regarding the need for subsequent operation after adequate abscess drainage as intractable disease or recurrent abscess occurs in at least 30% of these patients within a year.
- If percutaneous drainage is unsuccessful, surgical drainage should be performed. The timing of surgery following percutaneous abscess drainage, when clinically indicated, occurs after clinical resolution of sepsis.
- Peritonitis is rare in Crohn's disease. Exploratory laparotomy with peritoneal lavage, with construction of a stoma is most commonly required. The decision whether to resect or not the bowel depends upon the operative findings and the patient's condition [26].
- Abdominal wall abscesses (psoas and rectus sheath) are less common and more difficult to control locally than intra-abdominal abscesses. In a retrospective review of 13 patients with an abdominal wall abscess treated by percutaneous and/or open operative drainage, all 13 required resection of the diseased segment even after successful drainage of the abscess [25].

4.3. Fistulas

Fistulas to adjacent organs (stomach, duodenum, bladder, vagina, and sigmoid colon) are treated by resection and anastomosis of the diseased segment of the bowel and closure of the fistula. Resection of the adjacent segment is necessary only when it is primarily involved with Crohn's disease. Bypasses should be avoided because persistent disease in the bypassed segment can lead to abscess formation, bleeding, perforation, bacterial overgrowth, and malignancy.

4.4. Strictures

Intestinal strictures can be relieved by resection; synchronous small bowel resection in patients with multiple strictures is common [27]. Strictureplasty or balloon dilation may be a suitable alternative for selected patients.

4.4.1. Strictureplasty

Strictureplasty is performed by longitudinal incision across the stricture and a transversal closure that enlarges the lumen. Indication is represented by the patients that have isolated areas of short stricture and are at risk for short bowel syndrome due to previous surgery or extension of enterectomy. Strictureplasty can relieve obstruction, and is often performed in association with a small bowel resection [27, 28]. It can also be performed without excision of bowel [29, 30]. It should not be performed in acutely inflamed bowel.

To avoid large enterectomy for extensive and/or multiple strictures occurring over long intestinal segments, a side-to-side isoperistaltic or other type of nonconventional strictureplasty is safe and effective [31, 32].

Strictureplasty has been associated with excellent results, including relief of obstruction, the ability to withdraw steroids, and improvement in symptoms [31, 33] the risk of fistula or recurrent stricture formation is low and comparable to resection. Whether preservation of diseased bowel increases the long-term risk of malignancy is unknown, although case reports have documented adenocarcinoma arising from sites of previous strictureplasty [34].

The following examples illustrate the range of findings in two of the largest series

In a series of 1124 procedures of strictureplasty on 314 patients there was a synchronous bowel resection in 66% of cases, overall morbidity was 18%, septic complications in 5%, morbidity was higher in patients with preoperative weight loss and older age, recurrence after surgery was met in 34% during a median follow-up of 7.5 years, recurrence was higher in younger patients [30]:

Another study included 479 procedures of strictureplasty performed in 100 patients with a follow-up of 7 years in average [35]. Overall morbidity was 22% and included sepsis – 11%, obstruction 4%, hemorrhage - 4% percent, and mortality – 3%. After a first strictureplasty the reoperation rate were 52% at 40 months, 56% at 26 months after a second, 86% at 27 months after a third, 63% at 26 months after a fourth. The major risk factor for reoperation was young age. The early relaparotomy rate was 8 percent. One patient developed cancer after many years of disease. The authors biopsied suspicious lesions, rather than going for routine biopsy of all lesions.

http://dx.doi.org/10.5772/53057

4.4.2. Balloon dilation

Another method to dilate intestinal strictures is with a hydrostatic balloon Experience is relatively limited compared with strictureplasty or resection, and the long-term efficacy and safety is therefore less well-established. A meta-analysis of 13 studies (with a total of 347 patients) reported overall technical success in 86 % of cases and long-term efficacy in 58 percent, with up to 33 months of follow-up [36]. On multivariate analysis, a stricture length of ≤4 cm was associated with better surgery-free outcomes. The outcome of balloon dilatation to relieve obstruction from intestinal strictures in Crohn's disease is not influenced by the type of concomitant medical therapy [37].

Couckuyte et al performed 78 dilatation procedures for 59 ileocolonic strictures in 55 patients, all procedures were carried out endoscopically under general anesthesia. Succes was registered in 90% with 11% perforations from which 30% needed surgery and 60% were solved only with medical treatment. Mean period of time to recurrence of obstruction was up to 11 months for 62% of patients. [38]

In pediatric patients injections of corticosteroids into strictures after balloon dilatations were followed by fewer redilatations than in placebo group. [39]. For adults it didn't work the same [40]

4.4.3. Stenting

Placement of an expandable metal stent within colonic strictures has been described, but experience is limited, and the safety of this approach is uncertain [41].

4.5. Colorectal disease

Options for surgery range from temporary diverting ileostomy to resection of segments of diseased colon or even the entire colon and rectum. Same conservative principles applied to disease involving the small intestine should also be applied to the surgical management of Crohn's colitis

The optimal procedure depends in part upon the extent of the disease and the clinical setting:

- Segmental colectomy may be adequate for isolated areas of colonic involvement. An Ileorectal anastomosis can be carried out if the rectum is spared. A proctectomy will be required in half of the patients [42]. While no prospective randomized study has been undertaken to compare segmental colectomy and total colectomy with ileorectal anastomosis, both procedures appear to be equally effective as treatment options for colonic Crohn's disease. However, patients undergoing segmental resection may have earlier recurrence [43]. The choice of operation depends upon the extent of colonic disease; there may be better outcomes with ileorectal anastomosis in those who have two or more involved colonic segments.

- Total proctocolectomy is indicated for patients with extensive, diffuse colorectal disease.

- Subtotal colectomy with ileostomy is usually performed in emergency situations.

- An abdominoperineal resection with a permanent end-colostomy is indicated in patients with severe Crohn's disease limited to the anorectum. An intersphincteric proctectomy will minimize the risk of a nonhealing wound and sexual or urinary dysfunction, by avoiding dissection near the hipogastric plexuses. In the presence of anorectal disease and sepsis a Hartmann procedure can be carried out in the first place leaving a small stump of distal rectum, followed by a perineal proctectomy. [44].

4.6. Anorectal disease

The management of anorectal disease, present in 14–38% of patients, remains difficult despite advances in medical therapy. Perianal fistula or abscess is the initial presentation of Crohn's disease in approximately 30% of cases and has been associated with increased extra-intestinal symptoms and steroid resistance, resulting in significant disability [8].

The number of Crohn's patients who require surgery has, however, decreased with the advances in medical management.

Most of the abscesses are small, difficult to drain and can disappear with antibiotics alone. The antibiotic therapy should associate ciprofloxacin to metronidazole. Greater abscesses can be drained by placement of a seton or by ultrasound or CT guided large bore needle aspiration or drain placement.

Treatment of the perianal fistula depends on the type of fistula (simple vs. complex) and underlying rectal inflammation.

Simple fistulas are intersphincteric or transsphincteric below the dentate line in origin with a single opening and no associated stricture or abscess. Such fistulas have an excellent response to antibiotic and surgical therapy and heal 80–100% of the time with simple fistulotomy [8]

Complex fistulas on the contrary, involve the superficial, transsphincteric, or intersphincteric region below the dentate line, have multiple openings, and can be associated with rectal stricture or rectovaginal fistula.

Pelvic MRI provides the most accurate information (90% accuracy) about fistulous burden and underlying rectal inflammation and is instrumental in surgical planning and monitoring response to therapy. Accuracy approaches 100% when MRI is combined with examination under anesthesia. [45, 46]

Complex fistulas represent a challenge and require aggressive immunomodulating therapy in combination with surgical therapy. Many patients feel improvement in symptoms with antibiotic therapy (ciprofloxacin and metronidazole); however, symptom relief is transient with recurrence on withdrawal of antibiotics. Infliximab has proven to be the immunosuppressive drug of choice in treatment of complex perianal fistulas with two randomized trials showing decreased number of fistulas, increased disease-free period, and fewer required hospitalizations and surgeries.[47]

Surgical therapy has evolved for complex fistulas as well with the development of less invasive techniques for closure of high fistulas to prevent incontinence associated with damage

http://dx.doi.org/10.5772/53057

to the anal sphincters. Some of the newest approaches use fibrin glue and collagen plugs to occlude fistulous tracts without requiring incision.

A study from Chung et al comparing collagen fistula plug to fibrin glue, rectal advancement flap, and seton placement for treatment of 51 patients with complex perianal fistulas showed a 75% resolution rate with use of the plug compared with less than 30% for each of the other modalities. [48]

The systematic review by Soltani and Kaiserof evaluating the efficacy of endorectal flap advancement for complex perianal Crohn's disease found a 46% resolution [49].

The review by Lewis and Maron on anorectal Crohn's disease provides an algorithm for management of complex perianal fistulas, stressing that surgical therapy in excess of seton placement should not be attempted during active proctitis due to inflammation [50].

Postoperative medical treatment for prevention of Crohn's disease recurrence is controversial in light of data supporting increased incidence of complications with preoperative immunosuppressive therapy. However, a randomized, placebo-controlled clinical trial showed no difference in incidence of adverse events (anastomotic leak, wound complications, infection, obstruction, bleeding, death) between postoperative patients treated with infliximab within 4 weeks of surgery and those untreated. [51]

Bordeianou et al studied the effect of immediate vs. tailored medical prophylaxis on endoscopic and/or symptomatic recurrence in 199 patients who underwent ileocecectomy for Crohn's disease. The group found that there was no difference in recurrence rates between patients treated with medication immediately after surgery and those treated based on endoscopic finding, adding to the debate on whether perioperative and postoperative medical suppression is advantageous. [52]

5. Minimally invasive surgery for inflammatory bowel disease

The laparoscopic approach was already proven feasible both for UC and CD.

5.1. Minimally invasive surgery for chronic ulcerative colitis

A way to use laparoscopy is only for the mobilization of the colon (cecum, ascendent, descendent, sigmoid) and to perform the rest of the operation in open but with a smaller incision [53]

Laparoscopic subtotal colectomy performed in emergency conditions was followed by acceptable outcomes and shorter hospital stay, although in such cases is not usually recommended [54].

Another possibility is to perform colon and rectal mobilisation, section of the mesocolon and even the rectum with liniar ENDO-GIA. Some authors do that by hand assisted technique.

5.1.1. To divert or not after laparoscopic surgery

This is a question still under debate. Ky et al had a series of 32 laparoscopic IPAA (29 for UC) in which they didn't divert and had a morbidity of 34% and 3% leak rate [55]. Hasegawa et al performed 18 cases all with diversions and had 33% morbidity and 0% leak rate [56]. Others like Marcello et al from 20 cases (13 for UC) divert only in 60% of cases and had 5% leak rate.[57]

Is laparoscopy superior to open approach? In short term yes – as already proven by comparison between them, with faster recovery (including faster ambulation, less postoperative pain, faster return of bowel movement and time to first passage of flatus and feces).

Brown et al compared laparoscopic-assisted restorative proctocolectomy to open approach and found shorter operative time in open group, and similar functional outcome and recovery, only better cosmesis by shorter abdominal scar. The hand-assisted method seems to reduce the operative time with more than 30 minutes [58].

Postoperative morbidity is still relatively high duet o extensive procedure (25-34%) [55, 56, 57]

5.2. Minimally invasive surgery for Crohn's disease

Laparoscopic approach have the potential of decreasing morbidity, speeding recovery, and reducing costs, while decreasing the incidence of small bowel obstruction and ventral (abdominal wall) hernias [59,60].

A randomized comparative trial between open and laparoscopic ileo-colic resection found a conversion rate of 6% and no significant difference in immediate postoperative recovery (passage of flatus and length of hospital stay). The only benefice was a faster recovery of forced expiratory volume and forced expiratory vital capacity. [61]

Maartense et al performed a comparative randomized controlled trial between laparoscopic-assisted ileocolonic resection performed by experienced surgeons in laparoscopy with open resections in Crohn's disease [62]. Morbidity, hospital stay, and costs were lower in the laparoscopic group, although there were no significant differences in quality-of-life at three months follow-up.

Alves et al found that the need for conversion to an open procedure was predicted by the severity of disease; independent predictors of conversion including a history of recurrent medical episodes of Crohn's disease and the presence of intra-abdominal abscess or fistula at the time of laparoscopy [63].

Recurrences after laparoscopic surgery were similar after conventional surgery. Laparoscopic colectomy was found to be safe and effective in the hands of experienced surgeons for selected patients with Crohn's colitis [64].

In the review by Fichera et al on Crohn's disease, the author highlights three meta-analyses that compared laparoscopic with open ileocolic surgery that demonstrated earlier return of bowel function leading to shorter hospital stay, fewer late small bowel obstructions, and decreased early complications such as wound infections and bleeding with laparoscopic surgery. [20]

Two large studies on laparoscopic surgery for isolated colonic disease found similarly good outcomes with fewer complications. Holubar et al reported their outcomes for 92 patients who underwent laparoscopic colectomy, showing a total complication rate of 34%, reintervention rate of 7.6%, and anastomotic leak rate of 3.8%, all consistent with reported outcomes for open colectomy. Fifteen percent of laparoscopic cases were converted to open and presence of small bowel disease was the only predictive factor identified, independent of presence of phlegmonous or fistulous disease. [65]

Umanskiy et al compared outcomes of 125 patients who underwent laparoscopic vs. open colectomy and/or proctectomy for Crohn's disease. The most common procedure in both groups was total proctocolectomy with end ileostomy and the only statistically significant difference in procedures performed applied to completion proctectomies, which were more likely to be open. Patients in the laparoscopic group had earlier return of bowel function, reduced length of hospital stay, and decreased intraoperative blood loss. Interestingly, the reduced blood loss did not result in fewer transfusions, which were similar in both groups [66].

5.2.1. *Recurrence after laparoscopic surgery*

There was also no clinical recurrence at 20 months [60]. In a study by Tabet et al with 39 months follow up, there were similar rates of recurrence 48% vs 45%. [67]

Watanabe et al and Bemelman et al performed laparoscopic-assisted resection for Crohn's disease, including patients with enteric fistulas. Postoperative outcome was better in laparoscopic group [68, 69]. Same results were noted by Duepree et al., Tabet et al, and Young Fadok et al. (all comparative studies) who found short term outcome benefits associated with the minimally invasive approach [60, 67, 70].

5.2.2. *Costs*

For Duepree et al costs per case were higher for laparoscopic group.[70]. Young-Fadok et al reported an overall cost for laparoscopic cases significantly less than for the open ones [60].

There is a broad range of conversion rates (1.4-24 %), morbidity (10-29 %), length of stay (3.3-8.8 days), and leak rates (0-5%). Most of the series involve relatively small numbers of patients. [59, 69, 70]

5.2.3. *Long term benefits of laparoscopic approach*

Laparoscopic surgery is considered to generate less postoperative adhesions and less incisional hernias.

Bergamaschi et al reported the results of a comparative study with long term follow up between laparoscopic and open ileocecal resections. At 5 years, they found a rate of 11.1 % small bowel obstructions for laparoscopic group and 35.4 percent for the open group, and the result was statistically significant.[59]

Generally, laparoscopic colectomy is followed by lower incidence of incisional hernia and small bowel obstruction, with significant differences, as reported by Duepree et al [70].

Functional outcome [71], quality of life [71] are similar but cosmetic results [71] especially for women [72] are higher after laparoscopy.

6. Complications

6.1. Early complications

Are usual after restorative proctocolectomy.

The most frequent are bowel obstruction, pouch bleeding, pelvic and wound sepsis, transient urinary dysfunction, and dehydration from temporary loop ileostomy with high output. Surgery is not mandatory in many of those cases. Incidence of pelvic abscess after IPAA is estimated to 5% [73]. Pelvic abscesses lead to transabdominal or local surgery in most of the cases, failure of pouch in quarter of cases, incontinence, need for constipating or bulking medications was in the patients in whom the reservoir was preserved. There was also a decrease in the quality of life of those patients.

Portal vein thrombosis can occur after IPAA. Clinical manifestations may include pain, fever, vomiting, leukocytosis, and unexplained postoperative ileus. Diagnose is made with CT-scanner. Treatment with anticoagulation will lead to full resolution.

6.2. Late complications

- stricture of the anastomosis,
- poor postoperative anorectal function,
- anal fistula and abscess,
- reduced fertility [74],
- pouchitis - this is the most frequent. In one series, the cumulative probability of suffering at least one episode of clinical pouchitis was 18 and 48 % at 1 and 10 years, respectively [75],
- irritable pouch syndrome and anismus (anorectal dysfunction)[76].

Majority of the pouch related complication can be solved by medical treatment consisting mainly in local measures, surgery being required in a minority. In one series of almost 1000 patients who had undergone IPAA, reoperation for complications was necessary in only 12 % [77].

As an example, ileal pouch fistulas and strictures refractory to dilatation are difficult to treat and may require revision of the pouch if Crohn's disease can be excluded. A transvaginal repair is favored for a pouch-vaginal fistula [78]. A combined abdominal perineal repair may offer better results compared with a local procedure [79]. A controlled septic condition does not preclude salvage surgery. Although pouch failure occurs more often than with primary IPAA, high patient satisfaction and quality of life can be achieved [80]. Furthermore, excision of the pouch is associated with a high risk of complications, especially delayed perineal wound healing [81, 82].

A number of unusual late complications have been described including [83, 84, 85]:

- Solitary ileal ulcer
- Traumatic ileal ulcer perforation
- Superior mesenteric artery syndrome
- Mucosal prolapse with outlet obstruction
- Volvulus
- Sacral osteomyelitis
- Puborectal spasm
- Fibroid polyps
- Pharmacobezoar

6.3. Long-term results of surgery

The long-term success of surgery depends upon the type of operation, the clinical setting, and surgical expertise. Several studies have suggested that functional results are poor during the long-term follow-up in patients who had adverse personality factors before surgery (such as problems with sexual satisfaction, difficulty expressing emotions, perfectionist body ideals, and poor frustration tolerance) [79]. The following results were described in some of the largest series.

One series included 1885 patients who underwent an ileal pouch-anal anastomosis for ulcerative colitis and were followed for an average of 11 years. The mean number of stools was 5.7 per day at one year and 6.4 at 20 years, and also increased at night from 1.5 to 2.0. The incidence of frequent fecal incontinence increased from 5 to 11 percent during the day and from 12 to 21 percent at night. The overall rate of pouch success at 5, 10, 15, and 20 years was 96, 93, 92, and 92 percent, respectively. Quality of life remained unchanged and 92 percent remained in the same employment. [86]

In another report that included 486 patients who had undergone proctocolectomy and ileoanal anastomosis for ulcerative colitis or familial adenomatous polyposis, the cumulative probabilities of pouch failure were 1, 5, and 7 percent at 1, 5, and 10 years, respectively [87] The most common cause of pouch failure was fistula formation.

Tulchinsky et al reported 634 patients who underwent restorative proctocolectomy for IBD. Patients were followed for a mean of 85 months. Failure (defined as removal of the pouch or the need for an ileostomy) was divided into early (occurring within one-year) or late (occurring more than one-year postoperatively). Three patients died postoperatively while an additional 23 died (of a variety of causes) during follow-up. Of the remaining patients, there were a total of 61 failures (10 %) of which 24.6% were early and 75.4% late. Failures were due to pelvic sepsis (52 %), poor function (30 %), pouchitis (11 %), and miscellaneous causes (four patients, all early failures). Predictors of failure included a final diagnosis of Crohn's disease, a type J or S reservoir, female gender, postoperative pelvic sepsis, and a one-stage procedure. Failure rates increased with time from 9% at five years to 13% at 10 years. [88]

Another series showed that results in older patients (>65) are not as good; however, appropriate case selection was followed by acceptable function and quality of life to patients of all ages [89].

Anal canal strictures were described in up to 11 percent of 213 patients [82]. Strictures that were not fibrotic responded well after anal dilation while fibrotic strictures were more commonly associated with intra- or postoperative complications and frequently required surgical therapy.

A systematic review of 43 observational studies (with a total of 9317 patients) found a pouch failure rate of 6.8%, increasing to 8.5% in those with more than five-year follow-up [90]. Pelvic sepsis occurred in 9.5%. Severe, mild, and urge fecal incontinence was reported in 3.7, 17, and 7.3 percent, respectively. These results suggest that current techniques are associated with non-negligible complication rates and leave room for improvement and continued development of alternative procedures.

IPAA may have long-term effects:

- on female reproductive health [91],
- some women experience increased dyspareunia [92], although the ability to experience orgasm and coital frequency remain unchanged,
- female fertility is significantly decreased [93], possibly due to pelvic adhesions, although successful pregnancies occur regularly [94], patients may experience a transient increase in stool frequency (including incontinence) during pregnancy, which resolves after delivery, pregnancy and delivery are safe in patients with IPAA. Patients should not be discouraged from childbearing because of the pouch. Whether vaginal or cesarean delivery is better for women with a pelvic pouch remains controversial.

Satisfactory long-term functional outcome and excellent quality of life have also been described after stapled restorative proctocolectomy. In a series of 977 patients, quality of life increased for two years after surgery, with no deterioration thereafter [95]. The prevalence of perfect continence increased from 76 percent before surgery to 82 percent after surgery and, although continence deteriorated somewhat more than two years after surgery, it was no worse than preoperative values. Ninety-eight percent of patients would have recommended the surgery to others. In another prospective, observational study, patients who had a stapled anastomosis had higher rates of daytime, nighttime, and complete continence compared with patients who underwent a hand-sewn anastomosis [32].

6.4. Morbidity of operation due to use of biologic agents

Preoperative use of infliximab. The efficacy of the biologic agents must be balanced against the morbidity associated with their usage, and surgeons have been worried about the safety associated with the preoperative use of these medications in patients requiring elective or nonelective operations for their IBD.

Beddy et al believed the evidence showed that recent biologic agent administration in a patient with Crohn's disease should not cause the surgeon to delay surgery or employ fecal diversion proximal to an anastomosis. However, they felt that patients with ulcerative colitis preoperatively managed with infliximab and immunosuppressant medications should undergo a three-stage rather than two-stage restorative proctocolectomy and ileal pouch-anal anastomosis (IPAA); the first operation would be a total or subtotal colectomy and creation of ileostomy that allows patients to be withdrawn from medications prior to performing the IPAA procedure. They proposed this approach in hopes of improving long-term ileal pouch function by decreasing the risk of short-term infectious complications attributed to combination therapy.[83]

Gainsbury et al, remarked that there is an increased risk of septic complications associated with preoperative infliximab and elective surgery for ulcerative colitis, growing evidence appears to refute that notion. [99]

Whether immunosuppressive therapy increases the risk of postoperative complications is still controversy. For some authors [98, 99, 100, 101] it may not be responsible but for others [102, 103, 104] it is, increasing risk for sepsis, intraabdominal abscesses [102,104], and especially when associated with other immunomodulators (ciclosporin) [103]. In this conceptual area there is need for more controlled trials.

Ellis et al found that unlike surgical mortality for most disorders, the operative mortality associated with colectomy for ulcerative colitis has increased in recent years despite centralization of care. This finding raises considerable concern that patients potentially are not receiving prompt or appropriate surgical care because of alterations in medical therapy. [105]

6.5. Pouchitis

Outside of the perioperative period, the most common late complication of ileal pouch anal anastomosis is pouchitis, occurring in up to 60% of patients.[106] Pouchitis is thought to be the result of immunologic reaction to altered bowel flora. Symptoms range from mild diarrhea to severe abdominal pain and fistulization with neighboring organs. In a recent review from the Cleveland Clinic, multivariate analysis identified pulmonary co-morbidities, S-pouch reconstruction, disease proximal to the splenic flexure, and extraintestinal disease are the factors predictive of subsequent pouchitis. Patients who developed pouchitis had higher incidence of obstruction, fistula, and stricture and reported lower quality of life than controls [94]. Once identified, the treatment of pouchitis is primarily medical, with most patients showing excellent response to antibiotics and/or probiotics and immunomodulators. A Cochrane database review of trials through 2010 found that ciprofloxacin was more effective than metronidazole and budesonide enemas were equally effective to metronidazole in the treatment of acute pouchitis. The probiotic VSL#3 was more effective than placebo for prevention and treatment of chronic pouchitis[108]. Haveranet al reported complete resolution of symptoms in stricturing and antibiotic resistant pouchitis with azathioprine and 6-mercaptorpurine. However, fistulizing disease required the addition of infliximab, with 46% of such patients ultimately requiring diverting ileostomy for relief. Alternatives to ileostomy for pouch failure include pouch salvage techniques such as transanal mobilization or abdominoperineal revision of the pouch, with success rates ranging from 48 to 93%.[18] A small percentage of patients will ultimately be identified as having Crohn's disease as the cause of their fistulae and pouch complications.[109]

In a review of almost 1800 IPAA attempts from the Mayo Clinic, abandonment was required in 4.1 % [97].

7. Postoperative monitoring

Risk of dysplasia and cancer

All patients who undergo surgical procedures for ulcerative colitis should be monitored regularly for the development of long-term complications.

In addition to functional problems, complications can occur at any stage, including the development of dysplasia and possibly cancer.

However, in a study of potentially high-risk patients (eg, Kock pouch for ≥14 years, a pelvic pouch for ≥12 years, a history of dysplasia or cancer in the proctocolectomy specimen or troublesome pouchitis), the development of dysplasia was rare [98].

7.1. Dysplasia

The presence of inflammatory changes in a retained rectal stump, anal transitional zone, and ileal reservoir after stapled pouch-anal anastomosis is a cause of concern because of the long-term risk of dysplasia.

A systematic review of 23 observational and case control studies estimated that the prevalence of confirmed dysplasia in the pouch, anal transitional zone, or rectal cuff was 1.13 % (0-19%) The prevalence of high-grade, low-grade, or indefinite dysplasia was 0.15, 0.98, and 1.23 %, respectively. Dysplasia was equally frequent in the pouch and rectal cuff or anal transitional zone [112].

If dysplasia and cancer are identified before or at operation the risk for postoperative dysplasia is higher. The risk of neoplasia is not completely eliminated by colectomy and mucosectomy. A retrospective review of 3203 patients with a preoperative diagnosis of IBD who underwent restorative proctocolectomy found that the cumulative incidence for pouch neoplasia at 5, 10, 15, 20 and 25 years were 0.9, 1.3, 1.9, 4.2, and 5.1 %, respectively 11 patients developed adenocarcinoma of the pouch or at the anal transitional zone, one developed lymphoma in the pouch, three developed squamous cell carcinoma at the anal transitional zone, and 23 developed pouch dysplasia. The prognosis of pouch adenocarcinoma appeared to be poor [100].

If the rectal cuff becomes symptomatic or develops dysplasia, the retained rectal mucosa from the restorative proctocolectomy can be removed by a transanal completion mucosectomy and reconstructing the ileal pouch-anal anastomosis as an alternative to a complete anal rectal resection and permanent ileostomy. The mucosectomy removes all rectal mucosa, confers a highest likelihood of a surgical cure, and reduces the risk of future dysplasia. Short term results in a series of 27 patients included reduced pouchitis symptoms and 90 % of patients were moderately to very satisfy with the procedure. Incontinence was reduced by 70 percent at 12 months of observation [101].

The optimal frequency of pouch endoscopy and biopsy is not well established. It is recommended to perform an initial screening five years after creation of an ileal pouch in children or when the total disease duration exceeds seven years [102].

In patients that had severe villous atrophy or dysplasia in the resected colon or rectum the aforementioned interval may be reduced. In patients with pouch or anal high-grade dysplasia detected during surveillance, resection of the ileal pouch and anal canal should be considered.

In a retrospective review of 222 patients who required operative intervention for Crohn's colitis, there were 2.3% dysplasia and 2.7% adenocarcinoma. In this small cohort, the risk factors for the development of dysplasia or adenocarcinoma included longer disease duration (over 17 years), extensive disease, and older age at diagnosis (38 years of age or older). These findings support colonoscopic screening and surveillance of patients with Crohn's colitis. [116]

7.2. Recurrence

The postoperative recurrence rate for patients undergoing a resection and anastomosis is high in Crohn's disease. In most series up to 20 percent of patients will not have a clinical recurrence even at 15 years after surgery Those with severe endoscopic or radiologic findings are at increased risk to have or develop symptoms (72 versus 42%). An increased risk for reoperation has been associated with perforating disease and smoking [117].

A laparoscopic approach does not appear to decrease the risk of recurrence. A retrospective review of 89 patients undergoing laparoscopically resected primary ileocolonic Crohn's colitis found recurrent disease in 61 percent [118]. The median time to recurrence was 13 months (range 1.3 months to 8.7 years). Only the presence of granulomas in the resected specimen was identified as a risk factor for time to recurrence, and these patients were almost three times more likely to develop a recurrence.

The recurrence rate is lower in patients with Crohn's colitis who undergo a total colectomy and ileostomy compared to those with disease involving other segments of the digestive tract. We already know, from a study in 1985 by Goligher et al Such patients have only a 10 percent recurrence rate in the small intestine at 10 years [106]. A number of medical options are available that may reduce the risk of recurrence. A relatively aggressive approach should be considered in patients with diffuse and distal Crohn's colitis. Total proctocolectomy in properly selected patients is associated with low morbidity, a decreased risk of recurrence, and a longer time to recurrence [20]

Author details

V. Surlin[1], C. Copaescu[2] and A. Saftoiu[1]

1 Department of Surgery, University of Medicine and Pharmacy of Craiova, and Attending Surgeon in the 1st Clinic of Surgery, Clinical County Emergency Hospital of Craiova, Romania

2 University Of Medicine Carol Davila, Head General Surgery Department, Delta Hospital Bucharest, Romania

Department of Gastroenterology and Hepatology, University of Medicine and Pharmacy of Craiova and Attending Physician in Gastroenterology Clinic of Clinical County Emergency Hospital of Craiova, Romania

References

[1] Zmora O., Mahajna A., Bar-Zakail B., Hershko D., Shabtai M., Krausz M., Ayalon A. – Is mechanical bowel preparation mandatory for left-sided colonic anastomosis? Results of a prospective randomised trial. Tech coloproctol, 01 july 2006; 10(2): 131-5

[2] Schapira M, Henrion J, Ravoet C, et al. Thromboembolism in inflammatory bowel disease. Acta Gastroenterol Belg 1999; 62:182.

[3] Irving PM, Pasi KJ, Rampton DS. Thrombosis and inflammatory bowel disease. Clin Gastroenterol Hepatol 2005; 3:617.

[4] Cohen RD. How should we treat severe acute steroid-refractory ulcerative colitis? Inflamm Bowel Dis 2009; 15:150.

[5] Becker JM, Stucchi AF. Treatment of choice for acute severe steroid-refractory ulcerative colitis is colectomy. Inflamm Bowel Dis 2009; 15:146.

[6] Randall J, Singh B, Warren BF, et al. Delayed surgery for acute severe colitis is associated with increased risk of postoperative complications. Br J Surg 2010; 97:404.

[7] Heyries L, Bernard JP, Perrier H, et al. [Hemorrhagic rectocolitis and autoimmune hemolytic anemia]. Gastroenterol Clin Biol 1998; 22:741.

[8] Nandivada P, Poylin V, Nagle D, Advances in the Surgical Management of Inflammatory Bowel Disease, Curr Opin Gastroenterol. 2012;28(1):47-51.

[9] Goudet P, Dozois RR, Kelly KA, et al. Changing referral patterns for surgical treatment of ulcerative colitis. Mayo Clin Proc 1996; 71:743.

[10] Michelassi, F. Indications for surgical treatment in ulcerative colitis and Crohn's disease. In: Operative Strategies in Inflammatory Bowel Disease, Michelassi, F, Milson, JW (Eds), Springer, 1997. p.151.

[11] Ananthakrishnan AN, McGinley EL, Binion DG, Saeian K. A nationwide analysis of changes in severity and outcomes of inflammatory bowel disease hospitalizations. J Gastrointest Surg 2011; 15:267–276.

[12] Oussalah A, Evesque L, Laharie D, et al. A multicenter experience with infliximab for ulcerative colitis: outcomes and predictors of response, optimization, colectomy, and hospitalization. Am J Gastroenterol 2010; 105:2617–2625.

[13] Gustavsson A, Järnerot G, Hertervig E, et al. Clinical trial: colectomy after rescue therapy in ulcerative colitis - 3-year follow-up of the Swedish-Danish controlled infliximab study. Aliment Pharmacol Ther 2010; 32:984–989.Chaparro M, Burgueño P, Iglesias E, et al. Infliximab salvage therapy after failure of ciclosporin in corticosteroid-refractory ulcerative colitis: a multicentre study. Aliment Pharmacol Ther 2012; 35:275–283.Goudet P, Dozois RR, Kelly KA, et al. Characteristics and evolution of extraintestinal manifestations associated with ulcerative colitis after proctocolectomy. Dig Surg 2001; 18:51.

[14] Cima R, Pemberton JH. Medical and surgical management of chronic ulcerative colitis. Arch Surg 2005; 140:300–310.

[15] Heuschen UA, Hinz U, Allemeyer EH, et al. Risk factors for ileoanal J pouchrelated septic complications in ulcerative colitis and familial adenomatous polyposis. Ann Surg 2002; 235:207–216.

[16] da Luz Moreira A, Kiran RP, Lavery I. Clinical outcomes of ileorectal anastomosis for ulcerative colitis. Br J Surg 2010; 97:65.

[17] Farouk R, Pemberton JH,WolffBG, et al. Functional outcomes after ileal pouchanal anastomosis for chronic ulcerative colitis. Ann Surg 2000;

[18] Fichera A, Michelassi F. Surgical treatment of Crohn's disease. J Gastrointest Surg 2007; 11:791.

[19] Grucela A, Steinhagen RM. Current surgical management of ulcerative colitis. Mt Sinai J Med 2009; 76:606–612.

[20] Simillis C, Purkayastha S, Yamamoto T, et al. A meta-analysis comparing conventional end-to-end anastomosis vs. other anastomotic configurations after resection in Crohn's disease. Dis Colon Rectum 2007; 50:1674.

[21] Worsey MJ, Hull T, Ryland L, Fazio V. Strictureplasty is an effective option in the operative management of duodenal Crohn's disease. Dis Colon Rectum 1999; 42:596.

[22] Cellini C, Safar B, Fleshman J. Surgical management of pyogenic complications of Crohn's disease. Inflamm Bowel Dis 2010; 16:512.

[23] Neufeld D, Keidar A, Gutman M, Zissin R. Abdominal wall abscesses in patients with Crohn's disease: clinical outcome. J Gastrointest Surg 2006; 10:445.

[24] Fleshman JW. Pyogenic complications of Crohn's disease, evaluation, and management. J Gastrointest Surg 2008; 12:2160.

[25] Spencer MP, Nelson H, Wolff BG, Dozois RR. Strictureplasty for obstructive Crohn's disease: the Mayo experience. Mayo Clin Proc 1994; 69:33.

[26] Tjandra JJ, Fazio VW, Lavery IC. Results of multiple strictureplasties in diffuse Crohn's disease of the small bowel. Aust N Z J Surg 1993; 63:95.

[27] Yamamoto T, Keighley MR. Long-term results of strictureplasty without synchronous resection for jejunoileal Crohn's disease. Scand J Gastroenterol 1999; 34:180.

[28] Dietz DW, Fazio VW, Laureti S, et al. Strictureplasty in diffuse Crohn's jejunoileitis: safe and durable. Dis Colon Rectum 2002; 45:764.

[29] Tonelli F, Fedi M, Paroli GM, Fazi M. Indications and results of side-to-side isoperistaltic strictureplasty in Crohn's disease. Dis Colon Rectum 2004; 47:494.

[30] Michelassi, F. Indications for surgical treatment in ulcerative colitis and Crohn's disease. In: Operative Strategies in Inflammatory Bowel Disease, Michelassi, F, Milson, JW (Eds), Springer, 1997. p.151.

[31] Michelassi F, Taschieri A, Tonelli F, et al. An international, multicenter, prospective, observational study of the side-to-side isoperistaltic strictureplasty in Crohn's disease. Dis Colon Rectum 2007; 50:277.

[32] Menon AM, Mirza AH, Moolla S, Morton DG. Adenocarcinoma of the small bowel arising from a previous strictureplasty for Crohn's disease: report of a case. Dis Colon Rectum 2007; 50:257.

[33] Fearnhead NS, Chowdhury R, Box B, et al. Long-term follow-up of strictureplasty for Crohn's disease. Br J Surg 2006; 93:475.

[34] Hassan C, Zullo A, De Francesco V, et al. Systematic review: Endoscopic dilatation in Crohn's disease. Aliment Pharmacol Ther 2007; 26:1457.

[35] Thienpont C, D'Hoore A, Vermeire S, et al. Long-term outcome of endoscopic dilatation in patients with Crohn's disease is not affected by disease activity or medical therapy. Gut 2010; 59:320.

[36] Couckuyt H, Gevers AM, Coremans G, et al. Efficacy and safety of hydrostatic balloon dilatation of ileocolonic Crohn's strictures: a prospective longterm analysis. Gut 1995; 36:577.

[37] Di Nardo G, Oliva S, Passariello M, et al. Intralesional steroid injection after endoscopic balloon dilation in pediatric Crohn's disease with stricture: a prospective, randomized, double-blind, controlled trial. Gastrointest Endosc 2010; 72:1201.

[38] East JE, Brooker JC, Rutter MD, Saunders BP. A pilot study of intrastricture steroid versus placebo injection after balloon dilatation of Crohn's strictures. Clin Gastroenterol Hepatol 2007; 5:1065.

[39] Matsuhashi N, Nakajima A, Suzuki A, et al. Long-term outcome of non-surgical strictureplasty using metallic stents for intestinal strictures in Crohn's disease. Gastrointest Endosc 2000; 51:343.

[40] Horgan, AF, Dozois, RR. Management of colonic Crohn's disease. Problems in General Surgery 1999; 16:68.

[41] Tekkis PP, Purkayastha S, Lanitis S, et al. A comparison of segmental vs subtotal/ total colectomy for colonic Crohn's disease: a meta-analysis. Colorectal Dis 2006; 8:82.

[42] Sher ME, Bauer JJ, Gorphine S, Gelernt I. Low Hartmann's procedure for severe anorectal Crohn's disease. Dis Colon Rectum 1992; 35:975.

[43] Buchanan GN, Halligan S, Bartram CI, et al. Clinical examination, endosonography, and MR imaging in preoperative assessment of fistula in ano: comparison with outcome-based reference standard. Radiology 2004; 233:674–681.

[44] Schwartz DA, Wiersema MJ, Dudiak KM, et al. A comparison of endoscopic ultrasound, magnetic resonance imaging, and exam under anesthesia for evaluation of Crohn's perianal fistulas. Gastroenterology 2001; 121:1064– 1072.

[45] Present DH, Rutgeerts P, Targan S, et al. Infliximab for the treatment of fistulas in patients with Crohn's disease. N Engl J Med 1999; 340:1398–1405.

[46] Chung W, Ko D, Sun C, et al. Outcomes of anal fistula surgery in patients with inflammatory bowel disease. Am J Surg 2010; 199:609–613.

[47] Soltani A, Kaiser AM. Endorectal advancement flap for cryptoglandular or Crohn's fistula-in-ano. Dis Colon Rectum 2010; 53:486–495.

[48] Lewis RT, Maron DJ. Anorectal Crohn's disease. Surg Clin N Am 2010; 90:83–97.

[49] Regueiro M, El-Hachem S, Kip KE, et al. Postoperative infliximab is not associated with an increase in adverse events in Crohn's disease. Dig Dis Sci 2011; 56:3610–3615.

[50] Bordeianou L, Stein SL, Ho VP, et al. Immediate vs tailored prophylaxis to prevent symptomatic recurrences after surgery for ileocecal Crohn's disease. Surgery 2011; 149:72–78.

[51] Kienle P, Weitz J, Benner A, et al. Laparoscopically assisted colectomy and ileoanal-pouch procedure with and without protective ileostomy. Surg Endosc. 2003May; 17(5):716-20.

[52] Fowkes L, Krishna K, Menon A, et al. Laparoscopic emergency and elective surgery for ulcerative colitis. Colorectal Dis 2008; 10:373–378.-

[53] Ky AJ, Sonoda T, Milsom JW. One-stage laparoscopic restorative proctocolectomy:an alternative to the conventional approach? Dis Colon Rectum. 2002 Feb;45(2): 207-10;discussion 210-1.

[54] Hasegawa H, Watanabe M, Baba H, Nishibori H, Kitajima M.Laparoscopic restorative proctocolectomy for patients with ulcerative colitis. J Laparoendosc Adv Surg Tech A. 2002 Dec;12(6):403-6.

[55] Marcello PW, Milsom JW, Wong SK, et al. Laparoscopic restorative proctocolectomy:case-matched comparative study with open restorative proctocolectomy. Dis Colon Rectum. 2000 May;43(5):604-8.

[56] Brown SR, Eu KW, Seow-Choen F. Consecutive series of laparoscopic-assisted vs.minilaparotomy restorative proctocolectomies. Dis Colon Rectum. 2001 Mar;44(3): 397-400.

[57] Bergamaschi R, Pessaux P, Arnaud JP. Comparison of conventional and laparoscopicileocolic resection for Crohn's disease. Dis Colon Rectum. 2003 Aug;46(8):1129-33.

[58] Young-Fadok TM, Hall Long K, McConnell EJ et al. Advantages of laparoscopicresection for ileocolic Crohn's disease. Improved outcomes and reduced costs. SurgEndosc. 2001 May;15(5):450-4.

[59] Milsom JW, Hammerhofer KA, Bohm B, et al. Prospective, randomized trialcomparing laparoscopic vs. conventional surgery for refractory ileocolic Crohn'sdisease.Dis Colon Rectum. 2001 Jan;44(1):1-8.

[60] Maartense S, Dunker MS, Slors JF, et al. Laparoscopic-assisted versus open ileocolic resection for Crohn's disease: a randomized trial. Ann Surg 2006; 243:143.

[61] Alves A, Panis Y, Bouhnik Y, et al. Factors that predict conversion in 69 consecutive patients undergoing laparoscopic ileocecal resection for Crohn's disease: a prospective study. Dis Colon Rectum 2005; 48:2302.

[62] Lowney JK, Dietz DW, Birnbaum EH, et al. Is there any difference in recurrence rates in laparoscopic ileocolic resection for Crohn's disease compared with conventional surgery? A long-term, follow-up study. Dis Colon Rectum 2006; 49:58.

[63] Holubar SD, Dozois EJ, Privitera A, et al. Minimally invasive colectomy for Crohn's colitis: a single institution experience. Inflamm Bowel Dis 2010; 16:1940–1946.

[64] Umanskiy K, Malhotra G, Chase A, et al. Laparoscopic colectomy for Crohn's colitis. A large prospective comparative study. J Gastrointest Surg 2010; 14:658–663.

[65] Tabet J, Hong D, Kim CW et al. Laparoscopic versus open bowel resection forCrohn's disease. Can J Gastroenterol. 2001 Apr;15(4):237-42.

[66] Watanabe M, Hasegawa H, Yamamoto S, et al. Successful application of laparoscopic surgery to the treatment of Crohn's disease with fistulas. Dis Colon Rectum. 2002 Aug;45(8):1057-61.

[67] Bemelman WA, Slors JF, Dunker MS et al. Laparoscopic-assisted vs. open ileocolic resection for Crohn's disease. A comparative study. Surg Endosc. 2000 ug;14(8):721-5.

[68] Duepree HJ, Senagore AJ, Delaney CP, et al. Advantages of laparoscopic resectionfor ileocecal Crohn's disease. Dis Colon Rectum. 2002 May;45(5):605-10.

[69] Dunker MS, Bemelman WA, Slors JFM, et al. Functional outcome, quality of life, body image, and cosmesis in patients after laparoscopic-assisted and conventional restorative proctocolectomy: a comparative study. Dis Colon Rectum 2001; 44:1800–1807.

[70] Polle SW, Dunker MS, Slors JF, et al. Body image, cosmesis, quality of life, and functional outcome of hand-assisted laparoscopic versus open restorative proctocolectomy: long-term results of a randomized trial. Surg Endosc 2007; 21:1301.

[71] Farouk R, Pemberton JH,WolffBG, et al. Functional outcomes after ileal pouchanal anastomosis for chronic ulcerative colitis. Ann Surg 2000;

[72] Olsen KO, Joelsson M, Laurberg S, Oresland T. Fertility after ileal pouch-anal anastomosis in women with ulcerative colitis. Br J Surg 1999; 86:493.

[73] Hahnloser D, Pemberton JH, Wolff BG, et al. Pregnancy and delivery before and after ileal pouch-anal anastomosis for inflammatory bowel disease: immediate and long-term consequences and outcomes. Dis Colon Rectum 2004; 47:1127.

[74] Shen B, Remzi FH, Lavery IC, et al. A proposed classification of ileal pouch disorders and associated complications after restorative proctocolectomy. Clin Gastroenterol Hepatol 2008; 6:145.

[75] Galandiuk S, Scott NA, Dozois RR, et al. Ileal pouch-anal anastomosis. Reoperation for pouch-related complications. Ann Surg 1990; 212:446.

[76] Burke D, van Laarhoven CJ, Herbst F, Nicholls RJ. Transvaginal repair of pouch-vaginal fistula. Br J Surg 2001; 88:241.

[77] Johnson P, Richard C, Ravid A, et al. Female infertility after ileal pouch-anal anastomosis for ulcerative colitis. Dis Colon Rectum 2004; 47:1119.

[78] Baixauli J, Delaney CP, Wu JS, et al. Functional outcome and quality of life after repeat ileal pouch-anal anastomosis for complications of ileoanal surgery. Dis Colon Rectum 2004; 47:2.

[79] Karoui M, Cohen R, Nicholls J. Results of surgical removal of the pouch after failed restorative proctocolectomy. Dis Colon Rectum 2004; 47:869.

[80] Prudhomme M, Dozois RR, Godlewski G, et al. Anal canal strictures after ileal pouch-anal anastomosis. Dis Colon Rectum 2003; 46:20.

[81] Taylor WE, Wolff BG, Pemberton JH, Yaszemski MJ. Sacral osteomyelitis after ileal pouch-anal anastomosis: report of four cases. Dis Colon Rectum 2006; 49:913.

[82] Jain A, Abbas MA, Sekhon HK, Rayhanabad JA. Volvulus of an ileal J-pouch. Inflamm Bowel Dis 2010; 16:3.

[83] Mmeje C, Bouchard A, Heppell J. Image of the month. Pharmacobezoar: a rare complication after ileal pouch-anal anastomosis for ulcerative colitis. Clin Gastroenterol Hepatol 2010; 8:A28.

[84] Hahnloser D, Pemberton JH, Wolff BG, et al. Results at up to 20 years after ileal pouch-anal anastomosis for chronic ulcerative colitis. Br J Surg 2007; 94:333.

[85] Lepistö A, Luukkonen P, Järvinen HJ. Cumulative failure rate of ileal pouch-anal anastomosis and quality of life after failure. Dis Colon Rectum 2002; 45:1289. -

[86] Tulchinsky H, Hawley PR, Nicholls J. Long-term failure after restorative proctocolectomy for ulcerative colitis. Ann Surg 2003; 238:229.

[87] Delaney CP, Fazio VW, Remzi FH, et al. Prospective, age-related analysis of surgical results, functional outcome, and quality of life after ileal pouch-anal anastomosis. Ann Surg 2003; 238:221.

[88] Hueting WE, Buskens E, van der Tweel I, et al. Results and complications after ileal pouch anal anastomosis: a meta-analysis of 43 observational studies comprising 9,317 patients. Dig Surg 2005; 22:69.

[89] Wax JR, Pinette MG, Cartin A, Blackstone J. Female reproductive health after ileal pouch anal anastomosis for ulcerative colitis. Obstet Gynecol Surv 2003; 58:270.

[90] Cornish JA, Tan E, Teare J, et al. The effect of restorative proctocolectomy on sexual function, urinary function, fertility, pregnancy and delivery: a systematic review. Dis Colon Rectum 2007; 50:1128.

[91] Johnson P, Richard C, Ravid A, et al. Female infertility after ileal pouch-anal anastomosis for ulcerative colitis. Dis Colon Rectum 2004; 47:1119.Hahnloser D, Pemberton JH, Wolff BG, et al. Pregnancy and delivery before and after ileal pouch-anal anastomosis for inflammatory bowel disease: immediate and long-term consequences and outcomes. Dis Colon Rectum 2004; 47:1127.FAZIO

[92] Beddy D, Dozois EJ, Pemberton JH. Perioperative complications in inflammatory bowel disease. Inflamm Bowel Dis 2011; 17:1610–1619.

[93] Gainsbury ML, Chu DI, Howard LA, et al. Preoperative infliximab is not associated with an increased risk of short-term postoperative complications after restorative proctocolectomy and ileal pouch-anal anastomosis. J Gastrointest Surg 2011; 15:397–403.

[94] Subramanian V, Pollok RC, Kang JY, Kumar D. Systematic review of postoperative complications in patients with inflammatory bowel disease treated with immunomodulators. Br J Surg 2006; 93:793.

[95] Colombel JF, Loftus EV Jr, Tremaine WJ, et al. Early postoperative complications are not increased in patients with Crohn's disease treated perioperatively with infliximab or immunosuppressive therapy. Am J Gastroenterol 2004; 99:878.

[96] Marchal L, D'Haens G, Van Assche G, et al. The risk of post-operative complications associated with infliximab therapy for Crohn's disease: a controlled cohort study. Aliment Pharmacol Ther 2004; 19:749.

[97] Gaertner WB, Decanini A, Mellgren A, et al. Does infliximab infusion impact results of operative treatment for Crohn's perianal fistulas? Dis Colon Rectum 2007; 50:1754.

[98] Appau KA, Fazio VW, Shen B, et al. Use of infliximab within 3 months of ileocolonic resection is associated with adverse postoperative outcomes in Crohn's patients. J Gastrointest Surg 2008; 12:1738.

[99] Schluender SJ, Ippoliti A, Dubinsky M, et al. Does infliximab influence surgical morbidity of ileal pouch-anal anastomosis in patients with ulcerative colitis? Dis Colon Rectum 2007; 50:1747.

[100] Selvasekar CR, Cima RR, Larson DW, et al. Effect of infliximab on short-term complications in patients undergoing operation for chronic ulcerative colitis. J Am Coll Surg 2007; 204:956.

[101] Ellis MC, Diggs BS, Vetto JT, Herzig DO. Trends in the surgical treatment of ulcerative colitis over time: increased mortality and centralization of care. World J Surg 2011; 35:671–676.

[102] Lipman JM, Kiran RP, Shen B, et al. Perioperative factors during ileal pouchanal anastomosis predict pouchitis. Dis Colon Rectum 2011; 54:311–317.

[103] Holubar SD, Cima RR, Sandborn WJ, Pardi DS. Treatment and prevention of pouchitis after ileal pouch anal anastomosis for chronic ulcerative colitis. Cochrane Database Syst Rev 2010:CD001176. doi: 10.1002/14651858. CD001176.pub2.Simchuk EJ, Thirlby RC. Risk factors and true incidence of pouchitis in patients after ileal pouch-anal anastomoses. World J Surg 2000; 24:851–856.

[104] Haveran LA, Sehgal R, Poritz LS, et al. Infliximab and/or azathioprine in the treatment of Crohn's disease-like complications after IPAA. Dis Colon Rectum 2011; 54:15–20.Browning SM, Nivatvongs S. Intraoperative abandonment of ileal pouch to anal anastomosis--the Mayo Clinic experience. J Am Coll Surg 1998; 186:441.

[105] Thompson-Fawcett MW, Marcus V, Redston M, et al. Risk of dysplasia in long-term ileal pouches and pouches with chronic pouchitis. Gastroenterology 2001; 121:275.

[106] Scarpa M, van Koperen PJ, Ubbink DT, et al. Systematic review of dysplasia after restorative proctocolectomy for ulcerative colitis. Br J Surg 2007; 94:534.

[107] Kariv R, Remzi FH, Lian L, et al. Preoperative colorectal neoplasia increases risk for pouch neoplasia in patients with restorative proctocolectomy. Gastroenterology 2010; 139:806.

[108] Sarigol S, Wyllie R, Gramlich T, et al. Incidence of dysplasia in pelvic pouches in pediatric patients after ileal pouch-anal anastomosis for ulcerative colitis. J Pediatr Gastroenterol Nutr 1999; 28:429.

[109] Maykel JA, Hagerman G, Mellgren AF, et al. Crohn's colitis: the incidence of dysplasia and adenocarcinoma in surgical patients. Dis Colon Rectum 2006; 49:950.

[110] Avidan B, Sakhnini E, Lahat A, et al. Risk factors regarding the need for a second operation in patients with Crohn's disease. Digestion 2005; 72:248.

[111] Malireddy K, Larson DW, Sandborn WJ, et al. Recurrence and impact of postoperative prophylaxis in laparoscopically treated primary ileocolic Crohn disease. Arch Surg 2010; 145:42.

[112] Goligher JC. The long-term results of excisional surgery for primary and recurrent Crohn's disease of the large intestine. Dis Colon Rectum 1985; 28:51.

[113] Litzendorf ME, Stucchi AF, Wishnia S, et al. Completion mucosectomy for retained rectal mucosa following restorative proctocolectomy with double-stapled ileal pouch-anal anastomosis. J Gastrointest Surg 2010; 14:562.

Section 3

Future Therapeutic Directions in IDB

Chapter 7

Targeting Colon Drug Delivery by Natural Products

Hyunjo Kim

Additional information is available at the end of the chapter

http://dx.doi.org/10.5772/52346

1. Introduction

Inflammatory Bowel Disease (IBD) classified with Ulcerative Colitis (UC) and Crohn Disease (CD) is an idiopathic, life-long, destructive chronic inflammatory disease in gastrointestinal tract [1] and probably multi-factorial disease caused by interplay of the external and internal environment. Little is known about the mechanism of pathogenesis of the disease but it has been reported that immunological mechanisms are involved in etiology. Under normal situations, the intestinal mucosa is in a state of controlled inflammation regulated by a delicate balance of pro-inflammatory (tumor necrosis factor [TNF]-alpha, interferon [IFN]-gamma, interleukin [IL]-1, IL-6, IL-12 and anti-inflammatory cytokines (IL-4, IL-10, IL-11), where particularly, IL-6 stimulates T-cell and B-cell proliferation and differentiation.

Therefore, the mucosal immune system is the central effect or of intestinal inflammation and injury, with cytokines playing a central role in modulating inflammation [2,3].

During last a couple of decade, the therapeutic agents for IBD have been changed rapidly and anti-inflammatory agents such as corticosteroid and salicylates or its metabolite were used but recently biological agents are introduced. Emerging changes in IBD medications or their use for an instance, balsalazid, budesonide, 5-aminosalicylate (5-ASA) and purine analogues such as azathioprine are improvements in conventional application, additionally, mycophenolate mofetil (MMF), thalidomide and heparin are newly introduced into IBDtherapy [4-6].

On the contrary, advances in molecular technology have enabled the development of novel and potentially effective targeted therapies with anti-TNF particularly infliximab, interferon-gamma and interleukin [7, 8]. Nevertheless, biologically active agents have some problems in terms of long termstorage conditions and immune-toxicity, additionally biocompatibility against major histological complex (MHC) of immunoglobulin G, which may cause in inconvenience of patient compliance and more expenditure. Thus, the great interest has been focused to the interplay between the adaptive and innate natural sources not only to achieve a better understanding of the immune-pathogeneses of inflammatory bowel disease but to identify targets for even more potent intervention [9-11].

Furthermore, colonic drug delivery has gained increased importance not just for the treatment of local diseases associated with the colon but also for its potential improvement related with adverse events such as ileocecal junction (ICJ) barrier and small volume capacity.

The various strategies for targeting orally administered drugs to the colon are consisted of pH dependent polymers, azo-polymers, covalent linkage of a drug with a carrier, formulation of timed released systems, drug carriers that are degraded specially by colonic bacteria and, bio-adhesive.

2. Natural products with anti-inflammatory and anti-tumor activity

In the field of pharmaceutics, the synthetic chemistry is gradually made more efficient and precise, but also gradually changing into bio-technological applications and a return to the infinitely more variable and complex chemistry of Nature.

Organisms in Nature produce secondary metabolites with the specific purpose to gain evolutionary advantages in the competition for example living space and in the search for nutrients. With an estimated numbers of more than 300 thousands species of plants and probably close to two million species of various organisms, the biodiversity of Nature remains an unparalleled reservoir of biological and chemical diversity. However, most of the biodiversity is as yet unexplored.

Most important thing is the development of strategies for selection, isolation and characterization with the objective to discover unique bioactive chemical structures with drug potential, and to reveal unknown targets, by studying the evolutionary structure–activity optimization in Nature.

In addition to the possibility to discover new drug candidates for drug development, bioactive natural projects have potential as pharmacological tools, intermediates, or templates for synthesis of drugs.

The increased uses of herbal remedies, which contain complex mixtures of natural products, need intensified scientific studies to establish efficacy and safety of these types of products as well as clinical studies.

With the increasing interest for environmental aspects, green chemistry, and a sustainable use of natural products, this renewal could have a strategic position in bridging chemistry and biology.

The correlation between the chemical structures responsible for the shown bioactivity needs to be studied to understand the observation on a molecular level using both in vivo, in vitro and in silico methods [12].Explanatory model the interdisciplinary nature of pharmacognocy interpreted in an explanatory model presented by Larsson and co-workers [13]. In this model a clearly defined role is presented for aspects of informatics, includingbio- and chemo-informatics. The studies of pure natural products against colon cancer are now in focus. Another project is focused on bioengineering of circular proteins, so called cyclotides, to create new structure–activity relationships. Novel strategies are developed for efficient prediction and selection of organisms and molecules and bioinformatics tools to predict novel targets based on lateral gene transfer.

A scientific platform has been built in our long-term research on anti-inflammatory natural products as demonstrated in a number of publications and doctoral theses. Many differentchemical structures have been discovered, and chemically and pharmacologically characterized using bioassay-guided isolation procedures. *In vivo* methods such as rat paw and mouse ear edema was used and later followed by in vitro enzyme and cell based methods. Two systems have been established to enable investigations of the effects of natural compounds on COX-2. The first method developed was an in vitro method suitable for measuring inhibition of COX-2 catalyzed prostaglandin E2 biosynthesis, based on scintillation proximity assay technology [14]. The second system comprises acell model, suitable for studying the effects of compounds on COX-2 and inducible nitric oxide synthase (iNOS) at different cellular levels, including the effects on mRNA, protein, prostaglandin E2, and nitric oxide levels [15].

In later years the project has developed towards enzyme inhibitors related to anti-tumor activity, especially in colon cancer. It has been shown that the process of inflammation and expression of cyclooxygenase-2 is important in colon carcinogenesis.Another important factor is diet. Many food python-chemicals have been shown to exert anti-inflammatory activity in vitro, and may act as cancer chemo-preventive agents [16, 17]. A vegetarian diet rich in python-chemicals may prevent colon carcinogenesis by affecting biochemical processes in the colonic mucosa. It has been shown that intact fecal water (water phase) samples from human volunteers significantly decreased prostaglandin production and COX-2 expression in colonic cells. NMR spectroscopy and multivariate data analysis were later used for further analysis of the composition of the fecal waters and to trace the COX-2 inhibiting activity [18, 19]. The wealth of different natural products with experimentally demonstratedCOX inhibitory effects and an urge to understand and characterize their structural diversity was the starting point for the application of chirography in our natural products research.

The identification from chemo graphic analyses of some specific groups of compounds, including a set of cardiac glycosides, as being of prime importance was further established in a screening of a large number of natural products for activity against colorectal cancer where several cardiac glycosides showed significant activity. This activity was further confirmed in primary cells from colon cancer patients. Cardiac glycosides have been reported to exhibit cytotoxic activity against several different cancer types, but studies against colorectal cancer are lacking. Drugs for clinical treatment of colon cancer are usually used in combination to overcome the problem with drug resistance and to increase the activity. Therefore, selected cardiac glycosides were tested in combination with four clinically relevant standard cyto-toxic drugs (5-fluorouracil, oxaliplatin, cisplatin, irinotecan) to screen for synergistic effects.

The combination of digoxin and oxaliplatin exhibited synergism including the otherwise highly drug resistant HT29 cell line [20]. In depth studies are now in progress necessary to understand these effects on a molecular level.

A plant flavonoid fisetin induces apoptosis in colon cancer cells by inhibition of COX2 and Wnt/EGFR/NF-kappaB-signaling pathways, which provide evidence that the plant flavonoid fisetin can induce apoptosis and suppress the growth of colon cancer cells by inhibition of COX2- and Wnt/EGFR/NF-kappaB-signaling pathways and suggest that fisetin could be a useful agent for prevention and treatment of colon cancer [21].The contribution of plukenetione A to the antitumor activity of Cuban propolis was assumed that plukenetione A contributes to the antitumor effect of Cuban propolis mainly by targeting to poisomerase I as well as DNA polymerase[22].Aberrant Wnt/beta-catenin signaling has recently been implicated in tumor genesis. On the basis of screening program targeting inhibition of TCF/beta-catenin transcriptional activity, a plant extract of Eleutherine palmfolia was selected as a hit sample. Activity-guided fractionations led to the isolation of 15 naphthalene derivatives (1-15), including 4 new glycosides, eleutherinosides B-E (1-4), and 10 of the 15 compounds showed strong activities with high viability among 293T cells, whose data showed that 2 and 9 inhibited the transcription of TCF/beta-catenin in SW480 colon cancer cells in a dose-dependent manner and selective cytotoxicity against three colorectal cancer cell lines. In addition, treatment with 9 led to a significant decrease in the level of nuclear beta-catenin protein, suggesting this reduction to have resulted in the inhibitory effect of 9 on the transcription of TCF/beta-catenin [23].

Penta-cyclic triterpene acids are known mainly for their anti-antigenic effects as well as their differentiation inducing effects. In particular, lupane-type triterpenes, such as botulin, botulnic acid and lupeol, display anti-inflammatory activities which often accompany immune modulation. Tri-terpene acids as well as triterpene mono-alcohols and diols also show an anti-oxidative potential. The pharmacological potential of triterpenes of the lupane, oleanane or urbane type for cancer treatment seems high; although up to now no clinical trial has been published using these tri-terpenes in cancer therapy. They provide a multi-target potential for coping with new cancer strategies. Whether this is an effective approach for cancer treatment has to be proven. Because various triterpenes are an increasingly promising group of plant metabolites, the utilization of different plants as their sources is of interest. Parts of plants, for example birch bark, rosemary leaves, apple peel and mistletoe shoots are rich in triterpenes and provide different triterpene compositions [24].

Advanced cancer is a multi-factorial disease that demands treatments targeting multiple cellular pathways. Chinese herbal cocktail which contains various phytochemicals may target multiple dys-regulated pathways in cancer cells and thus may provide an alternative/ complementary way to treat cancers. Previously reported that the Chinese herbal cocktail Tien-Hsien Liguid (THL) can specifically induce apoptosis in various cancer cells and have immuno-modulating activity.Further, evaluated the anti-metastatic, anti-angiogenic and anti-tumor activities of THL [25]. Dietary grape seed extract (GSE) effectiveness in preventing azoxymethane (AOM)-induced aberrant crypt foci (ACF) formation. GSE-feeding inhibited AOM-induced cell proliferation but enhanced apoptosis in colon including ACF, together with a strong decrease in cyclin D1, COX-2, iNOS, and survivin levels and showed that GSE-feeding also decreased AOM-caused increase in beta-catenin and NF-kappaB levels in colon tissues[26].Grifolin, a secondary metabolite isolated from the fresh fruiting bodies of the mushroom Albatrellus confluens, has been shown to inhibit the growth of some cancer cell lines in vitro by induction of apoptosis An apoptosis-related gene expression profiling analysis provided a clue that death-associated protein kinase 1 (dapk1) gene was up-regulated at least twofold in response to grifolin treatment in nasopharyngeal carcinoma cell CNE1. Further,investigated the role of DAPK1 in apoptotic effect induced by grifolin and observed that protein as well as mRNA level of DAPK1 was induced by grifolin in a dose-dependent manner in nasopharyngeal carcinoma cell CNE1. It was found that grifolin increased both Ser392 and Ser20 phosphorylation levels of transcription factor p53 protein, which could promote its transcriptional activity. Moreover, induced by grifolin, the recruitment of p53 to dapk1 gene promoter was confirmed to enhance markedly using EMSA and ChIP assays analysis. The involvement of DAPK1 in grifolin-induced apoptosis was supported by the studies that introducing siRNA targeting DAPK1 to CNE1 cells remarkably interfered grifolin-caused apoptotic effect as well as the activation of caspase-3. Grifolin induced up-regulation of DAPK1 via p53 was also observed in tumor cells derived from human breast cancer and human colon cancer. Up-regulation of DAPK1 via p53-DAPK1 pathway is an important mechanism of grifolin contributing to its ability to induce apoptotic effect. Since growing evidence found a significant loss of DAPK1 expression in a large variety of tumor types, grifolin may represent a promising candidate in the intervention of cancer via targeting DAPK1[27]. Five derivatives of the natural product sansalvamide A that are potent against multiple drug-resistant colon cancer cell lines were identified. These analogs share no structural homology to current colon cancer drugs, are cytotoxic at levels on par with existing drugs treating other cancers, and demonstrate selectivity for drug-resistant colon cancer cell lines over noncancerous cell lines. Thus, we have established sansalvamide A as a privileged structure for treating multiple drug-resistant colon cancers [28]. Anti-cancer activities of the ethanol extract of Ka-mi-kae-kyuk-tang (KMKKT) targeting angiogenesis, apoptosis and metastasis without any adverse effect on the body weight. This formula merits serious consideration for further evaluation for the chemoprevention and treatment of cancers of multiple organ sites[29].The effect of aged garlic extract (AGE) on the growth of colorectal cancer cells and their angiogenesis, which are important microenvironmental factors in carcinogenesis. AGE (aged garlic extract) could prevent tumor formation by inhibiting angiogenesis through the suppression of endothelial cell motility, proliferation, and tube formation. AGE would be a good chemo-preventive agent for colorectal cancer because of its anti-proliferative action on colorectal carcinoma cells and inhibitory activity on angiogenesis. Aged garlic extract (AGE) has manifold biological activities including immune-modulated and anti-oxidative effects. It is used as a major component of nonprescription tonics and cold-prevention medicines or dietary supplements [30, 31].

Transcription factor NF-kappaB is constitutively active in many human chronic inflammatory diseases and cancers. Epoxy quinone A monomer (EqM), a synthetic derivative of the natural product epoxyquinol A, has previously been shown to be a potent inhibitor of tumor necrosis factor-alpha (TNF-alpha)-induced activation of NF-kappaB [32]. EqM also effectively inhibits the growth of human leukemia, kidney, and colon cancer cell lines in the NCI's tumor cell panel. Among six colon cancer cell lines, those with low amounts of constitutive NF-kappaB DNA-binding activity are generally more sensitive to growth inhibition by EqM. Therefore, EqM inhibits growth and induces cell death in tumor cells through a mechanism that involves inhibition of NF-kappaB activity at multiple steps in the signaling pathway.

Colorectal cancer, the second most frequent diagnosed cancer in the US, causes significant morbidity and mortality in humans. Over the past several years, the molecular and biochemical pathways that influence the development of colon cancer have been extensively characterized. Since the development of colon cancer involves multi-step events, the available drug therapies for colorectal cancer are largely ineffective. The radiotherapy, photodynamic therapy, and chemotherapy are associated with severe side effects and offer no firm expectation for a cure. Thus, there is a constant need for the investigation of other potentially useful options. One of the widely sought approaches is cancer chemoprevention that uses natural agents to reverse or inhibit the malignant transformation of colon cancer cells and to prevent invasion and metastasis [33]. Curcumin (diferuloylmethane), a natural plant product, possesses such chemopreventive activity that targets multiple signaling pathways in the prevention of colon cancer development [34].Colon-targeting delivery of rhubarb extract, as a purgative, may prevent absorption of free anthraquinones in the upper gastrointestinal tract, thus improving clinical effects and lowering dosage [35, 36].Chemopreventive effects of arctiin, a lignin isolated from Arctium lappa (burdock) seeds, on the initiation or post initiation period of 2-amino-1-methyl-6-phenylimidazo [4,5-b]pyridine (PhIP) induced mammary carcinogenesis in female rats and on 2-amino-3, 8-dimethylimidazo[4,5-f]quinoxaline (MeIQx)-associated hepatocarcinogenesis [37].

3. Plant peptides and proteins

Plant peptides and proteins may be considered an overlooked source for new chemical entities and novel bioactivities compared to low molecular natural products. The reason for this seems to be based on tradition and biased by the most commonly used techniques for natural products. However, during the last decades, the number of reported plant peptides has grown substantially, and the field is about to mushroom. In the form of Professor Gunnar Samuelsson's' pioneering studies of mistletoe toxins was reported [38]. In the mid 1990san attempt to assess plant peptides more broadly, with the design of an isolation protocol directly designed for their isolation [39]. One of the results of this effort was the discovery of a set of macrocyclic peptides in the plant family Violaceae [40]. Strikingly, the peptides we characterized in Violaceae were found to be nearly identical with one of the most intriguing examples of pharmacognostic research in general, and plant peptides in particular, namely the peptide Kalata B1. The discovery of Kalata B1 was based on the ethno-pharmacological use of the plant Oldenlandia affinis. It was experienced a high frequency of complicated deliveries due to the use of this plant, which was locally known as ''Kalata-Kalata'' [41]. Native women secretly used a decoction of this plant to facilitate childbirth, which they sipped as a tea but also applied directly at the birth canal [42]. It induced extremely strong uterine contractions, which sometimes developed into cervical spasms necessitating acute caesarean section.

The complete sequence and the cyclic structure was however not determined for more than 20 years later [43].At the time of our report of the first cocktail of "palate-like" peptides in Violaceae, four similar peptides had been reported in the literature as the serendipitous discoveries of three independent groups. When including those peptides in a sequence comparison, i.e. the anti-HIV circulins A and B, the neurotensin binding inhibitor cyclo-psychotride A and the partially characterized violapeptide I, it was clear that they fell in two subgroups based on sequencesimilarity. Today, around 150 cyclotides have been reported from species of three plant families, Violaceae, Rubiaceae and Cucurbitaceae. The family Violaceae seems to be particularly rich in these proteins [44-47] and a single Violaceae species may contain more than 60 different cyclotides. It has been suggested that there might be 9,000 cyclotides in the Violaceae alone[48].

In addition to the amide bond that cyclizes the backbone, cyclotides contain three stabilizing disulfide bonds in a knotted arrangement, i.e. two disulfides form a ring together with their connecting protein backbone, which is threaded by the third disulfide [49-51].

CCK motif, and make cyclotides extraordinary stable protein structures [52]. Besides being uterotonic,anti-HIV, hemolytic and neurotensin binding inhibitory, the list now includes antimicrobial [53], antifouling [54], antihelmintic, molluscicidal, cytotoxic [55, 56]) and insecticidal activities. The latter effects are some of the most well studied and interesting effects: the cytotoxic effect together with the haemolytic effect have been the focus for detailed structure activity studies [57, 58], and the discovery of their insecticidal effect likely revealed cyclotides' role in planta. Cyclotides' mechanism of action is however yet unknown, but evidence is accumulating showing that membrane interactions followed by membrane pore or fissure formation are involved [59-61], which could provide an explanation to several of the reported effects.

Combined with the extraordinary CCK motif—with its conserved scaffold that can be dressed with variable loop sequences—the demonstrated biological activity of the cyclotides make them a first class target for protein engineering. To this end, inherent activities of native cyclotides can be reinforced or abolished, or new biologically active peptide epitopes can begrafted into the scaffold. For example, reinforcing the cytotoxic effect could potentially provide us with leads for anticancer drugs, or to completely remove that effect could provide us with an inert scaffold ideal for grafting. The first successful grafting of a biologicallyactive epitope was reported just recently, showing proof of concept [62].

The success of these strategies relies on the ability of efficient methods for production of cyclotides and cyclotide mutants. Being gene products, cell based production systems seem promising, but although cyclotide producing plant cell cultures have been established [63], solid phase peptide synthesis is still the method of choice [64, 65].Our knowledge about their biosynthesis is yet scarce. We know the structural arrangement of the cyclotide precursor from cDNA, and that an asparaginyl endo-peptidase has a likely role for cleaving at the N terminal side of the mature peptide and that protein disulfide isomerases seem to play a role for their successful folding. However, the order of the events to produce mature cyclotides is not yet known, i.e. if disulfide bonds are formed before or after excision and ligation, and nothing is known about how these processes are controlled. In the perspective of exploiting the cyclotide scaffold for engineering of bioactive peptides, the possibility of farming designed molecules in plantar promises to be the optimal solution; the way there is still long though.

Matrix metalloproteinase (MMP) are zinc-dependent endopeptidases that mediate numerous physiologic and pathologic processes, including matrix degradation, tissue remodeling, inflammation, and tumor metastasis. To develop a vaccine targeting stromal antigens expressed by cancer-associated fibroblasts, it was focused on MMP11 (or stromelysin 3). MMP11 expression correlates with aggressive profile and invasiveness of different types of carcinoma [66]. Overexpression of IL-12 and IL-23, which share the p40 subunit, has been implicated in the pathogenesis of Crohn's disease. Targeting these cytokines with monoclonal antibodies has emerged as a new and effective therapy, but one with adverse reactions [67]. Intestinal fibrosis and stricture formation are major complications of inflammatory bowel disease (IBD), for which there are currently few effective treatments. It was investigated whether targeting transforming growth factor-beta1 (TGF-beta1), a key profibrotic mediator, with a peptide-based virus-like particle vaccine would be effective in suppressing intestinal fibrosis by using a mouse model of 2,4,6-trinitrobenzene sulfonic acid (TNBS)-induced chronic colitis [68]. Neutralization of macrophage migration inhibitory factor (MIF) by anti-MIF antibody reduces intestinal inflammation in mice. Anti-MIF autoantibody induced by DNA vaccine targeting MIF protects mice against experimental colitis [69].

Overexpression of the proto-oncogene c-Myb occurs in more than 80% of colorectal cancer (CRC) and is associated with aggressive disease and poor prognosis. To test c-Myb as a therapeutic target in CRC, which devised a DNA fusion vaccine to generate an anti-CRC immune response. c-Myb, like many tumor antigens, is weakly immunogenic as it is a "self" antigen and subject to tolerance [70].Four novel oral DNA vaccines provide protection against melanoma, colon, breast, and lung carcinoma in mouse models. Vaccines are delivered by attenuated Salmonella typhimurium to secondary lymphoid organs and respectively target vascular endothelial growth factor receptor-2, transcription factor Fos-related antigen-1, anti-apoptosis protein survivin and Legumain, an asparaginyl endopeptidase specifically overexpressed on tumor-associated macrophages (TAMs) in the tumor microenvironment (TME). These vaccines are all capable of inducing potent cell-mediated protective immunity against self-antigens, resulting in marked suppression of tumor growth and dissemination. Key mechanisms induced by these DNA vaccines include efficient suppression of angiogenesis in the tumor vasculature and marked activation of cytotoxic T cells, natural killer cells, and antigen-presenting dendritic cells [71]. Shigellosis is a major form of bacillary dysentery caused by Shigella infection. Shigella ribosome-based vaccines (SRV), considered among the potent vaccine candidates, are composed of O-antigen and ribosome isolated from S. flexneri 2a. The immunogenicity and protective efficacy of SRV was investigated and mice were vaccinated with SRV via the intranasal route. Interestingly, robust levels of Shigella-derived LPS-specific IgG and IgA Abs and antibody-forming cells were elicited in systemic and mucosal compartments following two intranasal administrations of SRV. Groups of mice receiving intranasal SRV developed milder pulmonary pneumonia upon challenge with virulent S. flexneri 2a than did those receiving parenteral SRV [72].

Over the past several years it has become apparent that the tumor stroma represents a significant target for anti-cancer therapies. Therefore we evaluated the strategy of targeting the tumor stroma with a novel DNA vaccine encoding murine platelet derived growth factor receptor-beta (mPDGFRbeta). Immunization with this vaccine induced cytotoxic lysis of mPDGFRbeta-expressing target cells and protected mice from the growth and dissemination of murine colon, breast and lung carcinoma. Furthermore, this novel vaccine suppresses angiogenesis in vivo and reduces the numbers of tumor-associated, mPDGFRbeta-expressing pericytes as suggested by a decrease in intra-tumor expression of mPDGFRbeta and NG2 [73].Viral vectors are under development for anticancer therapy. As they can infect tumors and activate the immune system, viral vectors may directly destroy cancers (oncolysis), deliver genes with antitumor activity directly to the cancer cells, or act as cancer vaccines. Better insights into the biology of the various vectors in use (e.g., poxvectors, adenovirus, adeno-associated virus, retrovirus, Newcastle disease virus) are making it possible to engineer viruses that are more tumor-specific, efficient at tumor infection, and which have enhanced safety due to incorporation of safeguards should dissemination occur [74].

Colorectal carcinoma is a leading cause of cancer-related mortality. Despite the introduction of new cytotoxic drugs, improved surgical and radiotherapeutic techniques, a large proportion of colorectal carcinomas remain incurable. New targeted therapeutic strategies, including immunotherapy, are being explored as complementary treatments. Recent advances in immunology and molecular biology have opened new avenues for the clinical testing of rationally designed vaccination strategies against cancer [75].The use of retrogen plasmid-based vaccine technology to break tolerance and to generate a robust, dose-dependent antibody response against the self cancer antigen, survivin. This phenomenon is due to the incorporation of the survivin antigen into the retrogen system rather than to some peculiarity unique to survivin. In contrast to other genetic immunization methods designed to produce antibody responses, the retrogen system results in a broad range of antibody isotypes, indicative of both a Th-1 and a Th-2 CD4+ response. Additional evidence of a Th-1 response is demonstrated by tumor growth inhibition in a mouse model of colon cancer metastasis [76].

An efficient strategy based on a fully synthetic dendrimeric carbohydrate display (multiple antigenic glycolpeptide; MAG) to induce anti carbohydrate antibody responses for therapeutic vaccination against cancer was developed. The superior efficacy of the MAG strategy over the traditional keyhole limpet hemocyanin glycolconjugate to elicit an anticarbohydrate IgG response against the tumor-associated Tn antigen was shown. The influence of the glycolic carrier elements of such a tumor antigen for their recognition by the immune system was influenced. Finally, we additionally developed the MAG system by introducing promiscuous HLA-restricted T-helper epitopes and performed its immunological evaluation in nonhuman primates. MAG:Tn vaccines induced in all of the animals strong tumor-specific anti-Tn antibodies that can mediate antibody-dependent cell cytotoxicity against human tumor [77].

Overcoming immune tolerance of tumor angiogenesis should be useful for adjuvant therapy of cancer, which hypothesized that vaccination with autologous endothelium would induce an autoimmune response targeting tumor angiogenesis.The effect of autologous with a vaccine of glutaraldehyde-fixed murine hepatic sinusoidal endothelial cells (HSEs) was more pronounced than that of xenogeneic human umbilical vein endothelial cells (HUVECs), which were tested in the same experimental setting. Its results suggest that vaccination with autologous endothelium can overcome peripheral tolerance of self-angiogenic antigens and therefore should be useful for adjuvant immunotherapy of cancer [78].Tumor cells are elusive targets for immunotherapy due to their heterogeneity and genetic instability. Here, a novel, oral DNA vaccine that targets stable, proliferating endothelial cells in the tumor vasculature rather than tumor cells was described. Targeting occurs through upregulated vascular-endothelial growth factor receptor 2 (FLK-1) of proliferating endothelial cells in the tumor vasculature. This vaccine effectively protected mice from lethal challenges with melanoma, colon carcinoma and lung carcinoma cells and reduced growth of established metastases in a therapeutic setting. CTL-mediated killing of endothelial cells indicated breaking of peripheral immune tolerance against this self antigen, resulting in markedly reduced dissemination of spontaneous and experimental pulmonary metastases. Angiogenesis in the tumor vasculature was suppressed without impairment of fertility, neuromuscular performance or hematopoiesis, albeit with a slight delay in wound healing [79]. The HER-2/neu oncogenic protein is a well-defined tumor antigen. HER-2/neu is a shared antigen among multiple tumor types. Patients with HER-2/neu protein-overexpressing breast, ovarian, non-small cell lung, colon, and prostate cancers have been shown to have a pre-existent immune response to HER-2/neu. No matter what the tumor type, endogenous immunity to HER-2/neu detected in cancer patients demonstrates two predominant characteristics. First, HER-2/neu-specific immune responses are found in only a minority of patients whose tumors overexpress HER-2/neu. Secondly, immunity, if detectable, is of low magnitude. These observations have led to the development of vaccine strategies designed to boost HER-2/neu immunity in a majority of patients. HER-2/neu is a non-mutated self-protein, therefore vaccines must be developed based on immunologic principles focused on circumventing tolerance, a primary mechanism of tumor immune escape [80].Listeria monocytogenes is an intracellular organism that has the unusual ability to live in the cytoplasm of the cell. It is thus a good vector for targeting protein antigens to the cellular arm of the immune response. Here, a model system, consisting of colon and renal carcinomas that express the influenza virus nucleoprotein and a recombinant L. monocytogenes that secrets This antigen, to test the potential of this organism as a cancer immunotherapeutic agent, which show that this recombinant organism can not only protect mice against lethal challenge with tumour cells that express the antigen, but can also cause regression of established macroscopic tumours in an antigen-specific T-cell-dependent manner.

An efficient strategy for the targeting of anti-tumor effector cells were prepared bispecific antibody (BsAb) containing anti-CD3 and an anti-c-erbB-2 proto-oncogene product.A trophoblast cell surface antigen has been characterized by a monoclonal antibody (mAb) 5T4, raised following immunization with solubilized wheat germ agglutinin binding glycoproteins from human syncytiotrophoblast plasma membrane (StMPM) [81].

4. Plant peptides and proteins targets and regulation of this important pathway

Aberrant activation of the canonical Wnt/beta-catenin pathway occurs in almost all colorectal cancers and contributes to their growth, invasion and survival. Phospholipase D (PLD) has been implicated in progression of colorectal carcinoma However, an understanding of the targets and regulation of this important pathway remains incomplete and besides, relationship between Wnt signaling and PLD is not known [82].Fibroblast activation protein is a product overexpressed by tumor-associated fibroblasts (TAF) and is the predominant component of the stoma in most types of cancer. Tumor-associated fibroblasts differ from normal adult tissue fibroblasts, and instead resemble transient fetal and wound healing-associated fibroblasts. Tumor-associated fibroblasts are critical regulators of tumor genesis, but differ from tumor cells by being more genetically stable [83]. Capability of human adipose tissue-derived mesenchyme stem cells (AT-MSC) to serve as cellular vehicles for gene-directed enzyme prodrug molecular chemotherapy. Yeast fusion cytosine deaminize : uracil phosphorribosyltransferase expressing AT-MSC (CD y-AT-MSC) combined with systemic 5-fluorocytosine (5FC) significantly inhibited growth of human colon cancer xenografts [84].

Dendritic cells (DCs), pulsed with the respective endothelium lysates significantly inhibited the growth of subcutaneous tumors as well as pulmonary metastases in mice, and their anti-tumor effect was superior to that of unparsed DCs. Immunohistopathological analysis showed significant decrease in the mean vascular density of tumors, correlating well with the extent of tumor inhibition. In vitro analysis of splenocytes isolated from immunized mice revealed an induction of cytotoxic T lymphocytes and activation of natural killer cells, with a lytic activity against activated endothelium but not tumor cells. In addition, antibodies reacting with activated endothelium [85]. Crohn's disease (CD) is an inflammatory bowel disease that is associated with several changes in the immune system, including an increased number of infiltrating macrophages. These macrophages release a variety of pro-inflammatory cytokines, such as tumor necrosis factor-alpha (TNF-alpha) which are critically involved in the onset and the development of CD. The present study was performed to explore the initial involvement of macrophages in the development of T-cell-mediated chronic colitis [86].

Tumor-associated fibroblasts are key regulators of tumor genesis. In contrast to tumor cells, which are genetically unstable and mutate frequently, the presence of genetically more stable fibroblasts in the tumor-stromal compartment makes them an optimal target for cancer immunotherapy. These cells are also the primary source of collagen type I, which contributes to decreased chemotherapeutic drug uptake in tumors and plays a significant role in regulating tumor sensitivity to a variety of chemotherapies [87].

Conventional anticancer therapy using cytotoxic drugs lacks selectivity and is prone to toxicity and drug resistance. Anticancer therapies targeting aberrant growth factor receptor signaling are gaining interest. The erbB receptor family belongs to the type I, the receptor tyrosine kinases class, and comprises EGFR, HER-2, HER-3, and HER-4. It has been targeted for solid tumor therapy, including breast, ovarian, colon, head-and-neck, and non-small-cell lung cancers. Structural aspects of this class of growth factor receptors, their oncogenic expression, and various pharmacological interventions including biological products and small molecules that inhibit these enzymes [88].

Recent reports of tumor regression following delivery of autologous tumor antigen-pulsed DCs suggest that defective antigen presentation may play a key role in tumor escape. Here, it is shown in two different murine tumor models, CT26 (colon adenocarcinoma) and B16 (melanoma), that the number and activation state of intratumor DCs are critical factors in the host response to tumors [89].Epidermal growth factor receptor (EGFR), a member of a family of membrane receptors with tyrosine kinase activity, is emerging as a target candidate for anti-cancer therapy, due to its overexpression in many carcinomas and its relationship with several hallmark properties of malignant behavior such as continuous cell proliferation, escape from apoptosis, cell migration and angiogenesis. Specially appealing is the overexpression of EGFR in tumors such as lung, colon, kidney and head and neck carcinomas which are mostly resistant to current chemotherapy [90].

It was identified an organic solute transporter (OST) that is generated when two novel gene products are co-expressed, namely human OSTalpha and OSTbeta or mouse OSTalpha and OSTbeta. The results also demonstrate that the mammalian proteins are functionally complemented by evolutionarily divergent OST alpha-OST beta proteins recently identified in the little skate, Raja erinaceous, even though the latter exhibit only 25-41% predicted amino acid identity with the mammalian proteins. Human, mouse, and skate OSTalpha proteins are predicted to contain seven trans membrane helices, whereas the OSTbeta sequences are predicted to have a single trans membrane helix. co-expression is not required for proper membrane targeting. Interestingly, OSTalpha and OSTbeta mRNAs were highly expressed and widely distributed in human tissues, with the highest levels occurring in the testis, colon, liver, small intestine, kidney, ovary, and adrenal gland [91].Human mucin 1 (MUC1) is an epithelial mucin glycoprotein that is overexpressed in 90% of all adenocarcinomas including breast, lung, pancreas, prostate, stomach, colon, and ovary. MUC1 is a target for immune intervention, because, in patients with solid adenocarcinomas, low-level cellular and humoral immune responses to MUC1 have been observed, which are not sufficiently strong to eradicate the growing tumor [92]. Efficient T cell priming by GM-CSF and CD40 ligand double-transduced C26 murine colon carcinoma is not sufficient to cure metastases in a therapeutic setting [93].

A new therapy against colon cancer was developed and investigated two kinds of strategy using a cancer-specific approach. First, employed the Cre/loxP regulation system to enhance the specific expression by carcinoembryonic antigen (CEA) promoter in CEA-producing tumor cells, and examined whether sufficient enhancement to transcriptional activity of CEA promoter, which maintains its specificity in vitro and in vivo, could be obtained. Next, using dendritic cells pulsed with HLA-A24 epitope peptides of CEA, we performed a Phase I study of active immunotherapy in patients with advanced colon cancer. These results suggest that the newly developed therapy for colon cancer is a promising strategy; however, minor modification may be necessary [94].Serum gastrin is known to be elevated in patients with liver-metastasizing colon cancer; thus, cholecystokinin (CCK) B/gastrin receptors may also be up-regulated. A liver-invasive model of colon cancer was established with the human colonic cell line C170HM2, which expresses the CCKB/gastrin receptor at both the gene and protein level. An antiserum has been derived that is directed against the NH2-terminal 17 amino acids of the human CCKB/gastrin receptor coupled to diphtheria toxoid. The peptide was denoted gastrin receptor protein (GRP) 1[95].2B1 is a bispecific murine monoclonal antibody (BsMAb) with specificity for the c-erbB-2 and Fc gamma RIII extracellular domains. This BsMAb promotes the *targeted* lysis of malignant cells overexpressing the c-erbB-2 gene product of the HER2/neu proto-oncogene by human natural killer cells and mononuclear phagocytes expressing the Fc gamma RIII A isoform [96-98].

5. Methods of targeting colon drug delivery by natural products

The various targeting methods to the colon include coating with pH dependent polymers, degradation by bacteria, specially azo-cross linked polymers and certain polysaccharides such as pectin and guar gum are good carriers for formulation, which are presented in Table 1.To achieve successful colonic delivery, a drug needs to be protected from absorption and the environment of the upper gastrointestinal tract and then be released into the proximal colon, which is considered the optimum site for colon targeted delivery of natural compounds. Colon targeting is naturally of value for the treatment of diseases of colon such as Chron's disease, ulcerative colitis, and colorectal cancer.

6. Classification of targeting colon drug delivery system

Colon targeting drug delivery system is classified into three categories greatly and the relevant developed systems are published in many reports.

Firstly, Local Therapy - Higher local drug level can be achieved while minimizing side effects that occur due to the release in the upper GIT.The system can treat local disease effectively such as constipation, irritable bowel disease and colon cancer.

Secondly,DelayedOnset - Maximal plasmalevel can be achieved in the morning hours after bedtime administration by delayed onset of the system to adjust the circadian variations in the signs and symptoms of disease such asrheumatoid arthritis, hypertension and etc.

Thirdly,Protein and Peptide Delivery - The colon is a "friendlier" environment for proteins, peptides and vaccines compare to the upper GIT. Clinically relevant bioavailability may be achieved if the drugs can be protected from the upper GIT.

7. Local targeting colon drug delivery

It was evaluated that colon targeting characteristic of Kuikang colon targeted pellets (KCP) with determination of residual baicalin and baicalein concentration in gastrointestinal tract (GIT).The major challenges in targeting drug to various parts of the gastrointestinal tract include control of drug release with respect to its environment and transit time. These two variables should be taken into consideration in designing a rational colonic drug delivery system. To this end, a swelling matrix core containing pectin, hydroxylpropyl methylcellulose (HPMC), microcrystalline cellulose and 5-aminosalicylic acid was developed. This was subjected to a dual coating operation: an inner pH-sensitive enteric and an outer semi-permeable membrane coat with a pore former [99-101].

A pectin-hydroxylpropyl methylcellulose coating was compressed onto core tablets labeled with 4MBq (99m)Tc-DTPA. Prolonged residence at the ICJ is assumed to have increased hydration of the hydrogel layer surrounding the core tablet. Forces applied as the tablets progressed through the ICJ may have disrupted the hydrogel layer sufficiently to initiate radiolabel release. Inadequate prior hydration of the hydrogel layer preventing access of pectinolytic enzymes and reduced fluid availability in the TC may have retarded tablet disintegration and radiolabel diffusion.

8. Delayed onset for targeting colon drug delivery

A multiparticulate system having pH-sensitive property and specific enzyme biodegradability for colon-targeted delivery of metronidazole was developed [102]. Pectin microspheres were prepared using emulsion-dehydration technique. These microspheres were coated with Eudragit(R) S-100 using oil-in-oil solvent evaporation method. The *in vivo* studies were also performed by assessing the drug concentration in various parts of the GIT at different time intervals which exhibited the potentiality of formulation for colon targeting. Hence, it can be concluded that Eudragit coated pectin microspheres can be used for the colon specific delivery of drug.

Designing pH-sensitive, polymeric nanoparticles of curcumin, a natural anti-cancer agent, for the treatment of colon cancer, which enhance the bioavailability of curcumin, simultaneously reducing the required dose through selective targeting to colon [103]. Eudragit S100 was chosen to aid targeting since the polymer dissolves at colonic pH to result in selective colonic release of the entrapped drug. Solvent emulsion-evaporation technique was employed to formulate the nanoparticles. The combined influence of 3 independent variables in the compression coated tablet of mesalamine [104] for ulcerative colitis. A 3-factor, 3-level

Box-Behnken design was used to derive a second order polynomial equation and construct contour plots to predict responses. The independent variables selected were: percentage of polymers (pectin and compritol ATO 888) in compression coating (X(1)), coating mass (X(2)) and coating force (X(3)). Fifteen batches were prepared and evaluated for percent of drug released in 5 h (Y(5)), time required for 50 % mesalamine to dissolve (t(50)) with rat cecal (RC) content and without rat cecal content (t(50)), percent of drug released in 24 h in the presence of rat cecal content (Y(24) with RC) [105].

The colon specificity of novel natural polymer kaya gum and compare with guar gum. Release profile of tablets was carried out in presence and absence of rat cecal contents. The fast disintegrating core tablets of budesonide, were initially prepared by direct compression technique. Later, these tablets were coated with kaya gum or guar gum. After suitable pre compression and post compression evaluation, these tablets were further coated using Eudragit L-100 by dip coating technique [106].Enteric-coated calcium pectinase microspheres (MS) aimed for colon drug delivery have been developed, by using theophylline as a model drug. The influence of pectin type (animated or non-animated) and MS preparation conditions ($CaCl_2$) concentration and cross-linking time) was investigated upon the drug entrapment efficiency and its release behavior. Pectin/ethyl cellulose-film-coated pellets of 5-fluorouracil (5-FU) [107] for colonic targeting were characterized. The pellet cores were coated to different film thicknesses with three different pectinethyl cellulose formulations using a fluidized bed coater [108]. The gastrointestinal (GI) transit of coated pellets was determined by counting the percentage of coated pellets in the GI lumen by celiotomy at certain times after oral administration. 5FU was administered to rats at a dose of 15 mg kg(-1). The toxicity of 5-FU in the GI tract was evaluated using histological examination. The 1:2 ratio pectin:ethyl cellulose-coated pelletswith 30% total weight gain (TWG-30%) produced more satisfactory drug-release profiles in the simulated gastric, intestinal and colonic fluids [109]. Most of the coated pellets were eliminated from the stomach in 2 h, moved into the small intestine after 2-4 h, and reached the large intestine after 4 h.A novel colon targeted tablet formulation was developed using natural polysaccharides such as chitosan and guar gum as carriers and diltiazem hydrochloride as model drug [110]. The prepared blend of polymer-drug tablets were coated with two layers, inulin as an inner coat followed by shellac as outer coat and was evaluated for properties such as average weight, hardness and coat thickness. In vitro release studies of prepared tablets were carried out for 2 h in pH 1.2 HCl buffers, 3 h in pH 7.4 phosphate buffer and 6 h in simulated colonic fluid (SCF) in order to mimic the conditions from mouth to colon. Coated micro-pellets of pH-dependent and enzyme-dependent kangfuxin colon targeting delivery system were prepared; to make them go to colon, then release, educe partial effect [111].

The ingredients for preparing the micro-pellets are 125% starch +2% CMC-Na, and add 30% ethanol to be binder, pellets were coated with Eudragit S100 to prepare pH-dependent and pectin-HPMC to prepare enzyme-dependent colon targeting micro-pellets.

Guar gum/ethyl cellulose mix coated pellets for potential colon-specific drug delivery were designed [112, 113]. The coated pellets, containing 5-fluorouracil as a model drug, were prepared in a fluidized bed coater by spraying the aqueous/ethanol dispersion mixture of guar gum and ethyl cellulose. The lag time of drug release and release rate were adjustable by changing the ratio of guar gum to ethyl cellulose and coat weight gain. In order to find the optimal coating formulation that was able to achieve drug targeting to the colon and concluded that mixed coating of guar gum and ethyl cellulose is able to provide protection of the drug load in the upper gastrointestinal tract, while allowing enzymatic breakdown of the hybrid coat to release the drug load in the colon.A pectin-based colon specific delivery system bearing 5-fluorouracil (5-FU) was developed for effective delivery of drug to the colon. Calcium pectinate gel (CPG) beads were prepared by ion tropic gelation method followed by enteric coating with Eudragit S-100 [114, 115]. The CPG beads formed were spherical with smooth surfaces.Eudragit S-100 coated calcium pectinate beads delivered most of its drug load (93.2+/-3.67%) to the colon after 9 h, which reflects its targeting potential to the colon. It is concluded that orally-administered 5-FU loaded Eudragit S-100 coated calcium pectinate beads can be used effectively for the specific delivery of drug to the colon.Colon-targeted drug delivery systems for 5-fluorouracil using pectin combined with ethyl cellulose as a film coat with fluidized bed coater were de4veloped. Pellets (0.8-1.0 mm in diameter) containing 40% 5-fluorouracil and 60% microcrystalline cellulose were prepared by extrusion and spheronization.Eudragit-coating of pectin microspheres was performed by oil-in-oil solvent evaporation method using coat: core ratio (5:1). The release profile of FU from Eudragitcoated pectin microspheres was pH dependent. In acidic medium, the release rate was much slower; however, the drug was released quickly at pH 7.4. It is concluded from the present investigation that Eudragitcoated pectin microspheres are promising controlled release carriers for colon-targeted delivery of FU.

Guar gum-based matrix tablets of rofecoxib for their intended use in the chemoprevention of colorectal cancer were developed and evaluated [116]. Matrix tablets containing 40% (RXL-40), 50% (RXL-50), 60% (RXL-60) or 70% (RXL-70) of guar gum were prepared by wet granulation technique. Colon delivery of beta-lactamases by pectin beads aiming to degrade residual beta-lactam antibiotics, in order to prevent the emergence of resistant bacterial strains[115]. Pectin beads were prepared according to inotropic gelation method using $CaCl_2$ as a gelling agent[117]. Particles were then washed and soaked in polyethyleneimine (PEI). Coating beads with PEI considerably improved their stability in simulated intestinal medium.

9. Polysaccharides as a strategy for targeting colon drug delivery

A variety of delivery strategies and systems have been proposed for colonic targeting. These generally rely on the exploitation of one or more of the following gastrointestinal features for their functionality: pH, transit time, pressure or micro flora. Coated systems that utilise the pH differential in the gastrointestinal tract and prodrugs that rely on colonic bacteria for release have been commercialized. Both approaches have their own inherent limitations. Many systems in development have progressed no further than the bench, while others are expensive or complex to manufacture, or lack the desired site-specificity. The universal polysaccharide systems appear to be the most promising because of their practicality and exploitation of the most distinctive property of the colon, abundant micro flora.

Recent research into the utilization of the metabolic activity and the colonic microenvironment in the lower gastrointestinal tract has attained great value in the design of novel colon-targeted delivery systems based on natural biodegradable polymers. In the current articles, special emphasis has been placed on polysaccharide systems, with minimal chemical modification, that have been exploitedfor colon targeting. These polysaccharide based encapsulation and targeted delivery systems are envisaged to have an immense potential for the development of food/nutraceutical formulations for colon-based diseases, including colorectal cancer [118].Pectin-ketoprofen (PT-KP) prodrug with the potential for colon targeted delivery has been evaluated and showed KP distributes mainly in stomach, proximal small intestine and distal small intestine. However, KP released from PT-KP mainly distributes in cecum and colon. Therefore, this approach suggests that PT-KP prodrug has a good colon targeting property [119].

Compression coatings for target drug delivery to the colon using indometacin (a water insoluble drug) and paracetamol (a water soluble drug) as model drugs were evaluated. The core tablets were compression-coated with 300 and 400 mg of 100% kayas gum, 100% albizia gum and a mixture of kaya and albizia gum (1:1). Colon targeted drug delivery systems were developed for tinidazole using guar gum as a carrier in the treatment of amoebiasis. Fast-disintegrating tinidazole core tablets were compression-coated with 55, 65 and 75% of guar gum [120]. Colon-targeted drug delivery systems for ornidazole [121]using guar gum as a carrier are developed.The core formulation containing ornidazole was directly compressed. Compression-coated tablets of ornidazole containing various proportions of guar gum in the coat were prepared. Compression-coated ornidazole tablets with either 65% (OLV-65) or 75% (OLV-75) of guar gum coat are most likely to provide targeting of ornidazole for local action in the colon owing to its minimal release of the drug in the first 5 hr. The ornidazole compression-coated tablets showed no change in physical appearance, drug content, or in dissolution pattern after storage at 40 degrees C/75% relative humidity for 6 months [122-125].

Novel tablet formulations for site-specific delivery of 5-fluorouracil to the colon without the drug being released in the stomach or small intestine using guar gum as a carrier were developed. Fast-disintegrating 5-fluorouracil core tablets were compression coated with 60% (FHV-60), 70% (FHV-70) and 80% (FHV-80) of guar gum [126]. Oral colon-targeting drug delivery systems for celecoxib using guar gum as a carrier were developed. Matrix tablets containing various proportions of guar gum were prepared by wet granulation technique using starch paste as a binder.Colon targeted drug delivery systems for metronidazole using guar gum as a carrier were developed. Matrix, multilayer and compression coated tablets of metronidazole containing various proportions of guar gum were prepared [127].The influence of metronidazole and tinidazole on the usefulness of guar gum, a colon-specific drug carrier based on the metabolic activity of colonic bacteria, using matrix tablets of albendazole (containing 20% of guar gum) as a model formulation is reported.Colon targeted drug delivery systems for mebendazole using guar gum as a carrier were developed. Matrix tablets containing various proportions of guar gum were prepared by wet granulation technique using starch paste as a binder [128, 129].

Controlling the delivery of drugs to different regions of the colon remains an elusive goal-was to define the diurnal variation in colonic transit and show how this influences the colonic distribution and residence time of different formulations given either in the morning or evening. Colonic transit of small particulates and a large capsule was measured during nocturnal sleep and daytime wakefulness. Sleep delays colonic transit and large capsules travel faster than dispersed small particles. However, substantial inter-individual variability in transit makes targeting specific regions of the human colon unreliable with either dispersed or single unit formulations [130].

Targeting of drugs to the colon, following oral administration, can be accomplished by the use of modified, biodegradable polysaccharides as vehicles. In a previous study, a cross-linked low swelling guar gum (GG) hydrogel was synthesized by reacting it with trisodium trimetaphosphate (STMP). In the present study the functioning of GG crosslinked products (GGP) as possible colon-specific drug carriers was analyzed by studying (a) the release kinetics of pre-loaded hydrocortisone from GGP hydrogels into buffer solutions with, or without GG degrading enzymes (alpha-galactosidase and beta-mannanase) and (b) direct measurements of the polymers' degradation [131]. Calcium pectinate preparations for drug delivery to the colon were investigated and highlight the value of scintigraphy in focusing the development strategy for colonic targeting preparations.

One of the review articles concluded that polysaccharide-based colon-targeted drug delivery systems are effective when they are precisely activated by the physiological conditions of the colon. Absence of enzymes during colonic disorders might hinder the activation of the delivery system. To guarantee delivery of the drug to the colon, it is preferable to combine polysaccharides with enteric or cellulose polymers [132]. The approach that is based on the formulation of natural polysaccharides has been used as tools to deliver the drugs specially to the colon as described in Table 1 and Table 2.

These polysaccharides remain intact in the physiological environment of stomach and small intestine but once the dosage form enters into colon, it is acted upon by polysaccharides, which degrades the polysaccharide and release the drug into the vicinity of bio-environment of colon (Table 3).As shown in Figure 1 the designed drug delivery systems have been developed that are based on the principle to prevent release of drug until 3-4 h after leaving the stomach, which are correspond to blood concentration profile as illustrated in Figure 2.

With the respect to natural products improved drug delivery systems are required for drugs currently in use to treat localized disease of the colon. The advantages of targeting drugs specially to the diseased colon are reduced incidence of systemic side effects, lower dose of drug, supply of the drug to the bio phase only when it is required and maintenance of the drug its intact form as close as possible to target site. Thus, the natural and modified properties of polysaccharides that are responsible for their colon targeting abilities. Among the different approaches used, polysaccharides that are precisely activated by the physiological conditions of the colon hold great promise, as they provide improved site specificity and meet the desired therapeutic needs.

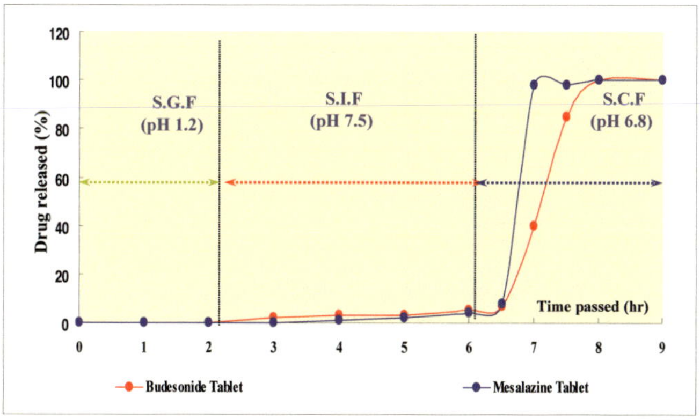

Figure 1. Dissolution profile from microbial degradable colon delivery system coated with polysaccharide.

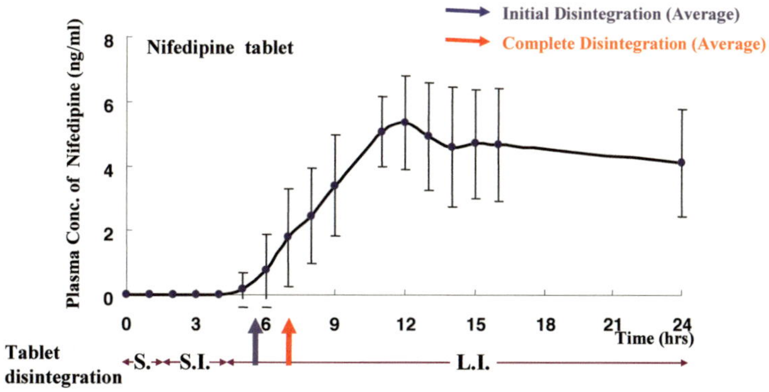

Figure 2. Blood plasma concentration profile of nifedipinetablet(top) and soft(bottom) capsule verse disintegration time

Polysaccharides	Main Chains	Side Chains	Bacterial Species
Pectin	1) α-1,4 D-garactouronicacid 2) 1,2 –L-rhamnose	D-galactose L-arabinose	Bacteroides , Bifidobacteria, Eubacteria
Guar Gum	1) α-1,4 D-mannose 2) α-1,3 or α-1,4 D-galactose	α-1,6 D-galactose	Bacteroides , Ruminococci
Amylose	α-1,4 D-glucose	-	
Chitosan	Deacetylated β-1,4 N-acetyl-D-glucosamine	-	
Chondroitin Sulfate	1) β-1,3 D-glucuronicacid 2) N-acetyl-D-glucosamine	-	Bacteroides
Cyclodextrine	α-1,4 D-glucose	-	Bacteroides
Dextran	α-1,6 D-glucose	α-1,3 D-glucose	Bacteroides
Xylan	β-1,4 D-xylose	β-1,3 L-arabinose	Bacteroides , Bifidobacteria

Table 1. Main Structural Features of Polysaccharides

System	CoLar ®		CSDS	Colon Delivery System
Developer	Allyzyme (U.K)		Samyang Co., (Korea)	Perio (Israel)
Composition	Amylose+Ethylcellulose Coating		Tablet or Soft capsule coated with Polysaccharide	1) Fast release: Ca.P + P 2) Slow release:Ca.P + GG
Dosage form	Coated Tablet		Coated Tablet Coated Soft Capsule	Matrix Tablet
Drug	Rensapride	Budesonide, Mesalazine Diclofenac	Prednisolone Theophylline	Diclofenac Insulin
Indication	Constipation Predominant I.B.S.	I.B.D. Rheumatoid Arthritis		Rheumatoid Arthritis Diabetes
Stage	PhaseI(Japan) PhaseII (U.K)	System Development	System Development	System Development
Licensee	S.K.B Now discontinuedfor internal reason			Alpharma Co.,

Table 2. Microbial Degradable Colon Delivery System.

http://dx.doi.org/10.5772/52346

System	Targit ®	Chronotopic ®	CTDC ®	Colon Delivery System
Developer	DanBio System (U.K)	Poli Chemical Industry (Italy)	Tanabe Seiyaku (Japan)	Chiesi (Italy)
Composition	Starch Capsule + Enteric Coating	1) 1st : Core Tablet 2)2nd:Low-Viscosity HPMC 3) 3rd : Eudragit	1) 1st layer: Eudragit L 2) 2nd layer: HPMC 3) 3rd layer: Eudragit E	Enteric(Eudragit–S) Coating
Dosage form	Coated Capsule	Coated tablet	Coated Capsule	Coated Tablet
Drug	Mesalazine	Mesalazine	Prednisolone Theophylline	Beclomethasone Dipropionate
Indication	I.B.D.	I.B.D.	-	I.B.D.
Stage	System Development	Phase II (Italy)	System Development	Phase III (Italy)
Licensee	Western Pharma.	-	-	-

Table 3. Time-Controlled &pH-Controlled Colon Delivery System

10. Protein and peptide drug targeting colon delivery

Targeted delivery to the gastrointestinal tract requires a multi-disciplinary approach to research involving contributions from polymer and material scientists, gastroenterologists, pharmaceutical scientists and technologists. Intestinal delivery is important not only for drugs that act locally, but also for those with systemic activity [133, 134]. In particular, there is considerable interest in the oral delivery of peptides and it is felt that the colon may provide an advantageous absorption site for such molecules. The different targeting mechanisms available to the pharmaceutical scientist to provide site-specific delivery in the gastrointestinal tract will be critically assessed. Delivery systems and targeting agents, which are being developed for the delivery of drugs, may also be exploited for the delivery of vaccines, since many of the delivery problems are common to both areas. Recent developments in the design of oral antigen formulations was discussed in this review [135-137].

Author details

Hyunjo Kim

Address all correspondence to: hyunjokim@hotmail.com

Pharmacy School of Sahmyook University, Seoul, Korea

References

[1] Fish, M., Kugathasan, S. Inflammatory bowel disease. *Adolesc Med Clin.*, 2004, 15(1), 67-90.

[2] Van Assche, G., Vermeire, S., Rutgeerts, P. Focus onmechanisms of inflammation in inflammatory bowel diseasesites of inhibition: current and future therapies. *Gastroenterol. Clin. North Am.*, 2006, 35(4), 743-56.

[3] Brown, S. J., Mayer, L. The immune response in inflammatorybowel disease. *Am. J. Gastroenteril.*, 2007, 102(9), 2058-69.

[4] Mutlu, E. A., Farhadi, A., Keshavarzian, A. New developmentsin the treatment of inflammatory bowel disease. *Expert Opin. Investig. Drugs.*, 2002, 11(3), 365-85.

[5] Sandborn, W. J. What's new: innovative concepts in inflammatorybowel disease. *Colorectal. Dis.*, 2006, 15(1), Suppl1:3-9.

[6] Haddish-Berhane N., Farhadi., A., Nyquist, C., Haghighi, K., Keshavarzian, A. Biological variability and targeteddelivery of therapeutics for inflammatory bowel disease:an silico approach. *Inflamm. Allergy Drug Targets.*, 2007, 6(1), 47-55.

[7] Su, C., Lichtenstein G. R. Recent developments in in-flammatory bowel disease. *Med. Clin. North Am*, 2002, 86(6), 1497-523.

[8] Ardizzone S., Bianchi Porro G. Biologic therapy forinflammatory bowel disease. *Drugs.*, 2005, 65(16), 2253-86.

[9] Jarnerot, G. Future aspects on inflammatory bowel disease. *Scand. J. Gastroenterol. Suppl.*, 1996, 220, 87-90.

[10] Robinson, M. Medical therapy of inflammatory boweldisease for the 21st century. *Eur. J. Surg. Suppl.*, 1998, 582, 90-8.

[11] Targan S. R. Current limitations of IBD treatment: wheredo we go from here? *Ann. N. Y. Acad. Sci.*, 2006, 1072, 1-8

[12] Larsson, S. Mistletoes and thionins. As selection modelsin natural products drug discovery. Acta Universitatis Upsaliensis. Comprehensive summaries of Uppsala dissertationsfrom the faculty of Pharmacy. 2007, 49, 1–65.

[13] Larsson, J., Gottfries, J., Muresan, S., Backlund, A. Chem-GPS-NP: tuned for navigation in biologically relevantchemical space. *J. Nat. Prod.* 2007, 70, 789–794.

[14] Huss, U., Ringbom, T., Perera, P., Bohlin, L., Vasänge, M. Screening of ubiquitous plant constituents for COX-2inhibition with a scintillation proximity based assay. *J Nat Prod.* , 2002, 65, 1571–1621.

[15] Huss, U. Studies on the effects of plant and food constituentson cyclooxygenase-2. Aspects in inflammation and cancer. Acta Universitatis Upsaliensis. Comprehensive summaries of Uppsala dissertations from the faculty of Pharmacy. 2003, 294, 1–56.

[16] Kim, D. J., Shin, D. H., Ahn, B., Kang, J. S., Nam, K. T., Park, C. B., Kim, C. K., Hong, J. T., Kim, T. B. Chemoprevention of coloncancer by Korean food plant components. *Mut Res.* 2003, 523(524), 99–107.

[17] Murakami, A., Ohigashi, H. Targeting NOX, INOS and COX-2 in inflammatory cells: chemoprevention usingfood phytochemicals. *Int J Cancer*, 2007, 121, 2357–2363.

[18] Pettersson, J., Karlsson, P. C., Choi, Y. H., Verpoorte. R., Rafter, J. J., Bohlin, L. NMR metabolomic analysis of fecal water from subjects on a vegetarian diet. *Biol Pharm Bull*, 2008a, 31, 1192–1198.

[19] Pettersson, J., Karlsson, P. C., Göransson, U., Rafter, J. J., Bohlin, L. The flavouring phytochemical 2-pentanone reducesprostaglandin production and COX-2 expression in colon cancer cells. *Biol Pharm Bull*, 2008b, 31, 534–537.

[20] Felth, J., Rickardson, L., Rosén, J., Wickström, M., Fryknäs, M., Lindskog, M., Bohlin, L., Gullbo, J. Cytotoxic effects of cardiac glycosides in colon cancer cells, alone and incombination with standard chemotherapeutic drugs. *J Nat Prod*, 2009, 72, 1969–1974.

[21] Suh, Y., Afaq, F., Johnson, J. J., Mukhtar, H. A plant flavonoid fisetin induces apoptosis in colon cancer cells by inhibition of COX2 and Wnt/EGFR/NF-kappaB-signaling pathways. *Carcinogenesis.* 2009, Feb; 30(2), 300-7.

[22] Díaz-Carballo, D., Malak, S., Bardenheuer, W., Freistuehler, M., Peter, Reusch, H. The contribution of plukenetione A to the anti-tumoral activity of Cuban propolis. *Bioorg Med Chem.* 2008, Nov 15, 16(22), 9635-43.

[23] Li, X., Ohtsuki, T., Koyano, T., Kowithayakorn, T., Ishibashi, M. New Wnt/beta-catenin signaling inhibitors isolated from Eleutherine palmifolia. *Chem Asian J.* 2009, 4(4), 540-7.

[24] Laszczyk, M. N. Pentacyclic triterpenes of the lupane, oleanane and ursane group as tools in cancer therapy. *Planta Med.* 2009, Dec;75(15), 1549-60.

[25] Chia, J. S., Du, J. L., Hsu, W. B., Sun, A., Chiang, C. P., Wang, W. B. Inhibition of metastasis, angiogenesis, and tumor growth by Chinese herbal cocktail Tien-Hsien Liquid. BMC Cancer. 2010, 30, 10-175.

[26] Velmurugan, B., Singh, R. P., Agarwal, R., Agarwal, C. Dietary-feeding of grape seed extract prevents azoxymethane-induced colonic aberrant crypt foci formation in fischer 344 rats. *Mol Carcinog.* 2010, 49(7), 641-52.

[27] Luo, X. J., Li, L. L., Deng, Q. P., Yu, X. F., Yang, L. F., Luo, F. J., Xiao, L. B., Chen, X. Y., Ye, M., Liu, J. K., Cao, Y. Grifolin, a potent antitumour natural product upregulates death-associated protein kinase 1 DAPK1 via p53 in nasopharyngeal carcinoma cells. *Eur J Cancer.* 2011, 47(2), 316-25.

[28] Otrubova, K., McGuire, K. L., McAlpine, S. R. Scaffold targeting drug-resistant colon cancers. *J Med Chem.* 2007, 50(9), 1999-2002.

[29] Lee, H. J., Lee, E. O., Rhee, Y. H., Ahn, K. S., Li, G. X., Jiang, C., Lü, J., Kim, S. H. An oriental herbal cocktail, ka-mi-kae-kyuk-tang, exerts anti-cancer activities by targeting angiogenesis, apoptosis and metastasis. *Carcinogenesis.* 2006, 27(12), 2455-63.

[30] Matsuura, N., Miyamae, Y., Yamane, K., Nagao, Y., Hamada, Y., Kawaguchi, N., Katsuki, T., Hirata, K., Sumi, S., Ishikawa, H. Aged garlic extract inhibits angiogenesis and proliferation of colorectal carcinoma cells. *J Nutr.* 2006, 136(3 Suppl), 842S-846S.

[31] Ishikawa, H., Saeki, T., Otani, T., Suzuki, T., Shimozuma, K., Nishino, H., Fukuda, S., Morimoto, K. Aged garlic extract prevents a decline of NK cell number and activity in patients with advanced cancer. *J Nutr.* 2006, 36(3 Suppl), 816S-820S.

[32] Liang, M. C., Bardhan, S., Pace, E. A., Rosman, D., Beutler, J. A., Porco, J. A., Jr, Gilmore, T. D. Inhibition of transcription factor NF-kappaB signaling proteins IKKbeta and p65 through specific cysteine residues by epoxyquinone A monomer: correlation with its anti-cancer cell growth activity. *Biochem Pharmacol.* 2006, 71(5), 634-45.

[33] Momin, M., Pundarikakshudu, K. In vitro studies on guar gum based formulation for the colon targeted delivery of Sennosides. *J Pharm Pharm Sci.* 2004, 7(3), 325-31.

[34] Narayan, S. Curcumin, a multi-functional chemopreventive agent, blocks growth of colon cancer cells by targeting beta-catenin-mediated transactivation and cell-cell adhesion pathways. *J Mol Histol.* 2004, 35(3), 301-7.

[35] Yang, C. X., Xu, X. H., Dong, Y. Advances in the research on targeted preparations of traditional Chinese medicine and natural drugs. *Zhongguo Zhong Yao Za Zhi.* 2003, 28(8), 696-700.

[36] Wu, X. A. Opinion of colon-targeting delivery about rhubarb extract as a purgative. *Zhongguo Zhong Yao Za Zhi.* 2002, 27(1), 72-4.

[37] Hirose, M., Yamaguchi, T., Lin, C., Kimoto, N., Futakuchi, M., Kono, T., Nishibe, S., Shirai, T. Effects of arctiin on PhIP-induced mammary, colon and pancreatic carcinogenesis in female Sprague-Dawley rats and MeIQx-induced hepatocarcinogenesis in male F344 rats. *Cancer Lett.* 2000, 155(1), 79-88.

[38] Samuelsson, G. Phytochemical and pharmacologicalstudies on Viscum album L. *Sve Farm Tidskr*. 1958, 62, 1–21.

[39] Claeson, P., Göransson, U., Johansson, S., Luijendijk, T., Bohlin, L. Fractionation protocol for the isolation of polypeptidesfrom plant biomass. *J Nat Prod*. 1998, 61, 77–81.

[40] Göransson, U., Luijendijk, T., Johansson, S., Bohlin, L., Claeson, P. Seven novel macrocyclic polypeptides from *Viola arvensis*. *J Nat Prod.* 1999, 62, 283–286.

[41] Gran, L. On the effect of a polypeptide isolated from"Kalata–kalata" (Oldenlandia affinis DC.) on the oestrogen dominated uterus. *Acta Pharmacol Toxicol.* 1973, 33, 400–408.

[42] Gran, L., Sandberg, F., Sletten, K. Oldenlandia affinis (R&S) DC—a plant containing uteroactive peptides used in African traditional medicine. *J Ethnopharmacol*. 2000, 70, 197–203.

[43] Saether, O., Craik, D. J., Campbell, I. D., Sletten, K., Juul, J., Norman, D. G. Elucidation of the primary and three-dimensional structure of the uterotonic polypeptide kalata B1. *Biochemistry*. 1995, 34, 4147–4158.

[44] Göransson, U., Craik, D. J. Disulfide mapping of thecyclotide kalata B1: chemical proof of the cyclic cysteineknot motif. *J Biol Chem*. 2003, 278, 48188–48196.

[45] Göransson, U., Svangärd, E., Claeson, P., Bohlin, L. Novelstrategies for isolation and characterization of cyclotides: the discovery of bioactive macrocyclic plant polypeptides in the Violaceae. *Curr Protein Pept Sci*. 2004, 5, 317–329.

[46] Herrmann, A., Burman, R., Mylne, J. S., Karlsson, G., Gullbo, J., Craik, D. J., Clark, R. J., Göransson, U. The alpine violet, *Viola biflora*, is a rich source of cyclotides with potent cytotoxicity. *Phytochemistry*. 2008, 69, 939–952.

[47] Ireland, D. C., Colgrave, M. L., Craik, D. J. A novel suite ofcyclotides from Viola odorata: sequence variation and theimplications for structure, function and stability. *BiochemJ*. 2006, 400, 1–12.

[48] Simonsen, S. M., Sando, L., Ireland, D. C., Colgrave, M. L., Bharathi, R., Göransson, U., Craik, D. J. A continent of plant defensepeptide diversity: cyclotides in Australian Hybanthus (Violaceae). *Plant Cell*. 2005, 17, 3176–3189.

[49] Wang, C. K., Hu, S. H., Martin, J. L., Sjögran, T., Hajdu, J., Bohlin, L., Claeson, P., Göransson, U., Rosengren, K. J., Tang, J., Tan, N. H., Craik, D. J. Combined X-ray and NMR analysis of the stability of the cyclotide cystine knot fold thatunderpins its insecticidal activity and potential use as adrug scaffold. *J Biol Chem*. 2009, 284(16), 10672–10683.

[50] Göransson, U., Broussalis, A. M., Claeson, P. Expression ofthe Viola cyclotides by LC/MS and MS–MS sequencing ofintercysteine loops after introduction of charges and cleavagesites by aminoethylation. *Anal Biochem*. 2003, 318, 107–117.

[51] Rosengren, K. J., Daly, N. L., Plan, M. R., Waine, C., Craik, D. J. Twists, knots, and rings in proteins. Structural definitionof the cyclotide framework. *J Biol Chem*. 2003, 278, 8606–8616.

[52] Colgrave, M. L., Kotze, A. C., Kopp, S., McCarthy, J. S., Coleman, G. T., Craik, D. J. Anthelmintic activity of cyclotides: in vitrostudies with canine and human hookworms. *Acta Trop*. 2009, 109, 163–166.

[53] Tam, J. P., Lu, Y. A., Yang, J. L., Chiu, K. W. An unusual structural motif of antimicrobial peptides containing endto-end macrocycle and cystine-knot disulfides. *Proc Natl Acad Sci*. 1999, 96, 8913–8918.

[54] Göransson, U., Sjo°gren, M., Svangärd, E., Claeson, P., Bohlin, L. Reversible antifouling effect of the cyclotidecycloviolacin O2 against barnacles. *J Nat Prod.* 2004, 67, 1287–1290.

[55] Lindholm, P., Göransson, U., Johansson, S., Claeson, P., Gullbo, J., Larsson, R., Bohlin, L., Backlund, A. Cyclotides: anovel type of cytotoxic agents. *Mol Cancer Ther.* 2002, 1, 365–369

[56] Svangärd, E., Göransson, U., Hocaoglu, Z., Gullbo, J., Larsson, R., Claeson, P., Bohlin, L. Cytotoxic cyclotides from *Viola tricolor*. *J Nat Prod.* 2004, 67, 144–147.

[57] Göransson, U., Herrmann, A., Burman, R., Haugaard-Jönsson, L. M., Rosengren, K. J., The conserved glu in the cyclotidecycloviolacin O2 has a key structural role. *Chem Biochem.* 2009, 10, 2354–2360.

[58] Herrmann, A., Svangärd, E., Claeson, P., Gullbo, J., Bohlin, L., Göransson, U. Key role of glutamic acid for the cytotoxic activity of the cyclotide cycloviolacin O2. *CellMol Life Sci.* 2006, 63, 235–245.

[59] Kamimori, H., Hall, K., Craik, D., Aguilar, M. Studies on the membrane interactions of the cyclotides kalata B1 and kalata B6 on model membrane systems by surface plasmon resonance. *Anal Biochem.* 2005, 337, 149–153.

[60] Shenkarev, Z. O., Nadezhdin, K. D., Sobol, V. A., Sobol, A. G., Skjeldal, L., Arseniev, A. S. Conformation and mode ofmembrane interaction in cyclotides. Spatial structure of kalata B1 bound to a dodecylphosphocholine micelle. *FEBS J.* 2006, 273, 2658–2672.

[61] Svangärd, E., Burman, R., Gunasekera, S., Lövborg, H., Gullbo, J., Göransson, U. Mechanism of action of cytotoxiccyclotides: cycloviolacin O2 disrupts lipid membranes. *J Nat Prod.* 2007, 70, 643–647.

[62] Gunasekera, S., Foley, F. M., Clark, R. J., Sando, L., Fabri, L. J., Craik, D. J., Daly, N. L. Engineering stabilized vascularendothelial growth factor-A antagonists: synthesis, structural characterization, and bioactivity of grafted analoguesof cyclotides. *J Med Chem.* 2008, 51, 7697–7704.

[63] Seydel, P., Dörnenburg, H. Establishment of in vitroplants, cell and tissue cultures from Oldenlandia affinis for the production of cyclic peptides. *Plant Cell Tissue Org Cult.* 2006, 85, 247–255.

[64] Gunasekera, S., Daly, N. L., Anderson, M. A., Craik, D. J. Chemical synthesis and biosynthesis of the cyclotidefamily of circular proteins. *IUBMB Life*, 2006, 58, 515–524.

[65] Leta Aboye, T., Clark, R. J., Craik, D. J., Göransson, U. Ultrastablepeptide scaffolds for protein engineering-synthesisand folding of the circular cystine knotted cyclotide cycloviolacin O2. *Chem Bioche*, 2008, 9, 103–113.

[66] Peruzzi, D., Mori, F., Conforti, A., Lazzaro, D., De Rinaldis, E., Ciliberto, G., La Monica, N., Aurisicchio, L. MMP11: a novel target antigen for cancer immunotherapy. *Clin Cancer Res.* 2009, 15(12), 4104-13.

[67] Guan, Q., Ma, Y., Hillman, C. L., Ma, A., Zhou, G., Qing, G., Peng, Z. Development of recombinant vaccines against IL-12/IL-23 p40 and in vivo evaluation of their effects in the down regulation of intestinal inflammation in murine colitis. *Vaccine.* 2009, 27(50), 7096-104.

[68] Ma, Y., Guan, Q., Bai, A., Weiss, C. R., Hillman, C. L., Ma, A., Zhou, G., Qing, G., Peng, Z. Targeting TGF-beta1 by employing a vaccine ameliorates fibrosis in a mouse model of chronic colitis. *Inflamm Bowel Dis.* 2010, 16(6), 1040-50.

[69] Ohkawara, T., Koyama, Y., Onodera, S., Takeda, H., Kato, M., Asaka, M., Nishihira, J. DNA vaccination targeting macrophage migration inhibitory factor prevents murine experimental colitis. *Clin Exp Immunol.* 2011, 163(1), 113-22.

[70] Williams, B. B., Wall, M., Miao, R. Y., Williams, B., Bertoncello, I., Kershaw, M. H., Mantamadiotis, T., Haber, M., Norris, M. D., Gautam, A., Darcy, P. K., Ramsay, R. G. Induction of T cell-mediated immunity using a c-Myb DNA vaccine in a mouse model of colon cancer. *Cancer Immunol Immunother.* 2008, 57(11), 1635-45.

[71] Xiang, R., Luo, Y., Niethammer, A. G., Reisfeld, R. A. Oral DNA vaccines target the tumor vasculature and microenvironment and suppress tumor growth and metastasis. *Immunol Rev.* 2008, 222, 117-28.

[72] Shim, D. H., Chang, S. Y., Park, S. M., Jang, H., Carbis, R., Czerkinsky, C., Uematsu, S., Akira, S., Kweon, M. N. Immunogenicity and protective efficacy offered by a ribosomal-based vaccine from Shigella flexneri 2a. *Vaccine.* 2007, 25(25), 4828-36.

[73] Kaplan, C. D., Krüger, J. A., Zhou, H., Luo, Y., Xiang, R., Reisfeld, R. A. A novel DNA vaccine encoding PDGFRbeta suppresses growth and dissemination of murine colon, lung and breast carcinoma. *Vaccine.* 2006, 24(47-48), 6994-7002.

[74] Morse, M. A. Virus-based therapies for colon cancer. *Expert Opin Biol Ther.* 2005 , 5(12), 1627-33.

[75] Mosolits, S., Nilsson, B., Mellstedt, H. Towards therapeutic vaccines for colorectal carcinoma: a review of clinical trials. *Expert Rev Vaccines.* 2005, 4(3), 329-50.

[76] Decker, W. K., Qiu, J., Farhangfar, F., Hester, J. H., Altieri, D. C., Lin, A. Y. A retrogen plasmid-based vaccine generates high titer antibody responses against the autologous cancer antigen survivin and demonstrates anti-tumor efficacy. *Cancer Lett.* 2006, 237(1), 45-55.

[77] Lo-Man, R., Vichier-Guerre, S., Perraut, R., Dériaud, E., Huteau, V., BenMohamed, L., Diop, O. M, ; Livingston, P. O., Bay, S., Leclerc, C. A fully synthetic therapeutic vaccine candidate targeting carcinoma-associated Tn carbohydrate antigen induces tumor-specific antibodies in nonhuman primates. *Cancer Res.* 2004, 64(14), 4987-94.

[78] Okaji, Y., Tsuno, N. H., Kitayama, J., Saito, S., Takahashi, T., Kawai, K., Yazawa, K., Asakage, M., Hori, N., Watanabe, T., Shibata, Y., Takahashi, K., Nagawa, H. Vaccination with autologous endothelium inhibits angiogenesis and metastasis of colon cancer through autoimmunity. *Cancer Sci.* 2004, 95(1), 85-90.

[79] Niethammer, A. G., Xiang, R., Becker, J. C., Wodrich, H., Pertl, U., Karsten, G., Eliceiri, B. P., Reisfeld, R. A. A DNA vaccine against VEGF receptor 2 prevents effective angiogenesis and inhibits tumor growth. *Nat Med.* 2002, 8(12), 1369-75.

[80] Bernhard, H., Salazar, L., Schiffman, K., Smorlesi, A., Schmidt, B., Knutson, K. L., Disis, M. L. Vaccination against the HER-2/neu oncogenic protein. *Endocr Relat Cancer.* 2002, 9(1), 33-44.

[81] Pan, Z. K., Ikonomidis, G., Lazenby, A., Pardoll, D., Paterson, Y. A recombinant Listeria monocytogenes vaccine expressing a model tumour antigen protects mice against lethal tumour cell challenge and causes regression of established tumours. *Nat Med.* 1995, 1(5), 471-7.

[82] Kang, D. W., Min, do S. Positive feedback regulation between phospholipase D and Wnt signaling promotes Wnt-driven anchorage-independent growth of colorectal cancer cells. *PLoS One.* 2010, 5(8), e12109.

[83] Wen, Y., Wang, C. T., Ma, T. T., Li, Z. Y., Zhou, L. N., Mu, B., Leng, F., Shi, H. S., Li, Y. O., Wei, Y. Q. Immunotherapy targeting fibroblast activation protein inhibits tumor growth and increases survival in a murine colon cancer model. *Cancer Sci.* 2010, 101(11), 2325-32.

[84] Kucerova, L., Matuskova, M., Pastorakova, A., Tyciakova, S., Jakubikova, J., Bohovic, R., Altanerova, V., Altaner, C. Cytosine deaminase expressing human mesenchymal stem cells mediated tumour regression in melanoma bearing mice. *J. Gene Med.* 2008, 10(10), 1071-82.

[85] Yoneyama, S., Okaji, Y., Tsuno, N. H., Kawai, K., Yamashita, H., Tsuchiya, T., Yamada, J., Sunami, E., Osada, T., Kitayama, J., Takahashi, K., Nagawa, H. A study of dendritic and endothelial cell interactions in colon cancer in a cell line and small mammal model. *Eur J Surg Oncol.* 2007, 33(10), 1191-8.

[86] Kanai, T., Uraushihara, K., Totsuka, T., Nemoto, Y., Fujii, R., Kawamura, T., Makita, S., Sawada, D., Yagita, H., Okumura, K., Watanabe, M. Ameliorating effect of saporin-conjugated anti-CD11b monoclonal antibody in a murine T-cell-mediated chronic colitis. *J Gastroenterol Hepatol.* 2006, 21(7), 1136-42.

[87] Loeffler, M., Krüger, J. A., Niethammer, A. G., Reisfeld, R. A. Targeting tumor-associated fibroblasts improves cancer chemotherapy by increasing intratumoral drug uptake. *J Clin Invest.* 2006, 116(7), 1955-62.

[88] Kamath, S., Buolamwini, J. K. Targeting EGFR and HER-2 receptor tyrosine kinases for cancer drug discovery and development. *Med Res Rev.* 2006, 26(5), 569-94.

[89] Furumoto, K., Soares, L., Engleman, E. G., Merad, M. Induction of potent antitumor immunity by in situ targeting of intratumoral DCs. *J Clin Invest.* 2004, 113(5), 774-83.

[90] Lage, A., Crombet, T., González, G. Targeting epidermal growth factor receptor signaling: early results and future trends in oncology. *Ann Med.* 2003, 35(5), 327-36.

[91] Seward, D. J., Koh, A. S., Boyer, J. L., Ballatori, N. Functional complementation between a novel mammalian polygenic transport complex and an evolutionarily ancient organic solute transporter, OSTalpha-OSTbeta. *J Biol Chem.* 2003, 278(30), 27473-82.

[92] Mukherjee, P., Madsen, C. S., Ginardi, A. R., Tinder, T. L., Jacobs, F., Parker, J., Agrawal, B., Longenecker, B. M., Gendler, S. J. Mucin 1-specific immunotherapy in a mouse model of spontaneous breast cancer. *J Immunother.* 2003, 26(1), 47-62.

[93] Gri, G., Gallo, E., Di Carlo, E., Musiani, P., Colombo, M. P. OX40 ligand-transduced tumor cell vaccine synergizes with GM-CSF and requires CD40-Apc signaling to boost the host T cell antitumor response. *J Immunol.* 2003, 170(1), 99-106.

[94] Nakamori, M., Iwahashi, M., Tani, M., Yamaue, H., Ueda, K., Matsuda, K., Tanimura, H. [New therapeutic strategy against colon cancer based on a tumor-specific approach. *Gan To Kagaku Ryoho.* 2000, 27(14), 2209-15.

[95] Watson, S. A., Clarke, P. A., Morris, T. M., Caplin, M. E. Antiserum raised against an epitope of the cholecystokinin B/gastrin receptor inhibits hepatic invasion of a human colon tumor. *Cancer Res.* 2000, 60(20), 5902-7.

[96] Weiner, L. M., Clark, J. I., Davey, M., Li, W. S., Garcia de Palazzo, I., Ring, D. B., Alpaugh, R. K. Phase I trial of 2B1, a bispecific monoclonal antibody targeting c-erbB-2 and Fc gamma RIII. *Cancer Res.* 1995 , 55(20), 4586-93.

[97] Nishimura, T., Nakamura, Y., Tsukamoto, H., Takeuchi, Y., Tokuda, Y., Iwasawa, M., Yamamoto, T., Masuko, T., Hashimoto, Y., Habu, S. Human c-erbB-2 proto-oncogene product as a target for bispecific-antibody-directed adoptive tumor immunotherapy. *Int J Cancer.* 1992, 50(5), 800-4.

[98] Nishimura, T., Nakamura, Y., Takeuchi, Y., Gao, X. H., Tokuda, Y., Okumura, K., Habu, S. Bispecific antibody-directed antitumor activity of human CD4+ helper/killer T cells induced by anti-CD3 monoclonal antibody plus interleukin 2. *Jpn J Cancer Res.* 1991, 82(11), 1207-10.

[99] Zhang, Y. J., Li, J. Y., Xu, L. Y. Evaluation of targeting property for Kuikang colon targeted pellets. *Zhongguo Zhong Yao Za Zhi.* 2008, 33(13), 1556-7, 1604.

[100] Talukder, R. M., Fassihi, R. Development and in-vitro evaluation of a colon-specific controlled release drug delivery system. *J Pharm Pharmacol.* 2008, 60(10), 1297-303.

[101] Hodges, L. A., Connolly, S. M., Band, J., O'Mahony, B., Ugurlu, T., Turkoglu, M., Wilson, C. G., , Stevens, H. N. Scintigraphic evaluation of colon targeting pectin-HPMC tablets in healthy volunteers. *J Pharm Pharmacol.* 2008, 60(10), 1304-309.

[102] Vaidya, A., Jain, A., Khare, P., Agrawal, R. K., Jain, S. K. Metronidazole loaded pectin microspheres for colon targeting. *J Pharm Sci.* 2009, 98(11), 4229-36.

[103] Prajakta, D., Ratnesh, J., Chandan, K., Suresh, S., Grace, S., Meera, V., Vandana, P. Curcumin loaded pH-sensitive nanoparticles for the treatment of colon cancer. *J Biomed Nanotechnol.* 2009, 5(5), 445-55.

[104] Andrews, C. N; Griffiths, T. A., Kaufman, J., Vergnolle, N., Surette, M. G., Rioux, K. P. Mesalazine (5-aminosalicylic acid) alters faecal bacterial profiles, but not mucosal proteolytic activity in diarrhoea-predominant irritable bowel syndrome. *Aliment Pharmacol Ther.* 2011, 34(3), 374-83.

[105] Patel, N. V., Patel, J. K., Shah, S. H. Box-Behnken experimental design in the development of pectin-compritol ATO 888 compression coated colon targeted drug delivery of mesalamine. *Acta Pharm.* 2010, 60(1), 39-54.

[106] Prabhu, P., Ahamed, N., Matapady, H. N., Ahmed, M. G., Narayanacharyulu, R., Satyanarayana, D., Subrahmanayam, E. Investigation and comparison of colon specificity of novel polymer khaya gum with guar gum. *J Pharm Sci.* 2010, 23(3), 259-65.

[107] Tamura, T., Kuwahara, A., Kadoyama, K., Yamamori, M., Nishiguchi, K., Inokuma, T., Takemoto, Y., Chayahara, N., Okuno, T., Miki, I., Fujishima, Y., Sakaeda, T. Effects of bolus injection of 5-Fluorouracil on steady-state plasma concentrations of 5-Fluorouracil in Japanese patients with advanced colorectal cancer. *Int J Med Sci.* 2011, 8(5), 406-12.

[108] Maestrelli, F., Cirri, M., Corti, G., Mennini, N., Mura, P. Development of enteric-coated calcium pectinate microspheres intended for colonic drug delivery. *Eur J Pharm Biopharm.* 2008, 69(2), 508-18.

[109] Wei, H., Qing, D., De-Ying, C., Bai, X., Li-Fang, F. In-vitro and in-vivo studies of pectin/ethylcellulose film-coated pellets of 5-fluorouracil for colonic targeting. *J Pharm Pharmacol.* 2008, 60(1), 35-44.

[110] Ravi, V., Siddaramaiah, Pramod Kumar T. M. Influence of natural polymer coating on novel colon targeting drug delivery system. *J Mater Sci Mater Med.* 2008, 19(5), 2131-6.

[111] Yang, M., Qiu, X. L., Xie, X. L., Lai, J., Chen, S. W. Preparation of kangfuxin colon targeting micro-pellets. *Zhongguo Zhong Yao Za Zhi.* 2007, 32(15), 1529-32.

[112] Ji, C. M., Xu, H. N., Sun, N. Y., Lu, Y. P., Wu, W. Guar gum/ethylcellulose coated pellets for colon-specific drug delivery. *Yao Xue Xue Bao.* 2007, 42(6), 656-62.

[113] Jain, A., Gupta, Y., Jain, S. K. Potential of calcium pectinate beads for target specific drug release to colon. *J Drug Target.* 2007, 15(4), 285-94.

[114] Wei, H., Qing, D., De-Ying, C., Bai, X., Fanli-Fang. Pectin/Ethylcellulose as film coatings for colon-specific drug delivery: preparation and in vitro evaluation using 5-fluorouracil pellets. *PDA J Pharm Sci Technol.* 2007, 61(2), 121-30.

[115] Paharia, A., Yadav, A. K., Rai, G., Jain, S. K., Pancholi, S. S., Agrawal, G. P. Eudragit-coated pectin microspheres of 5-fluorouracil for colon targeting. *AAPS PharmSciTech.* 2007, 8(1), 12.

[116] Al-Saidan, S. M., Krishnaiah, Y. S., Satyanarayana, V., Rao, G. S. In vitro and in vivo evaluation of guar gum-based matrix tablets of rofecoxib for colonic drug delivery. *Curr Drug Deliv.* 2005, 2(2), 155-63.

[117] Bourgeois, S., Laham, A., Besnard, M., Andremont, A., Fattal, E. In vitro and in vivo evaluation of pectin beads for the colon delivery of beta-lactamases. *J Drug Target.* 2005, 13(5), 277-84.

[118] Kosaraju, S. L. Colon targeted delivery systems: review of polysaccharides for encapsulation and delivery. *Crit Rev Food Sci Nutr.* 2005, 45(4), 251-8.

[119] Xi, M. M., Zhang, S. Q., Wang, X. Y., Fang, K. Q., Gu, Y. Study on the characteristics of pectin-ketoprofen for colon targeting in rats. *Int J Pharm.* 2005, 298(1), 91-7.

[120] Odeku, O. A., Fell, J. T. In-vitro evaluation of khaya and albizia gums as compression coatings for drug targeting to the colon. *J Pharm Pharmacol.* 2005, 57(2), 163-8.

[121] Krishnaiah, Y. S., Indira Muzib, Y., Bhaskar, P. In vivo evaluation of guar gum-based colon-targeted drug delivery systems of ornidazole in healthy human volunteers. *J Drug Target.* 2003, 11(2), 109-15.

[122] Krishnaiah, Y. S., Veer Raju, P., Dinesh Kumar, B., Jayaram, B., Rama, B., Raju, V., Bhaskar, P. Pharmacokinetic evaluation of guar gum-based colon-targeted oral drug delivery systems of metronidazole in healthy volunteers. *Eur J Drug Metab Pharmacokinet.* 2003, 28(4), 287-94.

[123] Krishnaiah, Y. S., Muzib, Y. I., Rao, G. S., Bhaskar, P., Satyanarayana, V. Studies on the development of colon targeted oral drug delivery systems for ornidazole in the treatment of amoebiasis. *Drug Deliv.* 2003, 10(2), 111-7.

[124] Krishnaiah, Y. S., Indira Muzib, Y., Srinivasa Rao, G., Bhaskar, P., Satyanarayana, V. Design and in vitro evaluation of oral colon targeted drug delivery systems for tinidazole. *DJ Drug Target.* 2002, 10(8), 579-84.

[125] Asane, G. S., Rao, Y. M., Bhatt, J. H., Shaikh, K. S. Optimization, Characterisation and Pharmacokinetic Studies of Mucoadhesive Oral Multiple Unit Systems of Ornidazole. *Sci Pharm.* 2011, 79(1), 181-196.

[126] Krishnaiah, Y. S., Satyanarayana, V., Dinesh Kumar, B., Karthikeyan, R. S. In vitro drug release studies on guar gum-based colon targeted oral drug delivery systems of 5-fluorouracil. *Eur J Pharm Sci.* 2002, 16(3), 185-92.

[127] Krishnaiah, Y. S., Satyanarayana, V., Kumar, B. D., Karthikeyan, R. S. Studies on the development of colon-targeted delivery systems for celecoxib in the prevention of colorectal cancer. *J Drug Target.* 2002, 10(3), 247-54.

[128] Krishnaiah, Y. S., Bhaskar Reddy, P. R., Satyanarayana, V., Karthikeyan, R. S. Studies on the development of oral colon targeted drug delivery systems for metronidazole in the treatment of amoebiasis. *Int J Pharm.* 2002, 236(1-2), 43-55.

[129] Krishnaiah, Y. S., Seetha Devi, A., Nageswara Rao, L., Bhaskar Reddy, P. R., Karthikeyan, R. S., Satyanarayana, V. Guar gum as a carrier for colon specific delivery; influence of metronidazole and tinidazole on in vitro release of albendazole from guar gum matrix tablets. *J Pharm Pharm Sci.* 2001, 4(3), 235-43.

[130] Krishnaiah, Y. S., Veer Raju, P., Dinesh Kumar, B., Bhaskar, P., Satyanarayana, V. Development of colon targeted drug delivery systems for mebendazole. *J Control Release.* 2001, 77(1-2), 87-95.

[131] Br J Nutr. 2001 Sep;86(3):341-8. The prebiotic effects of biscuits containing partially hydrolysed guar gum and fructo-oligosaccharides--a human volunteer study. Tuohy KM, Kolida S, Lustenberger AM, Gibson GR. *J Control Release.* 2001, 77(1-2), 87-95.

[132] Shah, N., Shah, T., Amin A. Polysaccharides: a targeting strategy for colonic drug delivery. *Expert Opin Drug Deliv.* 2011, 8(6), 779-96.

[133] Hebden, J. M., Gilchrist, P. J., Blackshaw, E., Frier, M. E., Perkins, A. C., Wilson, C. G., Spiller, R. C. Night-time quiescence and morning activation in the human colon: effect on transit of dispersed and large single unit formulations. *Eur J Gastroenterol Hepatol.* 1999, 11(12), 1379-85.

[134] Gliko-Kabir, I., Yagen, B., Baluom, M., Rubinstein, A. Phosphated crosslinked guar for colon-specific drug delivery. II. In vitro and in vivo evaluation in the rat. *J Control Release.* 2000, 63(1-2), 129-34.

[135] Nagamitsu, A., Konno, T., Oda, T., Tabaru, K., Ishimaru, Y., Kitamura, N. Targeted cancer chemotherapy for VX2 tumour implanted in the colon with lipiodol as a carrier. *Eur J Cancer.* 1998, 34(11), 1764-9.

[136] Adkin, D. A., Kenyon, C. J., Lerner, E. I., Landau, I., Strauss, E., Caron, D., Penhasi, A., Rubinstein, A., Wilding, I. R. The use of scintigraphy to provide "proof of concept" for novel polysaccharide preparations designed for colonic drug delivery. *Pharm Res.* 1997, 14(1), 103-7.

[137] Wilding, I. R., Davis, S. S., O'Hagan, D. T. Targeting of drugs and vaccines to the gut. *Pharmacol Ther.* 1994, 62(1-2), 97-124.

Chapter 8

Food Nanoparticles and Intestinal Inflammation: A Real Risk?

Alina Martirosyan, Madeleine Polet,
Alexandra Bazes, Thérèse Sergent and
Yves-Jacques Schneider

Additional information is available at the end of the chapter

http://dx.doi.org/10.5772/52887

1. Introduction

Nanotechnology is a rapidly evolving field of research and industrial innovation with many potentially promising applications in agriculture, healthcare, engineering, processing, packaging or delivery of drugs or food supplements. Engineered nanomaterials (ENMs) already became part of our daily life as food packaging agents, drug delivery systems, therapeutics, biosensors, etc. In 2011, according to the Woodrow Wilson Nanotechnology Consumer Products Inventory, Ag nanoparticles (Ag-NPs) were the most commonly consumed ENMs, followed by TiO_2, SiO_2, ZnO, Au, Pt, etc (http://www.nanotechproject.org). By the most recent definition of European Parliament and Council [1] 'nanomaterial' (NM) is any material that is characterized to have at least one dimension ≤ 100 nm, or that comprises of separate functional parts either internal or on the surface, which have one or more dimensions ≤ 100 nm, including structures, e.g. agglomerates or aggregates, which may be larger than 100 nm, but which retain the typical properties of nanoscale.

In many countries ENMs are already used as food supplements and in food packaging: (i) nanoclays as diffusion barriers [2]; (ii) Ag-NPs as antimicrobial agent [3,4]; (iii) silicates and aluminosilicates (E554, E556, E559) as anti-caking and anti-clumping agents and in toothpastes, cheeses, sugars, powdered milks, etc [5]; (iv) TiO_2 (E171) for whitening and brightening, e.g. in sauces and dressings, in certain powdered foods [6], etc. According to FAO/WHO report [7] the ENMs have several current or projected applications in the agro-food sector: nanostructured food ingredients; nanodelivery systems; organic and inorganic nanosized additives; nanocoatings on food contact surfaces; surface functionnalized NMs; nanofiltration; nanosized agrochemicals; nanosensors; water decontamination, …

With an increasing number of ENMs present in consumer and industrial products, the risk of human exposure increases and this may become a threat to human health and the environment [8]. Individual ENMs may lead to one or more endpoints, which are not unique to NMs, but which need to be taken into account, e.g. cytotoxicity, stimulation of an inflammatory response, generation of reactive oxygen species (ROS) and/or genotoxicity. Although the exact mechanism underlying NPs toxicity is yet to be elucidated, studies have suggested that oxidative stress and lipid peroxidation regulate the NP-induced DNA damage, cell membrane disruption and cell death [9-12]. It has been suggested that ROS, in turn, modulate intracellular calcium concentrations, activate transcription factors, induce cytokine production [13], as well as lead to increased inflammation [14,15]. Small sized metallic NPs, e.g. Ag-NPs, TiO_2, Co-NPs may also cause DNA damage [16-20]. *In vitro* studies with different types of NPs (metal/metal oxide, TiO_2, carbon nanotubes, silica) on various cell lines have demonstrated oxidative stress-related inflammatory reactions. It is believed that this response is largely driven by the specific surface area of the NPs and/or their chemical composition [21-25]. Typically, the biological activity of particles increases with the particle size decrease [26-29]. Moreover, depending on their chemistry, NPs show different cellular uptake, subcellular localization and ability to induce the ROS production [30]. On the contrary, there are also cases reported of NPs having anti-inflammatory properties, such as certain Ce oxide [31] and Ag-NPs [32]. Nanocrystalline Ag has been demonstrated to have antimicrobial and anti-inflammatory properties and was found to reduce colonic inflammation following oral administration in a rat model of ulcerative colitis, suggesting that nano-silver may have therapeutic potential for treatment of this condition [32].

To sum up, based on the information currently available, no generic assumptions can be made regarding the toxicity upon exposure to NMs, their endpoints and the implications of different organs and tissues.

2. Behavior and fate of ENMs in the GIT

The gastrointestinal tract (GIT) is a complex barrier-exchange system and is one of the most important routes for macromolecules to enter the body, as well as a key actor of the immune system. The epithelium of the small and large intestines is in close contact with ingested materials, which are absorbed by the villi. To date, studies on exposure, absorption and bioavailability are mainly focused on the inhalation and dermal routes, and little is known about the toxicokinetic and toxicodynamic processes following oral exposure, particularly in relation to ingestion of ENMs that are present in food.

ENMs can reach the GIT either after mucociliary clearance from the respiratory tract after being inhaled [33], or can be ingested directly in food, water, drugs, drug delivery devices, etc [8,34]. The dietary consumption of NPs in developed countries is estimated around 10^{12} particles/person per day, consisting mainly of TiO_2 and mixed silicates [35].

http://dx.doi.org/10.5772/52887

It has been shown that several characteristics, such as (*i*) the particle size [36], (*ii*) surface charge [37], (*iii*) attachment of ligands [38,39], (*iv*) coating with surfactants [40], as well as (*v*) the administration time and dose [41] affect the fate and extent of ENMs absorption in GIT. The published literature on the safety of oral exposure to food-related ENMs currently provides insufficient reliable data to allow a clear safety assessment of ENMs [42] that is connected primarily with inadequate characterization of ENMs [43]. For instance, it has been demonstrated that smaller particles cross the colonic mucus layer faster than larger ones [37]. The NPs kinetics in the GIT also depends strongly on their charge, *i.e.* positively charged latex particles remain trapped in the negatively charged mucus, while negatively charged ones diffuse across the mucus layer and their interaction with epithelial cells becomes possible [41].

NPs that pass the mucus barrier may be translocated through the intestinal epithelium, which will depend not only on physicochemical characteristics of NPs [36-41], but also on the physiological state of the GIT [44]. The translocation of NPs potentially used as food components through the GIT remains to be explored [45]. Much of the current knowledge concerning the potential toxicity of NPs has been gained from *in vitro* or *in silico* test systems. Following ingestion, translocation of particles across the GIT can occur via different pathways:

1. Endocytosis through 'regular' epithelial cells (NPs < 50 - 100 nm) [46].
2. Transcytosis via microfold (M) cell uptake at the surface of intestinal lymphoid tissue (NPs of 20 - 100 nm and small microparticles *i.e.* 100 - 500 nm) [47]. M cells are specialized phagocytic enterocytes that are localized in intestinal lymphatic tissue – Peyer's Patches (PP). This transcytotic pathway occurs via vesicle formation at the apical (*i.e.* luminal) cell membrane that engulfs some extracellular material, which then moves across the cell, escaping therefore to fusion with lysosomes, fuses with the basolateral membrane (*i.e.* serosal) and releases the material at the opposite side of the intestinal barrier. The mechanism is size-dependent - the smaller the particle, the easier is the passage through the epithelium [48-50].
3. Persorption, where 'old' enterocytes are extruded from the villus into the gut lumen, leaving 'holes' in the epithelium, which allow translocation of even large particles, such as starch and pollen [51-53].
4. Another possible route by which NPs can gain access to the gastrointestinal tissue is the paracellular route across tight junctions (TJs) of the epithelial cell layer. TJs are remarkably efficient at preventing paracellular permeation, although their integrity can be affected by diseases, e.g. inflammation, and/or by metabolites (e.g. glucose), calcium chelators (e.g. citrate) [54] and even particle endocytosis [55].

All above-mentioned routes could be involved in NPs translocation. There are a number of published reports stating the involvement of different types of endocytosis in the process of NPs internalization: clathrin-mediated pathway, caveolin-mediated endocytosis and macropinocytosis for TiO_2 [56], size-dependent endocytosis for Au-NPs [57]; endocytotic pathways were described for SiO_2 [58,59] and Ag-NPs [60], etc.

Several studies demonstrated that the phenomenon of persorption is also true for NPs, e.g. in the case of colloidal Au-NPs [36]. Small and large NPs gain potentially access to this route, nevertheless its quantitative relevance remains low, as it seems to be very inefficient compared to the active uptake of particles by M-cells. For instance, it was indicated that one lymphoid follicle dome of the rabbit PP could transport about 10^5 microparticles of 460 nm diameter in 45 min [61]. It could be assumed that for smaller particles this would be even more efficient.

Particulate uptake may occur not only via the M-cells of the lymphoid follicle-associated epithelium (FAE) in PP [49,62], but also via the normal intestinal enterocytes [46]. A number of reports on intestinal uptake of micro- and nanoparticles state that the uptake of inert particles occurs trans-cellularly through normal enterocytes and via M-cells [61,63-65], as well as, to a lesser extent, through paracellular pathway [66].

3. Appropriate *in vitro* model of the intestinal barrier

There are several recognized parameters currently used for *in vitro* cytotoxicity assessment of ENMs, such as cell viability, stress and inflammatory responses, genotoxicity, etc [67]. However, it should be noted that due to specific physicochemical properties of ENMs, currently existing *in vitro* toxicity assays may have limited use and the methods should be carefully designed in order to discard the influence of nano-sized materials on the assay itself [28]. The risk assessment is further impaired by the lack of standardized test systems that fulfil these criteria. According to the new European Chemicals Legislation (REACH), new test systems for toxicity screening of ENMs should be developed, e.g. cell culture systems that will better reflect *in vivo* toxicity parameters [68].

Human colon adenocarcinoma (Caco-2) cells reproducibly display a number of properties characteristic to differentiated enterocytes and are the most popular cell culture system for studying intestinal passage and transport [69,70]. Cultured Caco-2 cells differentiate spontaneously into polarized monolayers [71] that possess an apical brush border and express functional TJs, biotransformation enzymes and efflux pumps [72]. Caco-2 cells grow as a monolayer and fully differentiate also on semi-permeable membranes of bicameral inserts. This permits to separate the apical (AP) compartment from the basolateral (BL) one, reflecting the intestinal lumen and the serosal side, respectively [65]. Transport of molecules and ions from the AP to the BL side and vice versa requires the passage either through the cells (transcellular route) or between the cells through TJs (paracellular route).

The gut lining epithelium is for the most part impermeable to microorganisms and microparticles, except for the lymphoid FAE found in PP [49,73,74]. M cells are responsible for transport of antigens, bacteria, viruses, as well as micro- and NPs to the antigen presenting cells within and under the epithelial barrier as the first step in developing immune responses [75]. There is only an incomplete and inadequate understanding of the development and function of FAE, as well as of the genes and proteins responsible for their specialized functions. One potential approach to study such complex and specialized tissues is to use cell culture systems more precisely reproducing the features of the *in vivo* tissue. Kernéis *et al.* [76] demonstrated that co-culturing of Caco-2 cells with murine PP lymphocytes appears to convert Caco-2 cells into M-like cells, including enhanced transport of particles across the epithelium monolayer. The induction of this phenotype did not require direct cell contact, as it was also achieved via physically separated co-culturing of Caco-2 and human Burkitt's lymphoma (Raji B) cells in bicameral culture inserts [77]. Although it is not clear whether this model faithfully reproduces all of the features of *in vivo* M cell function, nevertheless studies have confirmed that Caco-2 cells co-cultivated with Raji B cells *in vitro* express several genes specifically expressed in FAE *in vivo* [78].

In an improved *in vitro* co-culture model in bicameral system Caco-2 cells were exposed to lymphocytes from the BL chamber. In a so-called 'inverted' model (Figure 1) the lymphocytes were shown to migrate into the monolayer and induce the conversion of the enterocyte phenotype into the M-cells one [76,79]. Recently, des Rieux *et al.* [65] characterized the inverted model and compared it with previously developed one [77]. According to these results, in the inverted model, the M cell conversion rate was estimated to range between 15 - 30% (for comparison it was <10% in the human FAE [80]). The comparison of the *in vitro* models revealed that the inverted model appears to be physiologically and functionally more reproducible and efficient than the normally oriented one [65]. Thus this improved model could be used to better characterize and understand the biological effects, absorption and transportation mechanisms of NPs in intestinal cells.

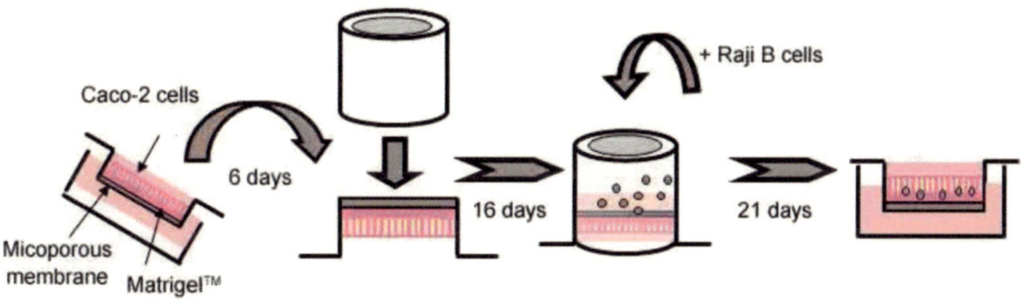

Figure 1. Co-culture model of Caco-2 and Raji B cells [63].

4. Epithelial barrier integrity and inflammatory response under the influence of NPs

During their differentiation epithelial cells develop junctional structures between the neighboring cells and form a tight protective barrier that restricts the absorption to some nutrients and substances while, in the meantime, provides a physical barrier impairing the permeation of pro-inflammatory molecules, e.g. pathogens, toxins, antigens and xenobiotics from the luminal environment into the mucosal tissues and circulatory system. This barrier comprises several structures [81], where the TJs are the most apical components of the junctional complex and are the main gatekeepers of the epithelial paracellular passage. TJ barrier disruption and increased paracellular permeability, followed by permeation of luminal pro-inflammatory molecules can activate the mucosal immune system, resulting in chronic inflammation and tissue damage [75]. Intestinal TJ barrier is evidenced to have a critical role in the pathogenesis of intestinal and systemic diseases [82-84]. Under physio-pathological conditions, pro-inflammatory cytokines, antigens and pathogens contribute to barrier impairment [85,86]. Considering the TJs integrity impairments under inflamed conditions, it could be assumed that NPs that lead to stress and/or inflammatory responses could also influence the TJs integrity.

Several methodological approaches allow measuring the barrier function in cell cultures, e.g. the evaluation of the transepithelial electrical resistance (TEER) and the passage of marker molecules, such as Lucifer Yellow (LY) [87]. Our results revealed that under the influence of Ag-NPs < 20 nm, a disruption of the barrier integrity occurs. In figure 2A the TEER values of both mono- and co-cultures of Caco-2 cells after 3h of incubation with different concentrations of Ag-NPs are shown. TEER values decreased as Ag-NPs concentration increased, even though the reduction was less obvious in co-culture conditions – a model that is closer to the physiological conditions of FAE.

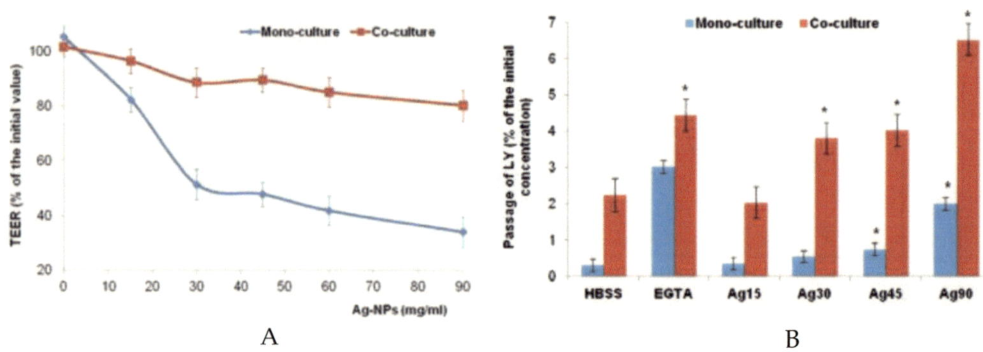

Figure 2. TEER values (A) and LY passage (B) of mono- and co-cultures of Caco-2 cells upon incubation with Ag-NPs (NM-300K, JRC repository, Ispra, IT) at 15 – 90 µg/ml. Experiments were conducted on mono- and co-cultures (*i.e.* Caco-2 cells with Raji B lymphocytes) cultivated for 21 days in polycarbonate bicameral inserts with 3 µm pore size (Transwell™, Corning Costar, NY) to reach a full differentiation and, for co-cultures, partial conversion into M like cells. TEER values were measured via Millicell-ERS volt-ohm meter (World Precision Instruments, Sarasota, FL) at the beginning and after 3h incubation period with Ag-NPs. The transport of LY was observed during 3h period with a 30 min sampling time from the BL compartment. Both the changes in TEER values ($P<0.0001$) and the LY passage ($P<0.003$) were calculated as a percentage from the initial value. Data represent the means ± SEM of 4 independent experiments. *Samples significantly different from the control (results were considered significant at $P<0,05$).

The passage of LY was evaluated by the amount of LY that passed from AP to BL compartment (Figure 2B). The presence of Ag-NPs increased the level of LY in the BL compartment that was dependent on the NP concentration. These results are in correlation with the NP-induced reduction of TEER values. Interestingly, in contrast to TEER results, the co-cultures had more elevated rate of LY passage than the corresponding mono-cultures.

To have an idea about the molecular mechanisms of the Ag-NPs-induced barrier integrity disruption, an immunostaining with confocal microscopy analysis of two TJs proteins occludin and ZO-1 was realized. As illustrated on Figure 3, in Ag-NP-treated cells the continuity of both occludin and ZO-1 was disrupted with the control comparison and the aggregation of both proteins was observed. It should further be noted that mono-cultures were more susceptible to the influence of Ag-NPs than co-cultures and the alterations in proteins distributions were more visible in mono-cultures. The immunostaining results in turn confirmed the TEER data, where a more obvious reduction was estimated in the case of mono-cultures (Figure 2).

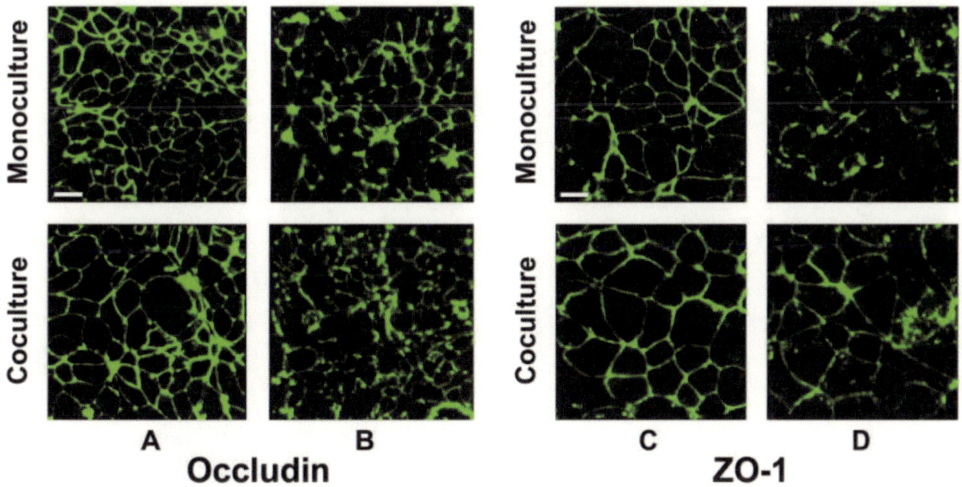

Figure 3. Subcellular localization of the occludin and ZO-1 TJs scaffolding proteins. Mono- and co-cultures of Caco-2 cells grown on bicameral inserts were treated with Ag-NPs (45 µg/ml) for 3h and then processed for immunostaining (B and D). Untreated cells were used as controls (A and C). In order to visualize the occludin and ZO-1 mouse anti-Occludin and mouse anti-ZO-1 (both from Invitrogen) were used as primary antibodies, as well as Alexa Fluor 488 goat anti-mouse (Invitrogen) as the secondary antibody. Images were collected by confocal laser scanning microscope; scale bars are 15 and 25 µm for occludin and ZO-1 staining, respectively.

The observed changes were reversible at low Ag-NPs concentrations (up to 30 µg/ml): the TEER values and TJs proteins distributions were recovered until the control level. Other NPs were also reported to possess the ability to open the TJs. For instance, the chitosan NPs were capable to open transiently and reversibly the epithelial TJs [88].

In contrast to Ag-NPs, we observed no change neither in TEER value and LY passage rate, nor TJs proteins distributions upon incubation of cell mono- and co-cultures with amorphous SiO_2 < 25 nm (NM-200, JRC repository, Ispra, IT) (results not shown). These findings provide additional evidence that the major input in the NPs-mediated barrier integrity disruption seems to belong to the charge of the NPs. Particularly, it has been previously reported that neutral and low concentrations of anionic NPs have no effect on blood-brain barrier integrity, in contrast to anionic NPs at high concentrations and cationic NPs [89]. A number of recent *in vitro* and *in vivo* studies highlight the importance of NPs surface charge for cellular uptake and biodistribution [90-92], indicating that for the majority of NPs the positive surface charge enhances cellular internalization [92-94]. The latter is likely linked to the adsorption of different bio-molecules at the surface of NPs, dependent on surface charge, as well as on chemical characteristics of NPs [95].

Another underlying condition in the TJs disruption is likely to be the cellular oxidative stress possibly induced by NPs [96]. Our results have shown that the fluorescence intensity of an oxidative stress indicator dichlorofluorescein was increased upon exposure of cells to Ag-NPs within a 3h time period (Figure 4). The ROS generation induction was dependent on NPs concentration reaching from about 1,5 to 3-fold increase, as compared with the untreated cells. Thus one mechanism of toxicity of Ag-NPs could likely be mediated by oxidative stress, already reported to be involved in the modulation of TJs integrity [97].

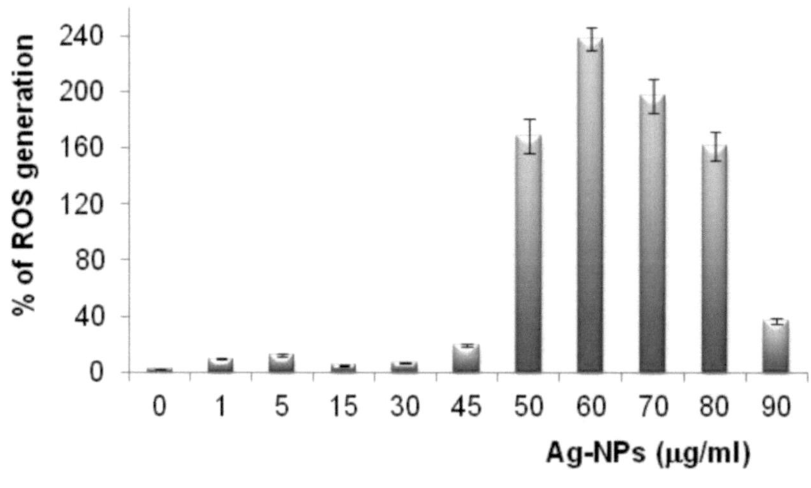

Figure 4. Effect of Ag-NPs (5 – 90 µg/ml) on intracellular ROS generation in Caco-2 cells. The ROS generation was investigated using the dichlorofluorescein (DCFH) assay. After being oxidized by intracellular oxidants, DCFH becomes DCF and emits fluorescence, quantification of which is a reliable estimation of overall oxygen species generation. The intracellular ROS level is presented as a percentage of the corresponding initial value after incubation together with NPs during 3h at 37°C. Data represent means ± SEM of 3 experiments with 3 different samples per condition, P<0.0001.

Altogether, the results reveal that some NPs, e.g. chitosan or Ag-NPs may enhance the epithelial barrier permeability and could therefore serve as an effective carrier for oral drug delivery [44]. However, it should be noted that the epithelial permeability increase in turn might favor the systemic absorption of ENMs, toxins and other xenobiotics, and would likely cause immune activation.

5. Potential toxicity of ENMs in the case of altered intestinal physiology

It has been reported that the exposure to some NPs is associated with the occurrence of autoimmune diseases, such as systemic lupus erythematosus, scleroderma, and rheumatoid arthritis [35]. Diseases, such as diabetes, may also lead to an increased absorption of particles in the GIT [41]. Furthermore, inflammation may lead to the uptake and translocation of particles of up to 20 nm [98]. Thus, an issue to be considered in relation to ENMs ingestion is a possible increase in their intestinal absorption in the case of systemic exposures, such as in Inflammatory Bowel Disease (IBD) and/or Crohn's disease (CD), which represent chronic disorders characterized by recurrent and serious inflammation of the GIT [99]. Crohn's disease affects primarily people in developed countries, where the highest incidence rates and prevalence for CD and ulcerative colitis (UC) have been reported from northern Europe, the United Kingdom and North America [100] with a frequency of 1 in 1,000 people in the Western world [5]. However, reports of increasing incidence and prevalence from other areas of the world, e.g. southern or central Europe, Asia, Africa, and Latin America state the progressive nature and worldwide rise of these diseases [100].

An abnormal intestinal barrier function plays a pivotal role in IBD [101]. Increased intestinal permeability has been reproducibly described in patients with CD, which is likely a predisposing factor to the pathogenesis and impaired epithelial resistance [102,103]. A barrier dysfunction has been reported in the colonic mucosa of patients with Irritable Bowel Syndrome (IBS), which results from increased paracellular permeability, presumably by an altered expression of ZO-1 [104]. Moreover, stress is believed to contribute to induction of IBS and recurrence of intestinal inflammation and can increase the paracellular permeability [105]. It should be noted that mediators of inflammation, such as ROS, endotoxins (lipopolysaccharides) and cytokines are able to provoke the disruption of TJs and thereby increase the paracellular permeability [97]. Significant changes in epithelial TJs structure and function were also observed in UC [106,107]. Thus the altered intestinal permeability could certainly be a result of disease progression, but there is evidence that it might also be the primary causative event.

Recently it was suggested that there could be an association between high levels of dietary NPs uptake and CD. Experimental results indicate that the accumulation of insoluble NPs in humans may be responsible for the compromised gastrointestinal functioning, as described in the case of CD and UC [5]. Microscopy studies have also shown that macrophages located in lymphoid tissue can uptake NPs, e.g. spherical anatase (TiO_2) with size of 100-200 nm from food additives, aluminosilicates of 100-400 nm typical of natural clay, and environmental silicates of 100-700 nm [108]. According to another study, some insoluble NPs, such as TiO_2, ZnO and SiO_2, upon their absorption and passage across the GIT, come into contact with and adsorb calcium ions and lipopolysaccharides. The resulting NPs–calcium–lipopolysaccharide conjugates activate both peripheral blood mononuclear cells and intestinal phagocytes, which are usually resistant to stimulation [109].

Despite the insufficiency of data linking the NPs consumption to the initiation of CD and UC, it seems that particles of 0.1 – 1.0 μm may be adjuvant triggers for the exacerbation of these diseases [110]. Micro and NPs have been constantly found in organs, e.g. in colon tissue and blood of patients affected by cancer, CD, and UC, while in healthy subjects NPs were absent [111]. Some evidence suggests that dietary NPs may exacerbate inflammation in CD [6]. More precisely, some members of the population may have a genetic predisposition where they are more affected by the intake of NPs, and therefore develop CD [9]. It has been also reported that micro- and NPs in colon tissues may lead to cancer and CD progression [111]. By contrast, a diet low in calcium and exogenous micro- and NPs has been shown to alleviate the symptoms of CD [5]. This analysis is still controversial, with some proposing that an abnormal response to dietary NPs may be the cause of this disease, and not an excess intake [6].

Although there is a clear association between particle exposure/uptake and CD, little is known of the exact role of the phagocytosing cells in the intestinal epithelium and particularly of the pathophysiological role of M cells. It has been shown that M cells are lost from the epithelium in the case of CD. Other studies found that endocytotic capacity of M cells is induced under various immunological conditions, e.g. a greater uptake of particles of 0.1 – 10 μm has been demonstrated in the inflamed colonic mucosa of rats compared to non-ulcerated tissue [109,112].

Thus more vulnerable members of the population, *i.e.* those with pre-existing digestive disorders, may potentially be more affected by the presence of ENMs, although, in contrast, ENMs may offer many potential routes to therapies for the same diseases. The diseases associated with gastrointestinal uptake of NPs, such as CD and UC have no cure and often require surgical intervention. Treatments are aimed at maintaining the disease in remission and mainly consist of anti-inflammatory drugs and specially formulated liquid meals [5]. If dietary NPs are conclusively shown to cause these chronic diseases, their use in food should be avoided or strictly regulated.

6. Potential health risks/benefits of nanotechnology-based food materials

The absorption, distribution, metabolism and excretion (ADME) parameters are likely to be influenced by the aggregation, agglomeration, dispersability, size, solubility, and surface area, charge and physico-chemistry of NPs [113]. Amongst these parameters the size, chemical composition and surface treatment appear to be the most critical ones for nanotoxicity issues [114]. Chemical composition, beside the chemical nature of the NP itself, also includes the surface coating of the NPs [115]. Coatings can be used to stabilize the NPs in solution, to prevent clustering or to add functionality to the NPs, depending on its intended use. Surface coatings can influence the reactivity of the NPs in various media, including water, biological fluids and laboratory test media [116,117]. From this point of view the interaction of NPs with food components is another aspect that may need consideration and about which little information is currently available. The possible interaction of food components may alter the physicochemical properties of ENMs that in turn may influence their passage through the GIT and their ADME properties.

ENMs, with their very large surface areas, may adsorb bio-molecules on their surface upon contact with food and/or biological fluids to form a bio-molecular "corona" [96,118]. Depending on the nature of the corona, the behavior of the NPs may differ, and there could be the potential for novel toxicities non-characteristic neither for the non-coated NPs, nor for the adsorbed biological material. These bio-molecules include proteins, lipids, sugars, different secondary metabolites and it is those interactions that may actually determine how ENMs will interact with living systems. Thus, the foregoing information on the food should be considered carefully, taking into account its major ingredients or components, which have physiological properties likely to influence the absorption/translocation of ENMs in the GIT.

Several studies have demonstrated that various food components provide beneficial anti-inflammatory and anti-mutagenic effects in the GIT. Although the information regarding these effects on intestinal TJ barrier integrity is limited, some results are available e.g. for glutamine [119,120] and fatty acids [121-123]. A growing number of data suggest the potential protective effect of phenolic compounds on the epithelial barrier function and their anti-inflammatory properties [124,125]. In particular, certain flavonoids that represent a part of human daily nutrition, e.g. epigallocatechin gallate, genistein, myricetin, quercetin and kaempferol are reported to exhibit promotive and protective effects on intestinal TJ barrier [124,126].

We have observed (unshown results) that quercetin attenuates the cytotoxic effect of Ag-NPs on Caco-2 cells, as well as allows recovering of the epithelial barrier function, which was evidenced by the recovery up to the initial value of the TEER and the LY passage rate in both mono- and co-cultures. The immunostaining analysis of occludin and ZO-1 also revealed the recovery of the protein distributions in the presence of quercetin, which additionally suggests the protective effect of the latter upon the harmful effects of Ag-NPs. In a similar study it was reported that positively charged Ni-NPs can efficiently enhance the permeation and uptake of quercetin into cancer cells, which can have important biomedical and chemotherapeutic applications [127].

A number of published reports indicate the potential application of antioxidants [10,128-130] and anti-inflammatory drugs [6,131] that are able to treat the adverse health effects caused by NPs. For instance, berberine, an alkaloid with a potential biomedical application, has been shown to attenuate TJ barrier defects induced by TNF-α, known to disrupt TJ integrity in IBD [132]. It has been reported that rats that underwent instillation of NPs into the lungs together with an antioxidant, *i.e.* nacystelin, showed an inflammation decrease up to 60% in comparison to those exposed to NPs alone [10].

To have an idea about the state of Ag-NPs in the presence of quercetin, NPs were characterized by transmission electron microscopy (TEM) (Figure 5). It could be seen that in the presence of quercetin a "capping" of Ag-NPs occurs, which confirms already existing data on Ag-NPs stabilization with reducing agents. Surface-active molecules, such as terpenoids and/or reducing sugars are believed to stabilize the NPs in the solutions, *i.e.* they are believed to react with the silver ions (Ag^+) and stabilize the Ag-NPs [133,134]. Flavonoids have been suggested to be responsible for the reduction of Ag^+ to Ag-NPs [135]. Fatty acids such as stearic, palmitic and lauric acids are used as agents for the formation and stabilization of Ag-NPs [136].

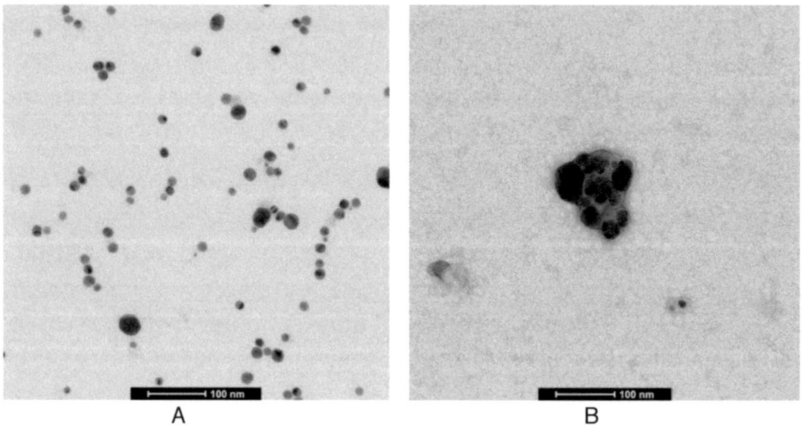

Figure 5. TEM analysis of Ag-NPs < 20 nm (NM-300K) alone (A) and in the presence of quercetin (B). The average size of Ag-NPs was about 20 nm, scale bar: 100 nm. NPs were characterized by transmission electron miscroscopy (TEM) (Technai Spirit TEM, FEI Company, Eindhoven, NL) by Dr. J. Mast at the Electron Microscopy Unit of the Veterinary and Agrochemical Research Centre VAR-CODA-CERVA, Uccle, BE.

Another major phenolic compound present in human diet is resveratrol, which possesses many beneficial health effects [137-141]. Considering abundance and health-promoting effects of resveratrol, we have also investigated its potential protective activity against the Ag-NP-induced cytotoxicity. The results indicated no protective effect of resveratrol and moreover, at a concentration of 100 μM, non-toxic by itself, it increased the toxic effect of Ag-NPs, illustrating a synergistic effect.

To conclude, it could be assumed that phenolic compounds, depending on the nature and concentration, may exhibit different effects on cells in the presence on NPs. This is not surprising, as it is known that these substances, depending on concentration, may exhibit both beneficial and toxic effects [141].

7. Future perspectives

Nanotechnology offers a wide range of opportunities for the development of innovative products and applications in agriculture, food production, processing, preservation and packaging. However, the present state of knowledge still contains many gaps preventing risk assessors from establishing the safety for many of the possible food related applications of nanotechnology [142]. Currently the routine assessment of ENMs *in situ* in the food or feed matrix is not possible, as well as equally impossible to determine physico-chemical state of ENMs, which increases the uncertainty in the exposure assessment. Complex matrices present in the food complicate the detection and characterization of

ENMs in final food/feed products, which itself contain a wide range of natural structures in the nano-size scale. The information on the potential of ENMs to cross the epithelial barriers, such as the GIT, blood-brain, placenta and blood-milk barriers are also important for hazard identification. It is also clear that the evaluation of the pro-inflammatory potential of ENMs is another issue of current importance, as the inflammation itself is associated with a number of high frequency diseases, e.g. cancer, diabetes, bowel diseases, etc.

From the above discussion and the research presented in this review, the need for more toxicology research on manufactured ENMs is clear. In addition to standard tests, there is a need to develop appropriate and rapid screening methods to be able to control the exposure level, as well as improved models that will permit to assess the toxicity and allow better understanding of the mechanisms that are involved. Employment of developed and well characterized *in vitro* cell culture systems may be relevant for evaluation of gut and immune responses to ENMs and to adapt conditions to specific health conditions or to consumer groups with special needs, such as in the case of bowel diseases. Further studies are necessary to assess whether the characteristic daily intake of ENMs may exacerbate or trigger disease symptoms in subjects with increased susceptibility, such as inflamed state of the GIT in the case of IBD, CD, UC, or even be its cause.

Another aspect deserving thorough investigation is the possible interaction of ENMs with food/feed components, which in turn could influence the overall behavior and effect of not only ENMs, but also the bioavailability of food components.

Acknowledgments

Authors thank to Dr. Jan Mast, head of the Electron Microscopy Unit in VAR-CODA-CERVA, Uccle, Belgium for scientific and technical support in the realization of Transmission Electron Microscopy analysis, as well as to the Biological Imaging Platform (IMAB) of the Université Catholique de Louvain (Louvain-la-Neuve, Belgium) for the realization of the confocal microscopy. This study was funded by the Belgian Federal Public Service and Belgian Federal Science Policy (BELSPO).

Author details

Alina Martirosyan, Madeleine Polet, Alexandra Bazes, Thérèse Sergent and Yves-Jacques Schneider

Institute of Life Sciences (Laboratory of Cellular, Nutritional and Toxicological Biochemistry) UCLouvain, Louvain-la-Neuve, Belgium

References

[1] Regulation (EU) No 1169/2011 of the European Parliament and of the Council of 25 October 2011 on the provision of food information to consumers. Official Journal of the European Union 2011;L304 18-63.

[2] Annual report of the Food Safety Authority of Ireland (FSAI) 2008. The relevance for food safety of applications of nanotechnology in the Food and Feed Industries. Available from http://www.fsai.ie/resources_and_publications/annual_reports.html.

[3] Sanguansri P, Augustin MA. Nanoscale materials development – a food industry perspective. Trends in Food Science & Technology 2006;17(10) 547-556.

[4] Chaudhry Q, Aitken R, Scotter R, Blackburn J, Ross B, Boxall A, Castle L, Watkins R. Applications and implications for nanotechnologies in the food sector. Food Additives and Contaminants 2008;25(3) 241-258.

[5] Lomer M, Thompson R, Powell J. Fine and ultrafine particles of the diet: influence on the mucosal immune response and association with Crohn's disease. Proceedings of the Nutrition Society 2002;61(1) 23-30.

[6] Lomer M, Hutchinson C, Volkert S, Greenfield S, Catterall A, Thompson R, Powell J. Dietary sources of inorganic microparticles and their intake in healthy subjects and patients with Crohn's disease. British Journal of Nutrition 2004;92(6) 947-955.

[7] Meeting report of the Food and Agriculture Organization of the United Nations and World Health Organization (FAO/WHO) expert meeting on the application of nanotechnologies in the food and agriculture sectors: potential food safety implications. 2010. Available from http://www.fao.org/docrep/012/i1434e/i1434e00.pdf.

[8] Oberdörster G, Maynard A, Donaldson K, Castranova V, Fitzpatrick J, Ausman K, Carter J, Karn B, Kreyling W, Lai D, Olin S, Monteiro-Riviere N, Warheit D, Yang H. Principles for characterizing the potential human health effects from exposure to nanomaterials: elements of a screening strategy. Particle and Fibre Toxicology 2005a; 2 8.

[9] Oberdörster E. Manufactured nanomaterials (Fullerenes, C60) induce oxidative stress in the brain of juvenile largemouth bass. Environmental Health Perspectives 2004;112(10) 1058-1062.

[10] Donaldson K, Stone V. Current hypotheses on the mechanisms of toxicity of ultrafine particles. Annali dell'Istituto Superiore di Sanita 2003;39(3) 405-410.

[11] Sayes C, Gobin A, Ausman K, Mendez J, West J, Colvina V. Nano-C60 cytotoxicity is due to lipid peroxidation. Biomaterials 2005;26(36) 7587–7595.

[12] Reeves J, Davies S, Dodd NJ, Jha A. Hydroxyl radicals (OH) are associated with titanium dioxide (TiO_2) nanoparticle-induced cytotoxicity and oxidative DNA damage in fish cells. Mutation Research 2008;640(1-2) 113-122.

[13] Brown D, Donaldson K, Borm P, Schins R, Dehnhardt M, Gilmour P, Jimenez L, Stone V. Calcium and ROS-mediated activation of transcription factors and TNF-alpha cytokine gene expression in macrophages exposed to ultrafine particles. Am. J. Physiology Lung Cellular and Molecular Physiology 2004;286(2) L344-L353.

[14] Brown D, Donaldson K, Stone V. Effects of PM10 in human peripheral blood monocytes and J774 macrophages. Respiratory Research 2004;5 29.

[15] Long H, Shi T, Borm P J, Määttä J, Husgafvel-Pursiainen K, Savolainen K, Krombach F. ROS-mediated TNF-alpha and MIP-2 gene expression in alveolar macrophages exposed to pine dust. Particle Fibre Toxicology 2004;1(1) 3.

[16] Kim S, Choi J, Choi J, Chung K, Park K, Yi J, Ryu D. Oxidative stress-dependent toxicity of silver nanoparticles in human hepatoma cells. Toxicology In Vitro 2009;(6) 1076-1084

[17] Gurr J, Wang A, Chen C, Jan K. Ultrafine titanium dioxide particles in the absence of photoactivation can induce oxidative damage to human bronchial epithelial cells. Toxicology 2005;213(1-2) 66-73.

[18] Mroz R, Schins R, Li H, Jimenez L, Drost E, Holownia A, MacNee W, Donaldson K. Nanoparticle-driven DNA damage mimics irradiation-related carcinogenesis pathways. European Respiratory Journal 2008;31(2) 241-251.

[19] Rahman Q, Lohani M, Dopp E, Pemsel H, Jonas L, Weiss D, Schiffmann D. Evidence that ultrafine titanium dioxide induces micronuclei and apoptosis in syrian hamster embryo fibroblasts. Environmental Health Perspectives 2002;110(8) 797-800.

[20] Papageorgiou I, Brown C, Schins R, Singh S, Newson R, Davis S, Fisher J, Ingham E, Case C. The effect of nano- and micron-sized particles of cobalt-chromium alloy on human fibroblasts in vitro. Biomaterials 2007;28(19) 2946-2958.

[21] Ghio A, Stonehuerner J, Dailey L, Carter J. Metals associated with both the water-soluble and insoluble fractions of an ambient air pollution particle catalyze an oxidative stress. Inhalation Toxicology 1999;11(1) 37-49.

[22] Hussain S, Hess K, Gearhart J, Geiss K, Schlager J. In vitro toxicity of nanoparticles in BRL3A rat liver cells. Toxicology In Vitro 2005;19(7) 975-983.

[23] Lin W, Huang Y-W, Zhou X-D, Ma Y. In vitro toxicity of silica nanoparticles in human lung cancer cells. Toxicology and Applied Pharmacology 2006;217(3) 252-259

[24] Pulskamp K, Diabaté S, Krug H. Carbon nanotubes show no sign of acute toxicity but induce cellular reactive oxygen species in dependence on contaminants. Toxicology Letters 2007;168(1) 58-74.

[25] Singh S, Shi T, Duffin R, Albrecht C, van Berlo D, Höhr D, Fubini B, Martra G, Fenoglio I, Borm P, Schins R. Endocytosis, oxidative stress and IL-8 expression in human lung epithelial cells upon treatment with fine and ultrafine TiO_2: Role of the specific

surface area and of surface methylation of the particles. Toxicology and Applied Pharmacology 2007;222(2) 141-151

[26] Borm P, Robbins D, Haubold S, Kuhlbusch T, Fissan H, Donaldson K, Schins R, Stone V, Kreyling W, Lademann J, Krutmann J, Warheit D, Oberdorster E. The potential risks of nanomaterials: a review carried out for ECETOC. Particle and Fibre Toxicology 2006;3 11.

[27] Card J; Zeldin D, Bonner J, Nestmann E. Pulmonary applications and toxicity of engineered nanoparticles. Am. Journal of Physiology, Lung Cellular and Molecular Physiology 2008;295(3) L400-411.

[28] Nel A, Xia T, Madler L, Li N. Toxic potential of materials at the nanolevel. Science 2006; 311(5761) 622-627.

[29] Oberdörster G, Oberdörster E, Oberdörster J. Nanotoxicology: an emerging discipline evolving from studies of ultrafine particles. Environmental Health Perspectives 2005b;113(7) 823-839.

[30] Xia T, Kovochich M, Brant J, Hotze M, Sempf J, Oberley T, Sioutas C, Yeh J, Wiesner M, Nel A. Comparison of the abilities of ambient and manufactured nanoparticles to induce cellular toxicity according to an oxidative stress paradigm. Nano Letters 2006;6(8) 1794-1807.

[31] Tsai Y, Oca-Cossio J, Agering K, Simpson N, Atkinson M, Wasserfall C, Constantinidis I, Sigmund W. Novel synthesis of cerium oxide nanoparticles for free radical scavenging. Nanomedicine 2007;2(3) 325-232.

[32] Bhol K, Schechter P. Effects of nanocrystalline silver (NPI 32101) in a rat model of ulcerative colitis. Digestive Diseases and Sciences 2007;52(10) 2732-4272.

[33] Takenaka S, Karg E, Roth C, Schulz H, Ziesenis A, Heinzmann U, Schramel P, Heyder J. Pulmonary and systemic distribution of inhaled ultrafine silver particles in rats Environmental Health Perspectives 2001;109(Suppl. 4) 547-551.

[34] Hagens W, Oomen A, de Jong W, Cassee F, Sips A. What do we (need to) know about the kinetic properties of nanoparticles in the body? Regulatory Toxicology and Pharmacology 2007;49(3) 217-219.

[35] Buzea C, Pacheco I, Robbie K. Nanomaterials and nanoparticles: sources and toxicity. Biointerphases 2007;4 MR17-71.

[36] Hillyer J, Albrecht R. Gastrointestinal persorption and tissue distribution of differently sized colloidal gold nanoparticles. Journal of Pharmaceutical Sciences 2001;90(12) 1927-1936.

[37] Jani P, Halbert GW, Langridge J, Florence A. The uptake and translocation of latex nanospheres and microspheres after oral administration to rats. Journal of Pharmacy and Pharmacology 1989;41(12) 809-812.

[38] Hussain N, Florence A. Utilizing bacterial mechanisms of epithelial cell entry: invasin-induced oral uptake of latex nanoparticles. Pharmaceutical Research 1998;15(1) 153-156.

[39] Hussain N, Jani P, Florence A. Enhanced oral uptake of tomato lectin conjugated nanoparticles in the rat. Pharmaceutical Research 1997;14(5) 613-618.

[40] Hillery A, Jani P, Florence A. Comparative, quantitative study of lymphoid and non-lymphoid uptake of 60 nm polystyrene particles. J of Drug Targeting 1994;2(2) 151-156

[41] Hoet P, Bruske-Hohlfeld I, Salata O. Nanoparticles - known and unkown health risks. Journal of Nanobiotechnology 2004;2(1) 12-27.

[42] Card J, Jonaitis T, Tafazoli S, Magnuson B. An appraisal of the published literature on the safety and toxicity of food-related nanomaterials. Critical Reviews in Toxicology 2011;41(1) 20-49.

[43] Magnuson B, Jonaitis T, Card J. A brief review of the occurrence, use, and safety of food-related nanomaterials. Journal of Food Science (2011;76(6) R126-133.

[44] Des Rieux A, Fievez V, Garinot M, Schneider Y-J, Preat V. Nanoparticles as potential oral delivery systems of proteins and vaccines: a mechanistic approach. Journal of Control Release 2006;116(1) 1-27.

[45] European Food Safety Authority (EFSA): Scientific Opinion of the Scientific Committee on the Potential Risks Arising from Nanoscience and Nanotechnologies on Food and Feed Safety. 2009. Available from http://www.efsa.europa.eu/EFSA/Scientific_Opinion/sc_op_ej958_nano_en,0.pdf?ssbinary=true

[46] Kalgaonkar S, Lonnerdal B. Receptor-mediated uptake of ferritin-bound iron by human intestinal Caco-2 cells. Journal of Nutritional Biochemistry 2009; 20(4) 304-311.

[47] Des Rieux A, Ragnarsson EG, Gullberg E, Preat V, Schneider Y-J, Artursson P. Transport of nanoparticles across an in vitro model of the human intestinal follicle associated epithelium. European Journal of Pharmaceutical Sciences 2005;25(4-5) 455-465.

[48] Seifert J, Haraszti B, Sass W. The influence of age and particle number on absorption of polystyrene particles from the rat gut. J of Anatomy 1996;189(Pt 3) 483-486.

[49] Gebert A, Rothkotter H, Pabst R. M cells in Peyer's patches of the intestine. International Review of Cytology 1996;167 91-159.

[50] Beier R, Gebert A. Kinetics of particle uptake in the domes of Peyer's patches. Am Journal of Physiology 1998;275(1 Pt 1) G130-137.

[51] Bockmann J, Lahl H, Eckert T, Unterhalt B. Blood titanium levels before and after oral administration titanium dioxide. Pharmazie 2000;55(2) 140-143.

[52] Volkheimer G. Passage of particles through the wall of the gastrointestinal tract. Environmental Health Perspectives 1974;9 215-225.

[53] Volkheimer G. Persorption of microparticles. Pathologe 1993;14(5) 247-252.

[54] Powell J, Whitehead M, Lee S, Thompson R. Mechanisms of gastrointestinal absorption: dietary minerals and the influence of beverage ingestion. Food Chemistry 1994;51(4) 381-388.

[55] Moyes S, Smyth S, Shipman A, Long S, Morris J, Carr K. Parameters influencing intestinal epithelial permeability and microparticle uptake in vitro. International Journal of Pharmacology 2007;337(1-2) 133-141.

[56] Thurn K, Arora H, Paunesku T, Wu A, Brown E, Doty C, Kremer J, Woloschak G. Endocytosis of titanium dioxide nanoparticles in prostate cancer PC-3M cells. Nanomedicine 2011;7(2) 123-130.

[57] Wang S, Lee C, Chiou A. Wei P. Size-dependent endocytosis of gold nanoparticles studied by three-dimensional mapping of plasmonic scattering images. Journal of Nanobiotechnology 2010;8 33

[58] Sun W, Fang N, Trewyn B, Tsunoda M, Slowing I, Lin V, Yeung E. Endocytosis of a single mesoporous silica nanoparticle into a human lung cancer cell observed by differential interference contrast microscopy. Analytical and Bioanalytical Chemistry 2008;391(6) 2119-2125.

[59] Hu L, Mao Z, Zhang Y, Gao C. Influences of size of silica particles on the cellular endocytosis, exocytosis and cell activity of HepG2 cells. Journal of Nanoscience Letters 2011;1(1)1-16.

[60] Kim S, Choi I. Phagocytosis and endocytosis of silver nanoparticles induce interleukin-8 production in human macrophages. Yonsei Medical Journal 2012;53(3) 654-657.

[61] Jepson M, Simmons N, Savidge T, James P, Hirst B. Selective binding and transcytosis of latex microspheres by rabbit intestinal M cells. Cell and Tissue Research 1993;271(3) 399-405.

[62] Seifert J, Sass W. Intestinal absorption of macromolecules and small particles. Digestive Diseases 1990;8(3) 169-178.

[63] Florence A, Hussain N. Transcytosis of nanoparticle and dendrimer delivery systems: evolving vistas. Advanced Drug Delivery Reviews 2001;50(Suppl.1) S69-S89.

[64] Hussain N, Jaitley V, Florence A. Recent advances in the understanding of uptake of microparticulates across the gastrointestinal lymphatics. Advanced Drug Delivery Reviews 2001;50(1-2) 107-142.

[65] Des Rieux A, Fievez V, Theate I, Mast J, Preat V, Schneider Y-J. An improved in vitro model of human intestinal follicle-associated epithelium to study nanoparticle transport by M cells. European Journal of Pharmaceutical Sciences 2007;30(5) 380-391.

[66] Aprahamian M, Michel C, Humbert W, Devissaguet J, Damge C: Transmucosal passage of polyalkylcyanoacrylate nanocapsules as a new drug carrier in the small intestine. Biology of the Cell 1987;61(1-2) 69-76.

[67] Kroll A, Pillukat M, Hahn D, Schnekenburger J. Current in vitro methods in nanoparticle risk assessment: limitations and challenges. European Journal of Pharmaceutics and Biopharmaceutics 2009;72(2) 370–377.

[68] Lilienblum W, Dekant W, Foth H, Gebel T, Hengstler J, Kahl R, Kramer P, Schweinfurth H, Wollin K. Alternative methods to safety studies in experimental animals: role in the risk assessment of chemicals under the new European Chemicals Legislation (REACH). Archives of Toxicology 2008;82(4) 211-236.

[69] Artursson P, Karlson J. Correlation between oral drug absorption in humans and apparent drug permeability coefficients in human intestinal epithelial (Caco-2) cells. Biochemical and Biophysical Research Communications 1991;175(3) 880-885.

[70] Artursson P, Borchardt R. Intestinal drug absorption and metabolism in cell cultures: Caco-2 and beyond. Pharmaceutical Research 1997;14(12) 1655-1658.

[71] Chantret I, Barbat A, Dussaulx E, Brattain MG, Zweibaum A. Epithelial polarity, villin expression, and enterocytic differentiation of cultured human colon carcinoma cells: a survey of 20 cell lines. Cancer Res 1988;48(7) 1936-1942.

[72] Pinto M, Robin-Leon S, Appay M, Kedinger M, Triadou N, Dussaulx E, Lacroix B, Simon-Assmann P, Haffen K, Fogh J, Zweibaum A. Enterocyte-like differentiation and polarization of the human colon carcinoma cell line Caco-2 in culture. Biology of the Cell 1983;47 323-330.

[73] Kraehenbuhl J, Neutra M. Epithelial M cells: differentiation and function. Annual Review of Cell and Developmental Biology 2000;16 301-332.

[74] Sansonetti P, Phalipon A. M cells as ports of entry for enteroinvasive pathogens: mechanisms of interaction, consequences for the disease process. Seminars in Immunology 1999;11(3) 193-203.

[75] Neutra M, Pringault E, Kraehenbuhl J. Antigen sampling across epithelial barriers and induction of mucosal immune responses. Annual Review of Immunology 1996;14 275-300.

[76] Kernéis S, Bogdonona A, Kraehenbuhl JP, Pringault E. Conversion by Peyer's patches lymphocytes of human enterocytes into M cells that transport bacteria. Science 1997;277(5328) 949-952.

[77] Gullberg E, Leonard M, Karlsson J, Hopkins A, Brayden D, Baird A, Artursson P. Expression of specific markers and particle transport in a new human intestinal M-cell model. Biochemical and Biophysical Research Communications 2000;279(3) 808-813.

[78] Lo D, Tynan W, Dickerson J, Scharf M, Cooper J, Byrne D, Brayden D, Higgins L, Evans C, O'Mahony DJ. Cell culture modeling of specialized tissue: identification of genes expressed specifically by follicle-associated epithelium of Peyer's patch by expression profiling of Caco-2/Raji co-cultures. International Immunology 2004;16(1) 91-99.

[79] Schulte R, Kerneis S, Klinke S, Bartels H, Preger S, Kraehenbuhl JP, Pringault E, Autenrieth IB. Translocation of Yersinia enterocoltica across reconstituted intestinal epithelial monolayers is triggered by Yersinia invasin binding to beta1 integrins apically expressed on M-like cells. Cell Microbiology 2000;2(2) 173-185.

[80] Owen R, Ermak T. Structural specializations for antigen uptake and processing in the digestive tract. Semininars in Immunopathology 1990;12(2-3) 139-152.

[81] Denker B, Nigam S. Molecular structure and assembly of the tight junctions. American Journal of Physiology 1998;274 (1 Pt2) F1-9.

[82] Turner J. Intestinal mucosal barrier function in health and disease. Nature Reviews Immunology 2009;9(11) 799-809.

[83] Clayburgh D, Shen L, Turner J. A porous defense: the leaky epithelial barrier in intestinal disease. Laboratory Investigation 2004;84(3) 282-291.

[84] Farhadi A, Banan A, Fields J, Keshavarzian A. Intestinal barrier: an interface between health and disease. Journal of Gastroenterology and Hepatology 2003;18(5) 479-497.

[85] Nusrat A, Turner J, Madara J. Molecular physiology and pathophysiology of tight junctions. IV. Regulation of tight junctions by extracellular stimuli: nutrients, cytokines, and immune cells. American Journal of Physiology, Gastrointestinal and Liver Physiology 2000;279(5) G851-857.

[86] Capaldo C, Nusrat A. Cytokine regulation of tight junctions. Biochimica et Biophysica Acta 2009;1788(4) 864-871.

[87] Bailey, C.. A., Bryla, P., Malick, A.W., The use of intestinal epithelial cell culture model, Caco-2, in pharmaceutical development. Advanced Drug Delivery Reviews 1996. 22(1-2) 85-103.

[88] Sonaje K, Lin K, Tseng M, Wey S, Su F, Chuang EY Hsu C, Chen C, Sung H. Effects of chitosan-nanoparticle-mediated tight junction opening on the oral absorption of endotoxins. Biomaterials 2011;32(33) 8712-8721.

[89] Lockman PR, Koziara JM, Mumper RJ, Allen DD. Nanoparticle surface charges alter blood-brain barrier integrity and permeability. J Drug Target. 2004;12(9-10) 635-41.

[90] He C, Hu Y, Yin L, Tang C, Yin C. Effects of particle size and surface charge on cellular uptake and biodistribution of polymeric nanoparticles. Biomaterials 2010;31(13) 3657-3666.

[91] Xiao K, Li Y, Luo J, Lee JS, Xiao W, Gonik AM, Agarwal RG, Lam KS. The effect of surface charge on in vivo biodistribution of PEG-oligocholic acid based micellar nanoparticles. Biomaterials 2011;32(13) 3435-3446.

[92] Yue Z, Wei W, Lv P, Yue H, Wang L, Su Z, Ma G. Surface charge affects cellular uptake and intracellular trafficking of chitosan-based nanoparticles. Biomacromolecules 2011;12(7) 2440-2446.

[93] Kelf T, Sreenivasan V, Sun J, Kim E, Goldys E, Zvyagin A. Non-specific cellular uptake of surface-functionalized quantum dots. Nanotechnology 2010;21(28) 285105.

[94] Chen L, McCrate J, Lee J, Li H. The role of surface charge on the uptake and biocompatibility of hydroxyapatite nanoparticles with osteoblast cells. Nanotechnology 2011;22(10) 105708.

[95] Lundqvist M, Stigler J, Elia G, Lynch I, Cedervall T, Dawson K. Nanoparticle size and surface properties determine the protein corona with possible implications for biological impact. Proceedings of the National Academy of Sciences of the USA 2008;105(38) 14265-14270.

[96] Schreibelt G, Kooij G, Reijerkerk A, van Doorn R, Gringhuis S, van der Pol S, Weksler B, Romero I, Couraud P, Piontek J, Blasig I, Dijkstra C, Ronken E, de Vries H. Reactive oxygen species alter brain endothelial tight junction dynamics via RhoA, PI3 kinase, and PKB signaling. FASEB Journal 2007;21(13) 3666-3676.

[97] Sheth P, Basuroy S, Li C, Naren A, Rao R. Role of phosphaditylinositol 3-kinase in oxidative stress-induced disruption of tight junctions. Journal of Biological Chemistry 2003, 278(49) 49239-49245.

[98] Ballestri M, Baraldi A, Gatti A M, Furci L, Bagni A, Loria P, Rapaa M, Carulli N, Albertazzi A. Liver and kidney foreign bodies granulomatosis in a patient with malocclusion, bruxism, and worn dental prostheses. Gastroenterology 2001;121(5) 1234-1238.

[99] Sheth P, Delos Santos N, Seth A, LaRusso N, Rao R. Lipopolysaccharide disrupts tight junctions in cholangiocyte monolayers by c-Scc-, TLR4-, and LPB-dependent mechanism. American Journal of Physiology, Gastrointestinal and Liver Physiology 2007;293(1) G308-318.

[100] Loftus EV Jr. Clinical epidemiology of inflammatory bowel disease: incidence, prevalence, and environmental influences. Gastroenterology 2004;126(6) 1504-1517.

[101] Laukoetter M, Nava P, Nusrat A. Role of intestinal barrier in inflammatory bowel disease. World Journal of Gastroenterology 2008;14(3) 401-407.

[102] Teahon K, Smethurst P, Levi A, Menzies I, Bjarnason I. Intestinal permeability in patients with Crohn's disease and their first degree relatives. Gut 1992;33(3) 320-323.

[103] Peeters M, Geypens B, Claus D, Nevens H, Ghoos Y, Verbeke G, Baert F, Vermeire S, Vlietinck R, Rutgeerts P. Clustering of increased small intestinal permeability in families with Crohn's disease. Gastroenterology 1997;113(3) 802-807.

[104] Piche T, Barabara G, Aubert P, Bruley dês Varannes S, Dainese R, Nano J, Cremon C, Strangellini V, de Giorgio R, Galmiche J, Neunlist M. Impaired intestinal barrier integrity in the colon of patients with irritable bowel syndrome: involvement of soluble mediators. Gut 2009;58(2) 196-201.

[105] Eutamene H, Bueno L. Role of probiotics in correction abnormalities of colonic flora induced by stress. Gut 2007;56(11) 1495-1497.

[106] Schmitz H, Fromm M, Bentzel C, Scholz P, Detjen K, Mankertz J, Bode H, Epple H, Riecken E, Schulzke J. Tumor necrosis factor-α (TNF-alpha) regulates the epithelial barrier in the human intestinal cell line HT-29/B6. Journal of Cell Science 1999;112(Pt 1) 137-146.

[107] Schulzke J, Ploeger S, Amasheh M, Fromm A, Zeissig S, Troeger H, Richter J, Bojarski C, Shumann M. Fromm M. Epithelial tight junctions in intestinal inflammation. Annals of the New York Academy of Sciences 2009;1165 294-300.

[108] Powell J, Ainley C, Harvey R, Manson I, Kendall M, Sankey E, Dhillon A, Thompson R. Characterization of inorganic microparticles in pigment cells of human gut associated lymphoid tissue Gut 1996;38(3) 390-395

[109] Powell J, Harvey R, Ashwood P, Wolstencroft R, Gershwin M, Thompson R. Immune potentiation of ultrafine dietary particles in normal subjects and patients with inflammatory bowel diseaseJournal of Autoimmunity 2000;14(1) 99-105.

[110] Lomer M, Grainger S, Ede R, Catterall A, Greenfield S, Cowan R, Vicary F, Jenkins A, Fidler H, Harvey R, Ellis R, McNair A, Ainley C, Thompson R, Powell J. Lack of efficacy of a reduced microparticle diet in a multi-centred trial of patients with active Crohn's disease. European Journal of Gastroenterology & Hepatology 2005;17(3) 377-384.

[111] Gatti A. Biocompatibility of micro- and nano-particles in the colon. Part II. Biomateials 2004;25(3) 385-392.

[112] Kucharzik T, Lugering A, Lugering N, Rautenberg K, Linnepe M, Cichon C, Reichelt R, Stoll R, Schmidt M, Domschke W. Characterization of M cell development during indomethacin-induced ileitis in rats. Alimentary Pharmacology and Therapeutics 2000;14(2) 247-256.

[113] Stone V, Nowack B, Baun A, van den Brink N, Kammer F, Dusinska M, Handy R, Hankin S, Hassellöv M, Joner E, Fernandes T. Nanomaterials for environmental studies: classification, reference material issues, and strategies for physico-chemical characterization. Science of the Total Environment 2010;408(7) 1745-1754.

[114] Bar-Ilan O, Albrecht R, Fako V, Furgeson D. Toxicity assessments of multisized gold and silver nanoparticles in zebrafish embryos. Small 2009;5(16) 1897-1910.

[115] Sayes C, Warheit D. Characterization of nanomaterials for toxicity assessment. Wiley interdisciplinary reviews. Nanomedicine and nanobiotechnology 2009;1(6) 660-670,

[116] Auffan M, Rose J, Wiesner M, Bottero J. Chemical stability of metallic nanoparticles: A parameter controlling their potential cellular toxicity in vitro. Environmental Pollution 2009;157(4) 1127-1133.

[117] Handy R, Henry T, Scown T, Johnston B, Tyler C. Manufactured nanoparticles: their uptake and effects on fish - a mechanistic analysis. Ecotoxicology 2008;17(5) 396-409.

[118] Lynch I, Cedervall T, Lundqvist M, Cabaleiro-Lago C, Linse S, Dawson K. The nanoparticle-protein complex as a biological entity; a complex fluids and surface science

challenge for the 21st Century. Journal of Colloid and Interface Science 2007;134-135 167-174.

[119] Li N, Lewis P, Samuelson D, Liboni K, Neu J. Glutamine regulates Caco-2 cell tight junction proteins. American Journal of Physiology, Gastrointestinal and Liver Physiology 2004;287(3) G726-733.

[120] Seth A, Basuroy S, Sheth P, Rao R. L-Glutamine ameliorates acetaldehyde-induced increase in paracellular permeability in Caco-2 cell monolayer. American Journal of Physiology, Gastrointestinal and Liver Physiology 2004;287(3) G510-517.

[121] Lindmark T, Nikkila T, Artursson P. Mechanisms of absorption enhancement by medium chain fatty acids in intestinal epithelial Caco-2 cell monolayers. Journal of Pharmacology and Experimental Therapeutics 1995;275(2) 958-964.

[122] Usami M, Muraki K, Iwamoto M, Ohata A, Matsushita E, Miki A. Effect of eicosapentaenoic acid (EPA) on tight junction permeability in intestinal monolayer cells. Clinical Nutrition 2001;20(4) 351-359.

[123] Usami M, Komurasaki T, Hanada A, Kinoshita K, Ohata A. Effect of gamma-linolenic acid or docosahexaenoic acid on tight junction permeability in intestinal monolayer cells and their mechanism by protein kinase C activation and/or eicosanoid formation. Nutrition 2003;19(2) 150-156.

[124] Suzuki T, Hara H. Role of flavonoids in intestinal tight junction regulation. Journal of Nutritional Biochemistry 2011;22(5) 401-408.

[125] Sergent T, Piront N, Meurice J, Toussaint O, Schneider Y-J. Anti-inflammatory effects of dietary phenolic compounds in an in vitro model of inflamed human intestinal epithelium. Chemico-Biological Interactions 2010;188(3) 659-667.

[126] Labbé D, Provençal M, Lamy S, Boivin D, Gingras D, Béliveau R. The flavonols quercetin, kaempferol, and myricetin inhibit hepatocyte growth factor-Induced medulloblastoma cell migration. Journal of Nutrition 2009;139(4) 646-652.

[127] Guo D, Wu C, Li J, Guo A, Li Q, Jiang H, Chen B, Wang X. Synergistic effect of functionalized nickel nanoparticles and quercetin on inhibition of the SMMC-7721 cells proliferation. Nanoscale Research Letters 2009;4(12) 1395-1402.

[128] Bosi S, da Ros T, Spalluto G, Prato M. Fullerene derivatives: an attractive tool for biological applications. European Journal of Medicinal Chemistry 2003;38(11-12) 913-923.

[129] Schubert D, Dargusch R, Raitano J, Chan S. Cerium and yttrium oxide nanoparticles are neuroprotective. Biochemical and Biophysical Research Communications 2006;342(1) 86-91.

[130] Romieu I. Nutrition and lung health. International Journal of Tuberculosis and Lung Disease 2005;9(4) 362-374

[131] Vermylen J, Nemmar A, Nemery B, Hoylaerts F. Ambient air pollution and acute myocardial infarction. Journal of Thrombosis and Haemostasis 2005;3(9) 1955-1961.

[132] Amasheh M, Fromm A, Krug SM, Amasheh S, Andres S, Zeitz M, Fromm M, Schulzke JD. TNFalpha-induced and berberine-antagonized tight junction barrier impairment via tyrosine kinase, Akt and NFkappaB signaling. Journal of Cell Science 2010;123(Pt 23) 4145-4155.

[133] Shankar S, Ahmad A, Sastry M. Geranium leaf assisted biosynthesis of silver nanoparticles. Biotechnology Progress 2003;19(6) 1627-1631.

[134] Tripathy A, Raichur M, Chandrasekaran N, Prathna T, Mukherjee A. Process variables in biomimetic synthesis of silver nanoparticles by aqueous extract of Azadirachta indica (Neem) leaves. Journal of nano research 2010;12(1) 237-246.

[135] Raut R, Jaya S, Niranjan D, Vijay B, Kashid S. Photosynthesis of silver nanoparticle using Gliricidia sepium (Jacq.). Current Nanoscience 2009;5(1) 117-122.

[136] Rao R, Basuroy S, Rao V, Karnaky Jr K, Gupta A. Tyrosine phosphorylation and dissociation of occluding-ZO-1 and E-caderin-beta-catenin coplexes from the cytoskeleton by oxidative stress. Biochemical Journal 2002;368(Pt 2) 471-481.

[137] Aggarwal B, Bhardwaj A, Aggarwal R, Seeram N, Shishodia S, Takada Y. Role of resveratrol in prevention and therapy of cancer: preclinical and clinical studies. Anticancer Research 2004;24(5A) 2783-2840.

[138] Jang M, Cai L, Udeani G, Slowing K, Thomas C, Beecher C, Fong H, Farnsworth N, Kinghorn A, Mehta R, Moon R, Pezzuto J. Cancer chemopreventive activity of resveratrol, a natural product derived from grapes. Science 1997;275(5297) 218-220.

[139] Fulda S, Debatin K. Resveratrol modulation of signal transduction in apoptosis and cell survival: a mini-review. Cancer Detection and Prevention 2006;30(3) 217-223.

[140] Donnelly L, Newton R, Kennedy G, Fenwick P, Leung R, Ito K, Russell R, Barnes P. Anti-inflammatory effects of resveratrol in lung epithelial cells: molecular mechanisms. American Journal of Physiology, Lung Cellular and Molecular Physiology 2004;287(4) L774-783.

[141] Martin K, Appel C. Polyphenols as dietary supplements: a double-edged sword. Nutrition and Dietary Supplements 2010;2 1-12.

[142] European Food Safety Authority (EFSA) Scientific Committee; Scientific Opinion on Guidance on the risk assessment of the application of nanoscience and nanotechnologies in the food and feed chain. EFSA Journal 2011;9(5) 2140-2176.